HANDBOOK OF NURSING DIAGNOSIS
Fourth Edition

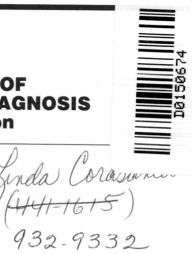

Linda Corasanti
(444-1615)
932-9332

Handbook of Nursing Diagnosis
Fourth Edition

Lynda Juall Carpenito, R.N., M.S.N.
Nursing Consultant, Mickleton, New Jersey

J. B. Lippincott Company   **Philadelphia**
New York London Hagerstown

Acquisition/Sponsoring Editor: Donna L. Hilton, R.N., B.S.N.
Coordinating Editorial Assistant: Susan Perry
Project Editor: Lorraine D. Smith
Manuscript Editor: Joy Perry
Indexer: Ellen Murray
Design Coordinator: Doug Smock
Production Manager: Helen Ewan
Production Coordinator: Kathryn Rule
Compositor: TAPSCO, Inc.
Printer/Binder: R. R. Donnelley & Sons Company
Cover Printer: New England Book Components

ISBN 0-397-54889-3

Any procedure or practice described in this book should be applied by the
health-care practitioner under appropriate supervision in accordance with
professional standards of care used with regard to the unique circumstances
that apply in each practice situation. Care has been taken to confirm the
accuracy of information presented and to describe generally accepted practices.
However, the author, editors, and publisher cannot accept any responsibility
for errors or omissions or for consequences from application of the information
in this book and make no warranty, express or implied, with respect to the
contents of the book.

Every effort has been made to ensure that drug selections and dosages are in
accordance with current recommendations and practice. Because of ongoing
research, changes in government regulations and the constant flow of information on drug therapy, reactions, and interactions, the reader is cautioned
to check the package insert for each drug for indications, dosages, warnings,
and precautions, particularly if the drug is new or infrequently used.

To Olen, my son

for your wisdom and commitment to justice
for our quiet moments and sudden hugs
for your unsolicited distractions
. . . I am grateful

for you are my daily reminder of what is
really important . . .
love, health, and human trust

Acknowledgments

I would like to thank the following people for their consultation during the development of the manual:

Rosalinda Alfaro-LeFevre, R.N., M.S.N.
Lecturer
Immaculata College
Immaculata, Pennsylvania
Per Diem Staff Nurse
Intensive Care Units
Paoli Memorial Hospital
Paoli, Pennsylvania

Cynthia Balin, R.N., M.S.N.
Doctoral Student
University of California, Los Angeles
Los Angeles, California

Martha Cress, R.N., B.S.N.
Nursing Education and Development
Duke University Medical Center
Durham, North Carolina

Ann Curtis, R.N., B.S.N.
Clinical Nurse Specialist
The Bryn Mawr Hospital
Bryn Mawr, PA

Mary Sieggreen, R.N., M.S.N., C.S.
Case Manager
Surgical Product Line
Harper Hospital
Detroit, Michigan

Acknowledgments

Joan Wagger, R.N., M.S.N.
Nursing Education and Development
Duke University Medical Center
Durham, North Carolina

Anne E. Willard, R.N., M.S.N.
Associate Professor
Cumberland County College
Vineland, New Jersey

A sincere "thank you" to Lippincott's Donna Hilton, Susan Perry, and Lorraine Smith for help in this undertaking, and once again, to my husband, Richard, for preparing the manuscript and his support on yet another project.

Contents

Section II
DIAGNOSTIC CLUSTERS
(Medical Conditions
With Associated Nursing Diagnoses and
Collaborative Problems) 311

Contents

Introduction

NURSING DIAGNOSES

In 1973, the North American Nursing Diagnosis Association (NANDA; formerly, the National Group for the Classification of Nursing Diagnosis) published its first list of nursing diagnoses. Since that time, the interest in nursing diagnosis and its application in clinical settings has grown substantially. In the 1970s, the main issue in nursing centered on the value of establishing a classification system for nursing diagnoses. Now that there is general agreement about the need for a formal taxonomy, the current issue is the implementation of nursing diagnoses. The challenge that nurses face today is one of identifying specific nursing diagnoses for those persons assigned to their care and of incorporating these diagnoses into a plan of care.

This handbook does not focus on teaching nurses about the concept of nursing diagnosis. For information describing the concept and specific instructions for clinical use the reader is referred to Carpenito LJ: Nursing Diagnosis: Application to Clinical Practice, 4th ed. Philadelphia, JB Lippincott, 1991.

This handbook is intended to supplement texts on nursing diagnosis in three ways:

- By providing a quick reference to each diagnostic category in terms of its definition, defining characteristics, and related factors
- By identifying possible nursing diagnoses and collaborative problems that could be associated with the major medical conditions
- By providing interventions and outcome criteria for each nursing diagnosis to serve as concise reminders of the indicated nursing care

Section I consists of 102 nursing diagnoses including 90 approved by NANDA and 10 additional categories. The following definition for a nursing diagnosis was approved at the ninth conference of NANDA:

- A nursing diagnosis is a clinical judgment about individual, family, or community responses to actual or potential health problems/life processes. Nursing diagnoses provide the basis for selection of nursing interventions to achieve outcomes for which the nurse is accountable.

In 1992, NANDA-approved diagnoses currently designated as Potential will be labeled High Risk for. This change has been incorporated into this edition.

Each nursing diagnosis is described in terms of

- Definition
- Defining characteristics or risk factors. Defining characteristics for actual nursing diagnoses are a single sign or symptom or a cluster of signs and symptoms. Diagnoses with clinical validation studies have major signs and symptoms that are present 80% of the time, minor signs and symptoms, 50% to 79% of the time. The *major* category includes those signs and symptoms that must be present to validate use of a diagnosis. The *minor* classification refers to characteristics that appear to be present in many but not all individuals experiencing the diagnosis. Minor characteristics are not less serious than the major ones; they are just not present in all individuals. Potential nursing diagnoses have risk factors.
- Related factors, which are examples of pathophysiological, treatment-related, situational, and maturational factors that can cause or influence the health status or contribute to the development of a problem

ACTUAL, HIGH RISK, POSSIBLE, AND WELLNESS NURSING DIAGNOSES

A nursing diagnosis can be actual, high risk, or possible.

Actual: An actual nursing diagnosis describes a clinical judgment that the nurse has validated because of the presence of major defining characteristics, or signs and symptoms.

High risk: A high risk nursing diagnosis describes a clinical judgment that an individual/group is more vulnerable to develop the problem than others in the same or similar situation.

Possible: A possible nursing diagnosis describes a problem that the nurse suspects may be present but that requires additional data collection in order to confirm or rule out its presence.

Wellness: A wellness nursing diagnosis is a clinical judgment about an individual, family, or community in transition from a specific level of wellness to a higher level of wellness (NANDA).

DIAGNOSTIC STATEMENTS

The diagnostic statement describes the health status of an individual or group and the factors that have contributed to the status.

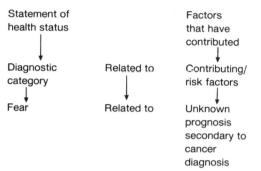

The diagnostic statement or the nursing diagnosis should consist of one, two or three parts.

One-part Statements

Wellness nursing diagnoses (proposed for 1992) will be written as one-part statements: Potential for Enhanced _____, e.g., Potential for Enhanced Parenting. Related factors are not present for wellness nursing diagnoses.

Two-part Statements

High risk and *possible* nursing diagnoses have two parts. The validation for a high risk nursing diagnosis is the presence of risk factors. The risk factors are the second part.

High risk nursing diagnosis   Related to   Risk factors

Possible nursing diagnoses are suspected because of the presence of certain factors. The nurse then either rules out or confirms the existence of an actual or a high risk diagnosis.

Examples of two-part statements are

High Risk for Impaired Skin Integrity related to immobility secondary to fractured hip

Possible Self-Care Deficit related to impaired ability to use left hand secondary to IV

Designating a diagnosis as possible provides the nurse with a method to communicate to other nurses that a diagnosis may be present. Additional data collection is indicated to rule out or confirm the tentative diagnosis.

Three-part Statements

An actual nursing diagnosis consists of three parts.

Diagnostic label + contributing factors +
signs and symptoms

The presence of major signs and symptoms (defining characteristics) validates that an actual diagnosis is present. It is not possible to have a third part for high risk or possible diagnoses because signs and symptoms do not exist.

Examples of three-part statements are

Anxiety related to unpredictable nature of asthmatic episodes as evident by statements of "I'm afraid I won't be able to breathe"

Urge Incontinence related to diminished bladder capacity secondary to habitual frequent voiding evident by inability to hold off urination after desire to void and report of voiding out of habit, not need

The presence of a nursing diagnosis is determined by assessing the individual's health status and his ability to function. To guide the nurse who is gathering this information, a Screening Assessment Tool is included in the Appendix at the end of the book. This guide directs the nurse to collect data according to the individual's functional health patterns. Functional health patterns and the corresponding nursing diagnoses are listed in Table 2, at the end of this introduction. If significant data are collected in a particular functional pattern, the next step is to check the related nursing diagnosis to see if any nursing diagnoses are substantiated by the data that are collected.

DIAGNOSTIC CLUSTERS

Section II of this handbook consists of seven parts: (1) Medical Conditions, (2) Surgical Procedures, (3) Obstetrical/Gynecological Conditions, (4) Neonatal Conditions, (5) Pediatric/Adolescent Disorders, (6) Psychiatric Disorders, and (7) Diagnostic and Therapeutic Procedures. Each of these subjects is represented by a series of diagnostic clusters under which groups of associated nursing diagnoses and collaborative problems are listed. A diagnostic cluster represents a set of collaborative problems and/or nursing diagnoses that are predicted to be present because of the situation. The intent of this section is to help the nurse identify possible nursing diagnoses and collaborative problems in each of these areas. It is important to note that each nursing diagnosis must be confirmed or ruled out on the basis of the data collected. The use of a nursing diagnosis without clinical validation based on defining characteristics is hazardous and unsound, and jeopardizes the effectiveness and validity of the nursing care plan. The listing of tentative nursing diagnoses under medical and surgical diagnoses was intended to facilitate the assessment, identification, and validation process, *not to replace it.*

In addition to the possible nursing diagnoses listed under each medical category, there is a list of collaborative problems or potential complications that may occur.

THE BIFOCAL CLINICAL PRACTICE MODEL

Nurses are accountable to treat two types of clinical judgments or diagnoses—nursing diagnoses and collaborative problems.

Nursing interventions are classified as nurse-prescribed or physician-prescribed. Nurse-prescribed interventions are those which the nurse can legally order for nursing staff to implement. Nurse-prescribed interventions treat, prevent, and monitor nursing diagnoses. Nurse-prescribed interventions manage and monitor collaborative problems. Physician-prescribed interventions represent treatments for collaborative problems that the nurse initiates and manages. Display 1 represents these relationships.

Collaborative problems are certain physiological complications that nurses monitor to detect onset or changes of status. Nurses manage collaborative problems utilizing physician-prescribed and nursing-prescribed interventions to minimize the complications of the events.

The nurse makes independent decisions regarding both collaborative problems and nursing diagnoses. The decisions differ in that, for nursing diagnoses, the nurse prescribes the definitive treatment for the situation; for collaborative problems the nurse monitors the patient's condition to detect onset or status of physiological complications and manages the events with nursing and physician-prescribed interventions. Collaborative

DISPLAY 1. RELATIONSHIP BETWEEN NURSING-PRESCRIBED INTERVENTIONS AND PHYSICIAN-PRESCRIBED INTERVENTIONS

NURSING-PRESCRIBED INTERVENTIONS	NURSING DIAGNOSES	PHYSICIAN-PRESCRIBED INTERVENTIONS
• Reposition q2h • Lightly massage vulnerable areas • Teach how to reduce pressure when sitting	High Risk for Impaired Skin Integrity related to immobility secondary to fatigue	None

NURSING-PRESCRIBED INTERVENTIONS	COLLABORATIVE PROBLEMS	PHYSICIAN-PRESCRIBED INTERVENTIONS

• Maintain NPO state
• Monitor:
  Hydration
  Vital Signs
  Intake/output
  Specific gravity
• Monitor electrolytes
• Maintain IV at prescribed rate
• Provide/encourage mouth care
	Potential Complication: Fluid and Electrolyte Imbalances	• IV (type, amount)
		• Laboratory studies

problems are labeled "Potential Complications:" (specify).
Examples:

> Potential Complication: Hemorrhage
> Potential Complication: Renal Failure

The physiological complications that nurses monitor are usually related to disease, trauma, treatments, and diagnostic studies. The following illustrates some collaborative problems

Situation	Collaborative Problem
Anticoagulant therapy	Potential Complication: Hemorrhage
Pneumonia	Potential Complication: Hypoxia

Outcome criteria or client goals are used to measure the effectiveness of nursing care. When a client is not progressing to goal achievement or has worsened, the nurse must reevaluate the situation. Display 2 represents the questions to be considered. If none of these options is appropriate, the situation probably is not a nursing diagnosis. For example:

Potential Fluid Volume Deficit related to the effects of prolonged PTT secondary to anticoagulant therapy

Goal: The client will have hemoglobin > 13

Examine the questions in Display 2; which option is appropriate? None. The nurse would initiate physician-prescribed orders if the client presented signs of bleeding. This situation is a collaborative problem, not a nursing diagnosis: e.g.,

Potential Complication: Bleeding with a nursing goal of:

The nursing goal will be to manage and minimize episodes of bleeding. Collaborative problems have nursing goals that represent the accountability of the nurse—to detect early and to manage. Nursing diagnoses have client goals that represent the accountability of the nurse—to achieve or maintain a favorable status after nursing care.

Table 1 is a list of frequently used collaborative problems.

DISPLAY 2.   EVALUATION QUESTIONS

Is the diagnosis correct?
Has the goal been mutually set?
Is more time needed for the plan to work?
Does the goal need to be revised?
Do the interventions need to be revised?

Table 1. Frequently Used Collaborative Problems

1. Potential Complication: Gastrointestinal/Hepatic/Biliary

PC: Paralytic Ileus/Small Bowel Obstruction
PC: Hepatorenal Syndrome
PC: Hyperbilirubinemia
PC: Evisceration
PC: Hepatosplenomegaly
PC: Curling's Ulcer
PC: Ascites
PC: Gastrointestinal Bleeding

2. Potential Complication: Metabolic/Immune/Hematopoietic

PC: Hypoglycemia, hyperglycemia
PC: Immunodeficiency
PC: Negative Nitrogen Balance
PC: Electrolyte Imbalances
PC: Thyroid Dysfunction
PC: Hypothermia (Severe)
PC: Hyperthermia (Severe)
PC: Septicemia
PC: Acidosis/Alkalosis
PC: Anemia
PC: Thrombocytopenia
PC: Hypothyroidism/Hyperthyroidism
PC: Allergic Reaction
PC: Sickling Crisis
PC: Adrenal Insufficiency

3. Potential Complication: Neurological/Sensory

PC: Increased Intracranial Pressure
PC: Stroke
PC: Seizures
PC: Spinal Cord Compression
PC: Autonomic Dysreflexia
PC: Retinal detachment
PC: Hydrocephalus
PC: Microcephalus
PC: Meningitis
PC: Cranial Nerve Impairment
PC: Paresis/Paresthesia/Paralysis

(Continued)

Table 1. Frequently Used Collaborative Problems
(*Continued*)

- PC: Peripheral Nerve Impairment
- PC: Increased Intraocular Pressure
- PC: Corneal Ulceration
- PC: Neuropathies

4. Potential Complication: Cardiac/Vascular

- PC: Dysrhythmias
- PC: Congestive Heart Failure
- PC: Cardiogenic Shock
- PC: Thromboemboli/Deep Vein Thrombosis
- PC: Hypovolemic Shock
- PC: Peripheral Vascular Insufficiency
- PC: Hypertension
- PC: Congenital Heart Disease
- PC: Decreased Cardiac Output
- PC: Cardiac Tamponade
- PC: Air Embolism
- PC: Compartmental Syndrome
- PC: Disseminated Intravascular Coagulation
- PC: Endocarditis
- PC: Septic Shock
- PC: Embolism
- PC: Spinal Shock
- PC: Ischemic Ulcers

5. Potential Complication: Respiratory

- PC: Atelectasis/Pneumonia
- PC: Tracheobronchial Constriction
- PC: Oxygen Toxicity
- PC: Pulmonary Embolism
- PC: Pleural Effusion
- PC: Tracheal Necrosis
- PC: Ventilator Dependency
- PC: Pneumothorax
- PC: Laryngeal Edema
- PC: Hypoxemia

(*Continued*)

Table 1. Frequently Used Collaborative Problems
(*Continued*)

6. Potential Complication: Renal/Urinary

PC: Acute Urinary Retention
PC: Renal Failure
PC: Bladder Perforation

7. Potential Complication: Reproductive

PC: Fetal Distress
PC: Postpartum Hemorrhage
PC: Pregnancy Associated Hypertension
PC: Prenatal Bleeding
PC: Preterm Labor
PC: Hypermenorrhea
PC: Polymenorrhea
PC: Syphilis

8. Potential Complication: Musculoskeletal

PC: Pathological Fractures
PC: Osteoporosis
PC: Joint Dislocation

Some physiological complications, such as pressure ulcers and infection from invasive lines, are problems that nurses can prevent. Prevention is different from detection. Nurses do not prevent paralytic ileus but, instead, detect its presence early to prevent greater severity of illness or even death. Physicians cannot treat collaborative problems without nursing knowledge, vigilance, and judgment.

Thus the type of intervention differentiates a nursing diagnosis from a collaborative problem and also differentiates an actual nursing diagnosis from a high risk or possible one. Below are definitions of each type and the corresponding intervention focus:

Type	*Focus of Nursing Interventions*
Actual (is present)	To reduce, eliminate, or promote (positive) and monitor
High Risk (may happen)	To prevent onset and monitor

Possible (may be present)	To rule out or confirm with additional data
Wellness	To teach higher level of wellness
Collaborative Problem	To monitor and manage

For example, for the diagnosis *Impaired Skin Integrity related to immobility as manifested by a 2-cm epidermal lesion on the left heel,* the nurse would order interventions to monitor the lesion while providing care to eliminate it. Monitoring is an intervention used for all diagnoses. If the outcome criteria for a problem necessitate medical interventions and the nursing focus is primarily on monitoring or surveillance, perhaps a nursing diagnosis is inappropriate because a collaborative problem is present. Nursing diagnoses are not more important than collaborative problems, and collaborative problems are not more important than nursing diagnoses. Rather, priorities are determined by the client's situation.

How to Use This Handbook

1. Collect data, both subjective and objective, from client, family, other health care professionals, and records. (Refer to Appendix: Adult Screening Admission Assessment.)
2. Identify a possible pattern or problem.
3. Refer to the medical diagnostic category and review the possible associated nursing diagnoses and collaborative problems. Select the possibilities.
4. After you have selected what physiological complications or collaborative problems are indicated to be monitored for, label them Potential Complications: (specify).
5. After you have determined which functional patterns are altered or at risk of altered functioning, review the list of nursing diagnostic categories under that pattern and select the appropriate diagnosis (refer to Table 2).
6. If you select an actual diagnosis,
   - Do you have signs and symptoms to support its presence? (Refer to Section I, Nursing Diagnostic Categories, under the selected diagnosis.)
   - Write the actual diagnosis in three parts:
     Category related to contributing factors as manifested by signs and symptoms
7. If you select a high risk diagnosis
   - Are risk factors present?
   - Write the high risk diagnosis in two parts:
     Category related to risk factors

8. If you suspect a problem but have insufficient data, gather the additional data to confirm or rule out the diagnosis. If this additional data collection must be done later or by other nurses, label the diagnosis *possible* on the care plan.*

* Specific focus assessment criteria questions, outcome criteria, and interventions for each nursing diagnosis category can be found in Carpenito LJ: Nursing Diagnosis: Application to Clinical Practice, 4th ed. Philadelphia, JB Lippincott, 1991.

Table 2. Nursing Diagnostic Categories Grouped Under Functional Health Patterns*

1. **Health Perception–Health Management**
   Growth and Development, Altered
   Health Maintenance, Altered
   Health Seeking Behaviors
   Noncompliance
   High Risk for Injury
     High Risk for Suffocation
     High Risk for Poisoning
     High Risk for Trauma

2. **Nutritional–Metabolic**
   Body Temperature, High Risk for Altered
     Hypothermia
     Hyperthermia
     Thermoregulation, Ineffective
   Fluid Volume Deficit
   Fluid Volume Excess
   Infection, High Risk for
   ‡Infection Transmission, High Risk for
   Nutrition, Altered: Less Than Body
     Requirements
   Nutrition, Altered: More Than Body
     Requirements
   Nutrition, Altered: Potential for More Than Body
     Requirements
   †Breastfeeding, Effective

(Continued)

Table 2. Nursing Diagnostic Categories Grouped Under Functional Health Patterns* (*Continued*)

Breastfeeding, Ineffective
Swallowing, Impaired
†Protection, Altered
Tissue Integrity, Impaired
Oral Mucous Membrane, Altered
Skin Integrity, Impaired

3. **Elimination**
‡Bowel Elimination, Altered
Constipation
Colonic Constipation
Perceived Constipation
Diarrhea
Bowel Incontinence
Urinary Elimination, Altered Patterns of
Urinary Retention
Total Incontinence
Functional Incontinence
Reflex Incontinence
Urge Incontinence
Stress Incontinence
‡Maturational Enuresis

4. **Activity–Exercise**
Activity Intolerance
Cardiac Output, Decreased
Disuse Syndrome, High Risk for
Diversional Activity Deficit
Home Maintenance Management, Impaired
Mobility, Impaired Physical
‡Respiratory Function, High Risk for Altered
Ineffective Airway Clearance
Ineffective Breathing Patterns
Impaired Gas Exchange
(Specify) Self-care Deficit: (Syndrome,‡ Feeding, Bathing/Hygiene, Dressing/Grooming, Toileting)
Tissue Perfusion, Altered: (Specify) (Cerebral, Cardiopulmonary, Renal, Gastrointestinal, Peripheral)

(*Continued*)

Table 2. Nursing Diagnostic Categories Grouped Under Functional Health Patterns (*Continued*)

5. **Sleep–Rest**
   Sleep Pattern Disturbance

6. **Cognitive–Perceptual**
   ‡Comfort, Altered
      Pain
      Chronic Pain
   Decisional Conflict
   Dysreflexia
   Knowledge Deficit: (Specify)
   High Risk for Aspiration
   Sensory–Perceptual Alteration: (Specify) (Visual,
      Auditory, Kinesthetic, Gustatory, Tactile,
      Olfactory)
   Thought Processes, Altered
   Unilateral Neglect

7. **Self-Perception**
   Anxiety
   Fatigue
   Fear
   Hopelessness
   Powerlessness
   ‡Self-Concept Disturbance
      Body Image Disturbance
      Personal Identity Disturbance
      Self-Esteem Disturbance
         Chronic Low Self-Esteem
         Situational Low Self-Esteem

8. **Role–Relationship**
   ‡Communication, Impaired
      Communication, Impaired Verbal
   Family Processes, Altered
   ‡Grieving
      Grieving, Anticipatory
      Grieving, Dysfunctional
   Parenting, Altered
   Parental Role Conflict
   Role Performance, Altered

(*Continued*)

Table 2. Nursing Diagnostic Categories Grouped Under Functional Health Patterns (*Continued*)

Social Interactions, Impaired
Social Isolation

9. **Sexuality–Reproductive**
   Sexual Dysfunction
   Sexuality Patterns, Altered

10. **Coping–Stress Tolerance**
    Adjustment, Impaired
    Coping, Ineffective Individual
      Defensive Coping
      Ineffective Denial
    Coping: Disabling, Ineffective Family
    Coping: Compromised, Ineffective Family
    Coping: Potential for Growth, Family
    Post-trauma Response
      Rape Trauma Syndrome
    ‡Self-harm, High Risk for:
    Violence, High Risk for:

11. **Value–Belief**
    Spiritual Distress

---

*The Functional Health Patterns were identified in Gordon M: Nursing Diagnosis: Process and Application. New York, McGraw–Hill, 1982, with minor changes by the author.

†These categories were accepted by the North American Nursing Diagnosis Association in 1990.

‡These diagnostic categories are not currently on the NANDA list but have been included for clarity and usefulness.

Please Note: In order to reflect a society where nurses are male and female and clients are male and female, the pronouns *she, her, he, his, him,* etc., will be used interchangeably throughout this book. The intent is to retain the use of gender pronouns without stereotyping.

Section I

Nursing Diagnoses

Activity Intolerance

DEFINITION

Activity Intolerance: A reduction in one's physiological capacity to endure activities to the degree desired or required. (Magnan)*

Author's Note:

Activity Intolerance is a diagnostic judgment that describes an individual who has compromised physical conditioning. This individual can engage in therapies that increase strength and endurance. Activity Intolerance differs from Fatigue because it is relieved by rest and the goal is to increase tolerance to activity. With the nursing diagnosis Fatigue, the goal is to assist the person to adapt to the fatigue, not to increase endurance.

DEFINING CHARACTERISTICS

Major (Must Be Present)

Altered response to activity
  Respiratory
    Dyspnea
    Shortness of breath

  Excessive increase in rate
  Decrease in rate

  Pulse
    Weak
    Decrease in rate
    Excessive increase in rate

  Failure to return to resting after 3 minutes
  Rhythm change

  Blood pressure
    Failure to increase with activity
    Increase in diastolic by 15 mm Hg

  Decrease

---

* Magnan MA. Activity intolerance: Toward a nursing theory of activity. Paper presented at the Fifth Annual Symposium of the Michigan Nursing Diagnosis Assn. Detroit, 1987.

Minor (May Be Present)

Pallor or cyanosis
Confusion
Vertigo
Weakness
Fatigue

RELATED FACTORS

Any factor that compromises oxygen transport can cause activity intolerance. Some common factors are listed below.

Pathophysiological

Alterations in the oxygen transport system
  Cardiac
    Idiopathic hypertrophic subaortic stenosis
    Congenital heart disease
    Cardiomyopathies
    Congestive heart   Angina
      failure   Myocardial infarction
    Dysrhythmias   Valvular disease
  Respiratory
    Chronic obstructive pulmonary disease
    Atelectasis   Bronchopulmonary
                   dysplasia
  Circulatory
    Anemia   Hypovolemia
    Peripheral arterial
      disease
  Acute infection
    Viral infection   Hepatitis
    Mononucleosis
  Acute or chronic infection
  Endocrine or metabolic disorders
  Chronic diseases
    Renal   Inflammatory
    Hepatic   Musculoskeletal
                Neurological
  Nutritional disorders
    Obesity   Inadequate diet
    Malnourishment

Hypovolemia
Electrolyte imbalance
Malignancies

Treatment-related

Surgery
Diagnostic studies
Treatment schedule/treatments (frequency)
Prolonged bed rest
Medications
    Antihypertensives   Antidepressants
    Minor tranquilizers   Antihistamines
    Hypnotics   Beta blockers

Situational (Personal, Environmental)

Depression
Lack of motivation
Sedentary life-style
Extreme stress
Pain
Sleep disturbances
Stressors
Fatigue
   Assistive equipment that requires strength (walkers, crutches, braces)
   Stress
Environmental barriers
Climatic extremes
Air pollution
Atmospheric pressure changes (*e.g.,* relocation to high altitude)

Maturational

Elderly (sensory-motor deficit)

OUTCOME CRITERIA

The person will

1. Identify factors that reduce activity tolerance
2. Progress to (specify the highest level of mobility possible)
3. Exhibit a decrease in hypoxic signs of increased activity (pulse, blood pressure, respirations)

INTERVENTIONS

1. Assess the individual's response to activity.
   a. Take resting pulse, blood pressure, and respirations.
   b. Consider rate, rhythm, and quality (if signs are abnormal—*e.g.,* pulse above 100—consult with physician about the advisability of increasing activity).
   c. Take vital signs immediately after activity; take pulse for 15 seconds and multiply by 4 instead of for a full minute.
   d. Have person rest for 3 minutes; take vital signs again.
   e. Discontinue the activity if the client responds to the activity with:
      • Complaints of chest pain, dyspnea, vertigo, or confusion
      • Decrease in pulse rate
      • Failure of systolic rate to increase
      • Decrease in systolic blood pressure
      • Increase in diastolic rate 15 mm Hg
      • Decrease in respiratory rate
   f. Reduce the intensity, frequency, or duration of the activity if:
      • The pulse takes longer than 3–4 minutes to return within 6 beats of the resting pulse rate
      • The respiratory rate increase is excessive after the activity
      • Other signs of hypoxia are present, *e.g.,* confusion, vertigo
2. Progress the activity gradually.
   a. For a person who is or has been on prolonged bed rest, begin range of motion (ROM) at least b.i.d.
   b. Plan rest periods according to the person's daily schedule (rest periods may occur between activities).
   c. Promote a sincere "can do" attitude to provide a positive atmosphere to encourage increased activity; convey to clients the belief that they can improve their mobility status. Acknowledge progress.
   d. Allow person to set activity schedule and functional activity goals (if the goal is too low, make a contract: *e.g.,* "If you walk halfway up the hall, I will play a game of cards with you.").

e. Increase tolerance for the activity by having the client perform the activity more slowly, or for a shorter period of time with more rest pauses, or with more assistance.

f. Gradually increase exercise tolerance by increasing the time out of bed by 15 minutes each day.

g. Allow the person to gauge the rate of the ambulation.

h. Encourage person to wear comfortable walking shoes (slippers do not support the feet properly).

3. Teach the person energy conservation methods for activities.

a. Take rest periods during activities, at intervals during the day, and 1 hour after meals.

b. Sit rather than stand when performing activities, unless this is not feasible.

c. When performing a task, rest every 3 minutes for 5 minutes to allow the heart to recover.

d. Stop an activity if fatigue or signs of cardiac hypoxia are present (↑ pulse, dyspnea, chest pain).

4. Instruct the person to consult his or her physician and physiatrist for a long-term exercise program, or to contact the American Heart Association for names of cardiac rehabilitation programs.

5. For persons with chronic pulmonary insufficiency:

a. Encourage conscious controlled breathing techniques during increased activity and times of emotional and physical stress (techniques include pursed-lip and diaphragmatic breathing).

b. For pursed-lip breathing, the person should breathe in through the nose, then slowly breathe out through partially closed lips while counting to seven and making a "pu" sound (often this is learned naturally by person with progressive lung disease).

c. Teach diaphragmatic breathing.
   • The nurse should place hands on the person's abdomen below the base of the ribs and keep them there while the client inhales.
   • To inhale, the person should relax the shoulders, breathe in through the nose, and push the stomach outward against the nurse's hands, holding breath for 1–2 seconds to keep the alveoli open.

- To exhale, the person should breathe out slowly through the mouth while the nurse applies slight pressure at the base of the ribs.
- This breathing technique should be practiced several times with the nurse; then the person should place his or her own hands at the base of the ribs and practice independently.
- Once learned, the client should practice this exercise a few times each hour.

d. Encourage gradual increase in daily activity to prevent "pulmonary crippling."

e. Encourage person to use adaptive breathing techniques to decrease the work of breathing.

f. Discuss physical barriers at home and at work (*e.g.,* number of stairs) and ways of alternating expenditure of energy with rest pauses (place a chair in bathroom near sink to rest during daily hygiene).

6. Refer to community nurse for follow-up if needed.

Adjustment, Impaired

DEFINITION

Impaired Adjustment: The state in which an individual is unable to modify his or her life-style/behavior in a manner consistent with a change in health status.

Author's Note:

The term *adjustment* describes an individual's psychosocial regulatory processes to establish equilibrium in a person-environment. This person is having difficulty adapting to a health status change. This diagnosis can apply to clients in varied settings: in-patient, rehabilitation, long-term care, community. Many other nursing diagnoses can co-exist or overlap with impaired adjustment, such as grieving, ineffective coping, anxiety, fear. This diagnosis may prove more clinically useful during the initial adjustment phase, *e.g.,* the first 3–4 months. Prolonged resistance to change may be more appropriately described as ineffective individual coping. At some point the nurse and client may agree that the choice is *not* to modify behavior.

DEFINING CHARACTERISTICS

Major (Must Be Present)

Verbalization of nonacceptance of health status change or inability to be involved in problem solving or goal setting

Minor (May Be Present)

Lack of movement toward independence; extended period of shock, disbelief, or anger regarding health status change; lack of future-oriented thinking

RELATED FACTORS

Adjustment impairment can result from a variety of situations and health problems. Some common sources are listed below.

Pathophysiological

Spinal cord injury
Paralysis
Loss of limb
Cerebrovascular accident (CVA)
Myocardial infarction
Progressive neurological diseases
Cancer
Chronic obstructive pulmonary disease (COPD)

Treatment-related

Dialysis

Situational (Personal, Environmental)

Inadequate support systems
Unavailable support systems
Impaired cognition
Depression
Loss (object, person, job)
Divorce

Maturational

Child/adolescent
Chronic disease
Disability

Adult
  Loss of ability to practice vocation
  Role reversal
Elderly
  Normal physiological aging changes

OUTCOME CRITERIA

The person will:

1. Identify the temporary and long-term demands of the situation
2. Differentiate coping behavior that is effective versus ineffective

INTERVENTIONS

1. Identify factors that interfere with or delay effective adjustment:
   a. Unmanageable level of stress (see *Anxiety*)
   b. Inability to identify the problem or ineffective problem solving
   c. Lack of mastery of developmental tasks for age
   d. History of patterns of ineffective coping and unresolved conflicts
   e. Inadequate or unavailable resources (*e.g.,* faith, knowledge about illness/disability, money, support system, skills to manage illness/disability)
2. Assist the family and significant others to cope:
   a. Explore with them their perception of how the situation will progress.
   b. Identify behaviors that facilitate adaptation.
   c. Stress the importance of trying to maintain usual roles and behavior.
   d. When appropriate, include the affected individual in family decision-making.
   e. Discuss the reality of everyday emotions: anger, guilt, jealousy; relate the hazards of denying these feelings.
   f. Discuss the hazards of trying to minimize the grief and trying to distract the grievers from grieving.
3. Establish an active relationship with the client and family by acknowledging the person's increased dependence

and initiating a collaborative approach to care (Friedman–Campbell).*
4. Identify dysfunctional coping mechanisms, *e.g.,* prolonged denial, use of chemical substances, avoidance, morbid preoccupation with the disability.
5. When appropriate, begin health teaching (Friedman–Campbell):*
   a. Share your perceptions of the injury and the person's response to it.
   b. Explain the nature of the illness or injury.
   c. Discuss the anticipated changes in life-style.
   d. Teach health behaviors that need to be learned to adapt to a new life-style.
6. Explore with clients their fears. Role-play fearful or stressful situations.
7. Initiate referrals as indicated.
   a. Identify resources available: community, financial, counseling, role models, self-help groups.
   b. Refer individuals and family to appropriate self-help literature.

Anxiety

DEFINITION

Anxiety: The state in which an individual/group experiences feelings of uneasiness (apprehension) and activation of the autonomic nervous system in response to a vague, nonspecific threat.

Author's Note:
Anxiety is a vague feeling of apprehension and uneasiness to a threat to one's value system or security pattern (May).* The
(Continued)

---

* Friedman–Campbell M, Hart CA: Theoretical strategies and nursing interventions to promote psychological adaptation to spinal cord injuries and disability. J Neurosurg Nurs 16(6):335–342, 1984

Author's Note (*Continued*)
individual may be able to identify the situation, *e.g.,* surgery, cancer, but in actuality the threat to self relates to the uneasiness and apprehension enmeshed in the situation. The situation is the source of the threats but it is not the threat.

In contrast fear is the feeling of apprehension to a specific threat or danger to which one's security patterns alert one, *e.g.,* flying, heights, snakes. When the threat is removed, the fearful feeling dissipates (May).*

Fear can exist without anxiety and anxiety can be present without fear. Clinically both may co-exist in a person's response to a situation. An individual who is facing surgery may be fearful of pain and anxious of a possible cancer diagnosis.

DEFINING CHARACTERISTICS

Major (Must Be Present)

Manifested by symptoms from three categories—physiological, emotional, and cognitive. Symptoms vary according to the level of anxiety.

Physiological

Increased heart rate
Insomnia
Elevated blood pressure
Fatigue and weakness
Increased respiratory rate
Flushing or pallor
Diaphoresis
Dry mouth
Dilated pupils
Body aches and pains (especially chest, back, neck)

Voice tremors/pitch changes
Trembling
Restlessness
Palpitations
Faintness/dizziness
Nausea and/or vomiting
Paresthesias
Frequent urination
Hot and cold flashes
Diarrhea

Emotional

Person admits to feelings of
Apprehension
Lack of self-confidence

Fear
Inability to relax

* May R: The Meaning of Anxiety. New York, WW Norton, 1987

11

Helplessness
Losing control
Nervousness
Tension, or being "keyed up"
Person exhibits
Irritability/impatience
Criticism of self and others
Angry outbursts
Withdrawal
Crying
Lack of initiative
Tendency to blame others
Self-deprecation
Startle reaction

Unreality
Anticipation of misfortune

Cognitive

Inability to concentrate
Lack of awareness of surroundings
Forgetfulness
Rumination
Orientation to past rather than to present or future
Blocking of thoughts (inability to remember)
Hyperattentiveness

RELATED FACTORS

Pathophysiological

Any factor that interferes with the basic human needs for food, air, comfort, and security

Situational (Personal, Environmental)

Actual or perceived threat to self-concept
Change in status and prestige
Failure (or success)
Lack of recognition from others

Loss of valued possessions
Ethical dilemmas

Actual or perceived loss of significant others
Death
Divorce
Cultural pressures

Moving
Temporary or permanent separation

Actual or perceived threat to biological integrity

Dying	Invasive procedures
Assault	Disease

Actual or perceived change in environment

Hospitalization	Safety hazards
Moving	Environmental
Retirement	pollutants

Actual or perceived change in socioeconomic status

Unemployment	Promotion
New job	

Transmission of another person's anxiety to the individual

Maturational (Threat to Developmental Task)

Infant/child
  Separation
  Mutilation
  Peer relationships
  Achievement
Adolescent
  Sexual development
  Peer relationships
  Independence
Adult
  Pregnancy
  Parenting
  Career development
  Effects of aging
Elderly
  Sensory losses
  Motor losses
  Financial problems
  Retirement

OUTCOME CRITERIA

The person will:

1. Describe his or her own anxiety and coping patterns
2. Relate an increase in psychological and physiological comfort
3. Use effective coping mechanisms in managing anxiety, as evidenced by (specify)

INTERVENTIONS

The nursing interventions for the diagnosis Anxiety apply to any person with anxiety regardless of the etiological and contributing factors.

1. Assess level of anxiety: Mild, moderate, severe, panic.
2. Provide reassurance and comfort.
   a. Stay with the person.
   b. Do not make demands or ask the person to make decisions.
   c. Speak slowly and calmly, using short, simple sentences.
   d. Be aware of your own concern and avoid reciprocal anxiety.
   e. Convey a sense of empathic understanding (*e.g.,* quiet presence, touch, allowing crying, talking, etc.).
3. Remove excess stimulation (*e.g.,* take person to quieter room); limit contact with others—patients or family—who are also anxious.
4. When anxiety is diminished enough for learning to take place, assist person in recognizing the anxiety in order to initiate learning or problem-solving.
   a. Encourage the person to recall and analyze similar instances of anxiety.
   b. Explore what alternative behaviors might have been used if coping mechanisms were maladaptive.
   c. Encourage the person to recall and analyze similar instances of anxiety.
5. Assist person with anger.
   a. Identify the presence of anger (*e.g.,* feelings of frustration, anxiety, helplessness, presence of irritability, verbal outbursts).
   b. Recognize your reactions to client's behavior; be aware of your own feelings in working with angry individuals.
   c. Assist in making connections between feelings of frustration and subsequent behavior.
   d. State limits clearly; tell person exactly what is expected (*e.g.,* "I cannot allow you to scream [throw objects, etc.]").
   e. When stating an unacceptable behavior, give an alternative (*e.g.,* suggest a quiet room, physical exertion, a chance for one-to-one communication).

    f. Develop behavior modification strategies; discuss with all personnel involved for consistency.

    g. Interact with the person when he is not demanding or manipulative.

6. Assist a child with anger.

    a. Encourage the child to share his or her anger (*e.g.,* "How did you feel when you had your injection?" "How did you feel when Mary would not play with you?").

    b. Tell the child that being angry is okay (*e.g.,* "I sometimes get angry when I can't have what I want.").

    c. Encourage and allow the child to express anger in acceptable ways (*e.g.,* loud talking, hitting a play object, or running outside around the house).

7. For patients identified as having chronic anxiety and maladaptive coping mechanisms, refer for ongoing psychiatric treatment.

Body Temperature, High Risk for Altered

Hypothermia

Hyperthermia

Thermoregulation, Ineffective

Author's Note:

High Risk for Altered Body Temperature represents a diagnosis that is difficult to differentiate from the other diagnoses that focus on body temperature: hypothermia, hyperthermia, ineffective thermoregulation. The risk factors listed could be used

(*Continued*)

Author's Note (*Continued*)

with each of the above diagnoses as a high risk for, *e.g.,* High Risk for Hyperthermia related to the effects of aging on ability to acclimatize to heat.

Usually when a nurse is inclined to use High Risk for Altered Body Temperature, it is with a client who has experienced a temperature elevation, but is presently afebrile. In this situation High Risk for Hyperthermia would be useful.

In acute case situations when an individual experiences fluctuations in temperature, the nursing diagnosis of Altered Comfort related to malaise, chills, and temperature fluctuations may more appropriately describe the nursing focus.

Hypothermia and Hyperthermia are abnormal temperature states that are treatable by nursing interventions by correcting the external causes, *e.g.,* inappropriate clothing, exposure to the elements (heat, cold), dehydration. The nursing focus for hypothermia and hyperthermia is prevention. I recommend that these diagnoses be used as High Risk for Hyperthermia and High Risk for Hypothermia to more appropriately describe the nursing role. Severe hypothermia and hyperthermia are life-threatening situations and require medical and nursing interventions for treatment. Such situations are collaborative problems and should be labeled Potential Complication: Hypothermia or Hyperthermia.

DEFINITION

High Risk for Altered Body Temperature: The state in which an individual is at risk of failing to maintain body temperature within normal range.

RISK FACTORS

Major (Must Be Present)

Presence of risk factors (see Related Factors)

RELATED FACTORS

Pathophysiological

Illness or trauma affecting temperature regulation
  Coma/increased intracranial pressure
  Brain tumor/hypothalamic tumor/head trauma

Cerebrovascular accident (CVA)
Infection
Integument (skin) injury
Anemia
Neurovascular disease/peripheral vascular disease
Pheochromocytoma (tumor of the adrenal
  medulla)
Altered metabolic rate

Treatment-related

Medications (*e.g.,* vasodilators/vasoconstrictors)
Sedation
Parenteral fluid infusion/blood transfusion
Dialysis
Surgery

Maturational

Extremes of age (*e.g.,* newborn, elderly)

Hypothermia

DEFINITION

Hypothermia: The state in which an individual has or is at risk
for a sustained reduction of body temperature below 35°C
(95°F) orally or 36°C (96°F) rectally.

DEFINING CHARACTERISTICS*

Major (80%–100%)

Reduction in body temperature below 35°C (95°F) orally
  or 36°C (96°F) rectally
Cool skin
Pallor (moderate)
Shivering (mild)

---

* Adapted from Carroll SM: Hypothermia: A Clinical Validation
Study. (Unpublished, 1987)

Minor (50%–79%)

Mental confusion/drowsiness/restlessness
Decreased pulse and respiration
Cachexia/malnutrition

RELATED FACTORS

Situational (Personal, Environmental)

Exposure to heat, cold, rain, snow, wind
Inappropriate clothing for climate
Poverty (inability to pay for shelter or heat)
Extremes of weight
Consumption of alcohol
Dehydration
Inactivity

Maturational

Extremes of age (*e.g.,* newborn, elderly)

OUTCOME CRITERIA

The person will

1. Identify risk factors for hypothermia
2. Relate methods of maintaining warmth/preventing heat loss
3. Maintain body temperature within normal limits

INTERVENTIONS (for High Risk for Hypothermia)

1. Teach client to reduce prolonged exposure to cold environment.
   a. Explain the importance of wearing a hat, gloves, and warm socks and shoes to prevent heat loss.
   b. Encourage the person to limit going outside when temperatures are very cold.
   c. Acquire an electric blanket, warm blankets, or down comforter for bed.
2. Consult with social service to identify sources of financial assistance/warm clothing/blankets.
3. Explain to family members that newborns, infants, and

the elderly are more susceptible to heat loss (see also
Ineffective Thermoregulation).
4. Teach the early signs of hypothermia:
    Cool skin
    Pallor, blanching, redness

Hyperthermia

DEFINITION

Hyperthermia: The state in which an individual has or is at
risk for a sustained elevation of body temperature greater than
37.8°C (100°F) orally or 38.8°C (101°F) rectally due to external factors.

DEFINING CHARACTERISTICS

Major (Must Be Present)

Temperature greater than 37.8°C (100°F) orally or
38.8°C (101°F) rectally

Minor (May Be Present)

Flushed skin
Warm to touch
Increased respiratory rate
Tachycardia
Shivering/goose pimples
Dehydration
Specific or generalized aches and pains (*e.g.,* headache)
Malaise/fatigue/weakness
Loss of appetite

RELATED FACTORS

Situational (Personal, Environmental)

Exposure to heat, sun
Inappropriate clothing for climate
Poverty
Extremes of weight
Dehydration
Inactivity or vigorous activity
Lack of knowledge

Maturational

Extremes of age (*e.g.,* newborn, elderly)

OUTCOME CRITERIA

The person will

1. Identify risk factors for hyperthermia
2. Relate methods of preventing hyperthermia
3. Maintain normal body temperature

INTERVENTIONS (for High Risk for Hyperthermia)

1. Teach the person the importance of maintaining an adequate fluid intake (at least 2000 ml a day unless contraindicated by heart or kidney disease) to prevent dehydration.
2. Monitor intake and output.
3. See also *Fluid Volume Deficit.*
4. Assess whether clothing or bedcovers are too warm for the environment or planned activity.
5. Teach the importance of increasing fluid intake during warm weather and exercise.
6. Teach the early signs of hyperthermia or heat stroke:
   Flushed skin   Headache
   Fatigue   Loss of appetite

Thermoregulation, Ineffective

DEFINITION

Ineffective Thermoregulation: The state in which an individual experiences or is at risk of experiencing an inability to effectively maintain normal body temperature in the presence of adverse or changing external factors.

Author's Note:
This diagnostic category is indicated when the nurse can maintain or assist a client to maintain a body temperature within normal limits by manipulating external factors (*e.g.*, clothing) and environmental conditions. Persons who are at high risk for this diagnosis are the elderly and neonates. For those with temperature fluctuations due to disease, infections, or trauma, see Altered Comfort.

DEFINING CHARACTERISTICS

Major (Must Be Present)

Temperature fluctuations related to limited metabolic compensatory regulation in response to environmental factors

RELATED FACTORS

Situational (Personal, Environmental)

Fluctuating environmental temperatures
Cold or wet articles (clothes, cribs, equipment)
Inadequate heating system
Inadequate housing
Wet body surface
Inadequate clothing for weather (excessive, insufficient)

Maturational

Neonate
  Large surface area relative to body mass
  Limited ability to produce heat (metabolic)
  Limited shivering ability
  Increased basal metabolism
Premature (same as neonate but more severe)
Elderly
  Decreased basal metabolism
  Loss of adipose tissue (limbs)

OUTCOME CRITERIA

The infant will

1. Have a temperature between 36.4° and 37°C

The parent will

1. Explain techniques to avoid heat loss at home

INTERVENTIONS

1. Reduce or eliminate the sources of heat loss.
    a. Evaporation
        - When bathing, provide a warm environment.
        - Wash and dry in sections to reduce evaporation.
        - Limit time in contact with wet clothing or blankets.
    b. Convection
        - Avoid drafts (air conditioning, fans, windows, open portholes on Isolette).
    c. Conduction
        - Warm all articles for care (stethoscopes, scales, hands of caregivers, clothes, bed linens).
    d. Radiation
        - Reduce objects in the room that absorb heat (metal).
        - Place crib or bed as far away from walls (outside) or windows as possible.
2. Monitor temperature.
    a. If temperature is below normal:
        - Wrap in two blankets.
        - Put on head cap.
        - Assess for environmental sources of heat loss.
        - If hypothermia persists over 1 hour, notify physician.
        - Assess for complications of cold stress: hypoxia, respiratory acidosis, hypoglycemia, fluid and electrolyte imbalances, weight loss.
    b. If temperature is above normal:
        - Loosen blanket.
        - Remove cap, if on.
        - Assess environment for thermal gain.
        - If hyperthermia persists over 1 hour, notify physician.

3. Teach caregiver why infant is vulnerable to temperature fluctuations (cold and heat).
   a. Demonstrate how to conserve heat during bathing.
   b. Instruct that it is not necessary to routinely check temperature at home.
   c. Teach to check temperature if infant is hot, sick, or irritable.

Bowel Elimination, Altered*

Constipation

Colonic Constipation

Perceived Constipation

Diarrhea

Bowel Incontinence

Author's Note:
Altered Bowel Elimination represents a broad category that is probably too broad for clinical use. It is recommended that more specific categories be used when possible. The three diagnostic categories relating to constipation represent one general constipation category and two specific types. The treatment of colonic constipation differs from the treatment of perceived constipation.

* This diagnostic category is not on the NANDA list but has been included for clarity or usefulness.

DEFINITION

Altered Bowel Elimination: The state in which an individual experiences or is at high risk of experiencing bowel dysfunction resulting in diarrhea or constipation.

DEFINING CHARACTERISTICS

Major (Must Be Present)

Reports or demonstrates one or more of the following:
Hard, formed stool
Painful defecation
Habitual use of laxatives/enemas
Bowel movements less than 3 times weekly
Loose, liquid stools
Increased frequency (more than 3 times a day)

Minor (May Be Present)

Painful defecation
Abdominal discomfort
Rectal fullness
Headache

Anorexia
Urgency
Abdominal cramping
Increased or decreased
bowel sounds

RELATED FACTORS

See Related Factors under Constipation and Diarrhea.

Constipation

DEFINITION

Constipation: The state in which an individual experiences or is at high risk of experiencing stasis of the large intestine, resulting in infrequent elimination and hard, dry feces.

DEFINING CHARACTERISTICS

Major (Must Be Present)

Hard, formed stool
and/or
Defecation occurs fewer than 3 times a week

Minor (May Be Present)

Decreased bowel sounds
Reported feeling of rectal fullness
Reported feeling of pressure in rectum
Straining and pain on defecation
Palpable impaction

RELATED FACTORS
Pathophysiological

Malnutrition
Sensory-motor disorders
    Spinal cord lesions   Cerebrovascular accident
    Spinal cord injury   (CVA, stroke)
    Spina bifida   Neurological diseases
Metabolic and endocrine disorders
    Anorexia nervosa   Hypothyroidism
    Obesity   Hyperpara-
                          thyroidism
Ileus
Pain (on defecation)
    Hemorrhoids
    Back Injury
Decreased peristalsis related to hypoxia (cardiac,
  pulmonary)
Megacolon

Treatment-related

Drug side effects
    Antacids   Anticholinergics
    Iron   Anesthetics
    Barium   Narcotics (codeine,
    Aluminum   morphine)
    Aspirin   Diuretics
    Phenothiazines   Antiparkinsonian agents
    Calcium
Surgery
Habitual laxative use

Situational (Personal, Environmental)

Immobility   Lack of privacy
Pregnancy   Inadequate diet (lack of
Stress   roughage/thiamine)

Lack of exercise	Dehydration
Irregular evacuation patterns	Fear of rectal or cardiac pain
Cultural/health beliefs	Faulty appraisal dementia

Maturational

Infant
  Formula
Child
  Toilet training (reluctance to interrupt play)
Elderly
  Decreased motility of gastrointestinal tract

OUTCOME CRITERIA

The person will

1. Relate less pain on defecation
2. Describe causative factors when known
3. Describe rationale and procedure for treatments

INTERVENTIONS

1. Assess causative factors:
    a. If caused by inadequate diet, fluids, exercise, medication side effects, environmental changes, stress, refer to *Colonic Constipation.*
    b. If caused by habitual laxative or enema use and faulty appraisal of normal bowel elimination, refer to *Perceived Constipation.*
    c. If cause is unknown, treat as colonic constipation and continue to assess for cause.
    d. If caused by painful defecation, use constipation related to painful defecation.
2. Reduce rectal pain, if possible, by instructing person in corrective measures:
    a. Gently apply a lubricant to anus to reduce pain on defecation.
    b. Apply cool compresses to area to reduce itching.
    c. Take sitz bath or soak in tub or warm water (43°–46°C) for 15-minute intervals if soothing.
    d. Take stool softeners or mineral oil as an adjunct to other approaches.

    e. Consult with physician regarding use of local anesthetics and antiseptic agents.
3. Protect the skin from contamination:
    a. Evaluate the surrounding skin area.
    b. Cleanse properly with nonirritating agent (*e.g.,* use gentle motion; use soft tissues following defecation).
    c. Suggest a sitz bath following defecation.
    d. Gently apply protective emollient or lubricant.
4. Initiate health teaching if indicated:
    a. Teach the methods to prevent rectal pressure that contributes to hemorrhoids.
    b. Avoid prolonged sitting and straining at defecation.
    c. Soften stools (*e.g.,* low roughage diet, high fluid intake).

Colonic Constipation

DEFINITION

Colonic Constipation: The state in which an individual experiences or is at risk of experiencing a delay in passage of food residue resulting in dry, hard stool.

DEFINING CHARACTERISTICS*

Major (80%–100%)

Decreased frequency
Hard, dry stool
Straining at stool
Painful defecation
Abdominal distention

Minor (50%–79%)

Rectal pressure
Headache, appetite impairment
Abdominal pain

---

* Adapted from McLane AM, McShane RE: Empirical validation of defining characteristics of constipation: A study of bowel elimination practices of healthy adults. In Hurley ME (ed): Classification of Nursing Diagnoses: Proceedings of the Sixth Conference, pp 448–455. St. Louis, CV Mosby, 1986

RELATED FACTORS
Pathophysiological

Malnutrition
Sensory-motor disorders
   Spinal cord lesions   Neurological diseases
   Spinal cord injury
   Cerebrovascular accident
    (CVA, stroke)
Metabolic and endocrine disorders
   Anorexia nervosa   Hypothyroidism
   Obesity   Hyperpara-
                    thyroidism
Ileus
Decreased peristalsis related to hypoxia (cardiac,
  pulmonary)
Megacolon

Treatment-related

Drug side effects
   Antacids   Anticholinergics
   Iron   Anesthetics
   Barium   Narcotics (codeine,
   Aluminum   morphine)
   Aspirin   Diuretics
   Phenothiazines   Antiparkinsonian agents
   Calcium
Surgery
Habitual laxative use

Situational (Personal, Environmental)

Immobility   Lack of privacy
Pregnancy   Inadequate diet (lack of
Stress   roughage/thiamine)
Lack of exercise   Dehydration
Irregular evacuation Fear of rectal or cardiac
  patterns   pain

Maturational

Infant
   Formula
Child
   Toilet training (reluctance to interrupt play)

Elderly
 Decreased motility of gastrointestinal tract

OUTCOME CRITERIA

The person will

1. Describe therapeutic bowel regimen
2. Relate or demonstrate improved bowel elimination
3. Explain rationale for interventions

INTERVENTIONS

1. Teach the importance of a balanced diet.
   a. Review list of foods high in bulk:
      - Fresh fruits with skins
      - Bran
      - Nuts and seeds
      - Whole grain breads and cereals
      - Cooked fruits and vegetables
      - Fruit juices
   b. Include approximately 800 g of fruits and vege-tables (about four pieces of fresh fruit and large salad) for normal daily bowel movement.
   c. Gradually increase amount of bran as tolerated (may add to cereals, baked goods, etc.). Explain the need for fluid intake with bran.
2. Encourage intake of at least 2 liters of fluids—8–10 glasses—unless contraindicated.
3. Recommend a glass of hot water to be taken 30 minutes before breakfast that may act as stimulus to bowel evac-uation.
4. Establish regular time for elimination.
5. Assist patient to normal semisquatting position to allow optimum usage of abdominal muscles and effect of force of gravity.
6. If fecal impaction is suspected, perform digital exami-nation of rectum: Have client assume position lying on left side. Don glove, lubricate forefinger, and insert; at-tempt to break up any hardened fecal mass and remove pieces.
7. If impaction is out of reach of gloved finger, consult physician.

Perceived Constipation

DEFINITION

Perceived Constipation: The state in which an individual self-prescribes the daily use of laxatives, enemas, or suppositories to ensure a daily bowel movement.

DEFINING CHARACTERISTICS*

Major (80%–100%)

Expectation of a daily bowel movement with the resulting overuse of laxatives, enemas, and suppositories
Expected passage of stool at the same time every day

RELATED FACTORS

Pathophysiological

Altered affect caused by change in
 Body chemistry
 Tumor
Obsessive-compulsive disorders
Central nervous system deterioration

Situational (Personal, Environmental)

Cultural/family health beliefs
Faulty appraisal

OUTCOME CRITERIA

The person will

1. Verbalize acceptance with bowel movement every 2–3 days

---

* McLane A, McShane R: Empirical validation of defining characteristics of constipation: A study of bowel elimination practices of healthy adults. In Hurley ME (ed): Classification of Nursing Diagnoses: Proceedings of the Sixth Conference, pp 448–455. St. Louis, CV Mosby, 1986

2. Not use laxatives regularly
3. Relate the causes of constipation
4. Describe the hazards of laxative use
5. Relate an intent to increase fiber, fluid, and exercise in daily life as instructed

INTERVENTIONS

1. Explain that bowel movements are needed every 2–3 days, not daily.
2. Explain the hazards of regular laxative use.
3. Teach the importance of a balanced diet.
   a. Review list of foods high in bulk:
      - Fresh fruits with skins
      - Bran
      - Nuts and seeds
      - Whole grain breads and cereals
      - Cooked fruits and vegetables
   b. Include approximately 800 g of fruits and vegetables (about four pieces of fresh fruit and large salad) for normal daily bowel movement.
   c. Gradually increase amount of bran as tolerated (may add to cereals, baked goods, etc.). Explain the need for fluid intake with bran.
   d. Suggest a commercial fiber product if fiber is inadequate in diet.
4. Encourage intake of at least 6–10 glasses of water (unless contraindicated).
5. Recommend a glass of hot water to be taken 30 minutes before breakfast that may act as stimulus to bowel evacuation.
6. Establish a regular time for elimination.
7. Emphasize the need for regular exercise.
   a. Suggest walking:
   b. If walking is prohibited:
      - Teach client to lie in bed or sit on chair and bend one knee at a time to chest (10–20 times each knee) three to four times a day.
      - Teach client to sit in chair or lie in bed and turn torso from side to side (20–30 times) six to ten times a day.

31

Diarrhea

DEFINITION

Diarrhea: The state in which an individual experiences or is at high risk of experiencing frequent passage of liquid stool or unformed stool.

DEFINING CHARACTERISTICS

Major (Must Be Present)

Loose, liquid stools
and/or
Increased frequency

Minor (May Be Present)

Urgency
Cramping/abdominal pain
Increased frequency of bowel sounds
Increase in fluidity or volume of stools

RELATED FACTORS
Pathophysiological

Nutritional disorders and malabsorptive syndromes
    Kwashiorkor   Crohn's disease
    Gastritis   Lactose intolerance
    Peptic ulcer   Spastic colon
    Diverticulitis   Celiac disease (sprue)
    Ulcerative colitis   Irritable bowel
Metabolic and endocrine disorders
    Diabetes mellitus   Thyrotoxicosis
    Addison's disease
Dumping syndrome
Infectious process
    Trichinosis   Shigellosis
    Dysentery   Typhoid fever
    Cholera   Infectious hepatitis
    Malaria
Cancer
Uremia
Tuberculosis

Arsenic poisoning
Fecal impaction

Treatment-related

Surgical intervention of the bowel
    Loss of bowel   Ileal bypass
Drug side effects
    Thyroid agents   Antibiotics
    Antacids   Cancer chemo-
    Laxatives   therapeutic agents
    Stool softeners
Tube feedings

OUTCOME CRITERIA

The person will

1. Describe contributing factors when known
2. Explain rationale for interventions
3. Report less diarrhea

INTERVENTIONS

1. Assess for causative/contributing factors: tube feedings, dietary indiscretions/contaminated foods, food allergies, foreign travel.
2. Reduce diarrhea.
    a. Discontinue solids.
    b. Ingest clear liquids (fruit juices, Gatorade, broth).
    c. Continue breastfeeding, discontinue formula.
    d. Avoid milk products, fat, whole grain, fresh fruits, and vegetables.
    e. Gradually add semisolids and solids (crackers, yogurt, rice, bananas, applesauce).
3. Increase oral intake to maintain a normal urine specific gravity (pale urine).
4. Encourage fluids high in potassium and sodium (orange and grapefruit juices, bouillon).
5. Caution against use of very hot or very cold liquids.
6. Explain to client and significant others the interventions required to prevent future episodes.

7. Teach precautions to take when traveling to foreign lands (Maresca).*
   a. Avoid foods served cold, salads, milk, fresh cheese, cold cuts and salsa.
   b. Drink carbonated or bottled beverages, avoid ice.
   c. Peel fresh fruits and vegetables.
8. Explain how to prevent transmission of infection (hand washing, proper storing, cooking, and handling of food).

Bowel Incontinence

DEFINITION

Bowel Incontinence: The state in which an individual experiences a change in normal bowel habits characterized by involuntary passage of stool.

Author's Note:

This diagnostic category represents a situation in which nurses have multiple responsibilities. Clients experiencing Bowel Incontinence have various responses that disrupt functioning, such as

Fear related to embarrassment over lack of control of bowels

High Risk for Impaired Skin Integrity related to irritative nature of feces on skin

For some spinal-cord injured persons, Bowel Incontinence related to lack of voluntary control over rectal sphincter would be descriptive.

DEFINING CHARACTERISTICS

Major (Must Be Present)

Involuntary passage of stool

* Maresca T: Assessment and management of acute diarrheal illness in adults. Nurse Pract 11(11):15–16, 1986

RELATED FACTORS
Pathophysiological

Loss of sphincter control
Progressive dementia
Progressive neuromuscular disorder, *e.g.,* multiple
  sclerosis
Inflammatory bowel disease

Situational

Depression
Cognitive impairment
Surgery
  Colostomy

OUTCOME CRITERIA

The person will

1. Evacuate a soft formed stool every day, every other day,
   or every third day

INTERVENTIONS

1. Assess previous bowel elimination patterns, diet, and
   life-style.
2. Determine present neurological and physical status,
   patient's functional level.
3. Plan a consistent, appropriate time for elimination.
   a. Daily bowel program for 5 days or until a pattern
      develops, then every other day bowel program;
      morning or evening
4. For persons with intact sacral reflex center:
   a. Position in an upright or sitting position if func-
      tionally able. If not functionally able (quadri-
      plegic) position in left side-lying position, use
      digital stimulation: gloves, lubricant, index finger
      (adults).
   b. For the functionally able, use assistive devices:
      dil stick, digital stimulator, raised commode seat,
      and lubricant and gloves as appropriate.
5. For persons with upper extremity mobility and those
   with abdominal musculature innervation, teach bowel
   elimination facilitation techniques as appropriate:

>   a. Valsalva maneuver
>   b. Forward bends
>   c. Sitting push-ups
>   d. Abdominal massage
>   6. For persons with absent sacral reflex center:
>   a. Plan daily evacuation schedule, either morning or evening with manual evacuation of rectal contents.
>   b. Position in upright or sitting position if functionally able.
>   c. Use assistive devices, raised commode seats, and lubricant as appropriate.
>   d. Teach bowel facilitation techniques:
>   • Valsalva maneuver
>   • Forward bends
>   • Abdominal massage
>   • Sitting push-ups if patient is functionally able
>   7. Maintain an elimination record of bowel schedule to include time, stool results, method(s) used, and number of involuntaries if any.
>   8. Teach the importance of diet high in fiber and optimal fluid intake.
>   9. Cleanse skin after each bowel movement. Protect intact skin with an ointment, *e.g.,* aluminum paste. If skin not intact, consult clinical nurse specialist or enterostomal therapist.
>   10. Provide physical activity and exercise appropriate to functional level, *e.g.,* abdominal exercises.
>   11. Teach appropriate use of stool softeners, suppositories, and hazards of enemas.
>   12. Teach signs and symptoms of fecal impaction and constipation.
>   13. Provide home care training for those who can be functionally independent with bowel program.

Breastfeeding, Effective

DEFINITION

Effective Breastfeeding: The state in which a mother–infant dyad exhibits adequate proficiency and satisfaction with the breastfeeding process.

Author's Note:

This diagnosis reportedly represents a wellness diagnosis. The newly proposed NANDA wellness diagnosis is defined as "a clinical judgment about an individual, family or community in transition from a specific level of wellness to a higher level of wellness" (NANDA Guidelines).* The above definition does not describe a mother–infant dyad seeking higher level breastfeeding. Instead it describes "adequate proficiency and satisfaction with the breastfeeding process."

In the management of breastfeeding experience the nurse will find three situations:

Ineffective Breastfeeding
High Risk for Ineffective Breastfeeding
Potential for Enhanced Breastfeeding

Effective Breastfeeding can be used to describe an evaluation of a mother-and-infant breastfeeding session for both *Ineffective* or *High Risk for Ineffective Breastfeeding.* This evaluation is the result of the nurse observing or the mother reporting those signs and symptoms listed as defining characteristics. In an acute setting, too little time has elapsed for the nurse to make a wellness nursing diagnosis concerning breastfeeding, given the recentness of the experience.

If the nurse, most likely in a community or private practice, has a mother who reports proficiency and satisfaction with the breastfeeding process and desires additional teaching to achieve even greater proficiency and satisfaction, the nursing diagnosis of *Potential for Enhanced Breastfeeding* is appropriate. The focus of this teaching and continued support would not be to prevent *Ineffective Breastfeeding* or to maintain adequate proficiency and satisfaction but rather to promote enhanced, higher quality breastfeeding.

I recommend that this diagnosis not be used in its present form but instead the nurse should use *Ineffective Breastfeeding* and *High Risk for Ineffective Breastfeeding.* Nurses who desire to use a wellness nursing diagnosis could use *Potential for Enhanced Breastfeeding.* Since this diagnosis is not on the NANDA list, nurses using it should send their experiences to NANDA.

* NANDA Guidelines: Taxonomy 1 Revised. St. Louis, North American Nursing Diagnosis Assn., 1990

DEFINING CHARACTERISTICS

Major

Mother able to position infant at breast to promote a
successful latch-on response
Infant is content after feeding
Regular and sustained suckling/swallowing at the breast
Appropriate infant weight patterns for age
Effective mother/infant communication patterns (infant
cues, maternal interpretation and response)

Minor

Signs and/or symptoms of oxytocin release (let down or
milk ejection reflex)
Adequate infant elimination patterns for age
Eagerness of infant to nurse
Maternal verbalization of satisfaction with the
breastfeeding process

Breastfeeding, Ineffective

DEFINITION

Ineffective Breastfeeding: The state in which a mother, infant,
or child experiences or is at risk of experiencing dissatisfaction
or difficulty with the breastfeeding process.

DEFINING CHARACTERISTICS

Major (Must Be Present)

Actual or perceived inadequate milk supply
Infant's inability to attach correctly onto maternal breast
No observable signs of oxytocin release
Observable signs of inadequate infant intake
Nonsustained suckling at the breast
Insufficient emptying of each breast at each feeding
Persistence of sore nipples beyond the first week of
breastfeeding
Insufficient opportunity for suckling at the breast

Infant exhibiting fussiness and crying within the first hour after breastfeeding; unresponsive to other comfort measures

Infant arching and crying at the breast, resisting latching on

RELATED FACTORS
Pathophysiological

Mastitis
Breast anomaly
    Inverted nipple(s)
Pain (breast, perineum, uterus)

Treatment-related

Previous breast surgery

Situational (Personal, Environmental)

History of breastfeeding difficulties/failure
Ambivalence (maternal, family)
Anxiety
Nonsupportive partner/family
Lack of knowledge
Interruption in breastfeeding
    Ill mother   Excess artificial nipple
    Ill infant   supplements
    Work schedule

Maturational

Neonate/infant
    Prematurity
    Poor sucking reflex

OUTCOME CRITERIA

The mother will

1. Make an informed decision related to method of feeding infant (breast or bottle)
2. Identify activities that deter or promote successful breastfeeding

Interventions

1. Assess knowledge, correct myths and misinformation.
2. Discuss advantages and disadvantages of breastfeeding.
3. Assist during first feedings.
   a. Position comfortably.
   b. Demonstrate different positions.
   c. Demonstrate and explain rooting reflex and show how it can be used to help infant latch on.
   d. Make sure baby grasps a good portion of areola and not just the nipple.
4. Advise mother to increase feeding times gradually, to start at 10 minutes per side and build up over next 3–5 days.
5. Instruct mother to offer both breasts at each feeding, alternating the beginning side each time.
6. Teach mother to wear well-fitting support brassiere day and night; apply warm compresses for 15–20 minutes before nursing for engorgement.
7. Teach management of sore nipples.
   a. Decrease nursing time to 5–10 minutes per side. Start baby on nontender side first. Allow for more frequent, short feedings. Suggest alternate positions to rotate infant's grasps. Allow breasts to dry after each feeding.
   b. Keep nursing pads dry.
   c. Use breast cream only after breasts are dry.
   d. Use breast shield as last measure and remove after milk has let down.
8. Provide breast pump or make patient aware of availability, if needed.
9. Encourage verbal expression of feelings.
10. Explore feelings and anticipation of problems. Older child may be jealous of contact with baby. Mother can use this time to read to older child.
11. Stress the need for rest.
    a. Encourage mother to make herself and infant a priority.
    b. Encourage mother to limit visits from relatives for first 4 weeks.
12. Initiate referrals as indicated (lactation specialist, La Leche League).

Cardiac Output,
Altered: Decreased: (Specify)

DEFINITION

Altered Cardiac Output: Decreased: The state in which an individual experiences a reduction in the amount of blood pumped by the heart, resulting in compromised cardiac function.

Author's Note:

This diagnostic category represents a situation in which nurses have multiple responsibilities. Individuals experiencing decreased cardiac output may present various responses that disrupt functioning, such as:

> Activity Intolerance
> Sleep Pattern Disturbance

Or they may be at risk for developing physiological complications, such as:

> Dysrhythmias
> Cardiogenic shock
> Congestive heart failure

I recommend that the nurse not use Altered Cardiac Output: Decreased but instead select another diagnostic category that better describes the situation. (Refer to Activity Intolerance.)

It is also recommended that the physiological complications for which nurses monitor in individuals with decreased cardiac output, and for which they collaborate with medicine for treatment, be labeled collaborative problems, such as

> Potential Complications:
> Dysrhythmias
> Cardiogenic shock
> Hypoxia

By not using Altered Cardiac Output: Decreased, the nurse can more specifically describe the situations that nurses either treat as a nursing diagnosis or co-treat as a collaborative problem.

DEFINING CHARACTERISTICS

Low blood pressure	Dysrhythmia
Rapid pulse	Oliguria
Restlessness	Fatigability
Cyanosis	Vertigo
Dyspnea	Edema (peripheral, sacral)
Angina	

Comfort, Altered*

Pain

Chronic Pain

DEFINITION

Altered Comfort: The state in which an individual experiences an uncomfortable sensation in response to a noxious stimulus.

Author's Note:

This diagnostic category, altered comfort, can represent a variety of uncomfortable sensations such as pruritus, immobility, or NPO status. When an individual experiences nausea and vomiting, the nurse should assess whether Altered Comfort or High Risk for Altered Nutrition is the appropriate category. Short-lived episodes of nausea and/or vomiting, *e.g.,* postoperatively, can be best described with Altered Comfort related to nausea/vomiting secondary to effects of anesthesia and/or analgesics. When the nausea/vomiting is at risk of compromising nutritional intake, use High Risk for Altered Nutrition: Less Than Body Requirements related to nausea and vomiting secondary to (specify).

---

* This diagnostic category is not currently on the NANDA list but has been included for clarity and usefulness.

DEFINING CHARACTERISTICS

Major (Must Be Present)

The person reports or demonstrates a discomfort.

Minor (May Be Present)

Autonomic response in acute pain
  Blood pressure increased
  Pulse increased
  Respirations increased
  Diaphoresis
  Dilated pupils
Guarded position
Facial mask of pain
Crying, moaning
Abdominal heaviness
Cutaneous irritation

RELATED FACTORS

Any factor can contribute to altered comfort. The most common are listed below.

Pathophysiological

Musculoskeletal disorders
  Fractures   Arthritis
  Contractures   Spinal cord disorders
  Spasms
Visceral disorders
  Cardiac   Intestinal
  Renal   Pulmonary
  Hepatic
Cancer
Vascular disorders
  Vasospasm   Phlebitis
  Occlusion   Vasodilation (headache)
Inflammation
  Nerve   Joint
  Tendon   Muscle
  Bursa
Contagious disease (rubella, chickenpox)

Treatment-related

Trauma (surgery, accidents)
  Diagnostic tests
    Venipuncture
    Invasive scanning (*e.g.,* intravenous pyelogram [IVP])
    Biopsy
  Medications

Situational (Personal, Environmental)

Immobility/improper positioning
Overactivity
Pressure points (tight cast, elastic bandage)
Pregnancy (prenatal, intrapartum, postpartum)
Allergic response
Chemical irritants
Stress

Pain

DEFINITION

Pain: The state in which an individual experiences and reports the presence of severe discomfort or an uncomfortable sensation.

Author's Note:

This diagnostic category represents an individual who is experiencing pain. Acute pain may be more useful as an etiology, *e.g.,* anxiety related to episodes of chest pain and unknown prognosis or Impaired Physical Mobility related to incisional pain.

DEFINING CHARACTERISTICS

Subjective
  Communication (verbal or coded) of pain descriptors

Objective

    Guarding behavior, protective

    Self-focusing

    Narrowed focus (altered time perception, withdrawal from social contact, impaired thought processes)

    Distraction behavior (moaning, crying, pacing, seeking out other people and/or activities, restlessness)

    Facial mask of pain (lackluster eyes, "beaten look," fixed or scattered movement, grimace)

    Altered muscle tone (may span from listless to rigid)

    Autonomic responses not seen in chronic stable pain (diaphoresis, blood pressure and pulse change, pupillary dilation, increased or decreased respiratory rate)

OUTCOME CRITERIA

The person will

1. Convey that others validate that the pain exists
2. Relate relief after a satisfactory relief measure as evidenced by (specify)

The child will, according to age and ability

1. Identify the source of the pain
2. Identify activities that increase and decrease pain
3. Describe comfort from others during the pain experience

INTERVENTIONS

1. Reduce lack of knowledge.
   a. Explain causes of the pain to the person, if known.
   b. Relate how long the pain will last, if known.
   c. Explain diagnostic tests and procedures in detail by relating the discomforts and sensations that will be felt and approximate the length of time involved (*e.g.,* "During the intravenous pyelogram you might feel a momentary hot flash through your entire body.").
2. Provide accurate information to reduce fear of addiction.
3. Relate your acceptance of patient's response to pain.
   a. Acknowledge the presence of the patient's pain.
   b. Listen attentively to patient concerning the patient's pain.

      c. Convey that you are assessing the pain because you want to better understand it (not determine if it is really present).

4. Assess the family for the presence of misconceptions about pain or its treatment.

5. Discuss the reasons why an individual may experience increased or decreased pain (*e.g.,* fatigue [increased] or presence of distractions [decreased]).

      a. Encourage family members to share their concerns privately (*e.g.,* fear that the person will use pain for secondary gains if they give the person too much attention).

      b. Assess whether the family doubts the pain and discuss the effects of this on the person's pain and on the relationship.

      c. Encourage the family to give attention also when pain is not exhibited.

6. Provide with opportunities to rest during the day and with periods of uninterrupted sleep at night (must rest when pain is ↓).

7. Discuss with the person and family the therapeutic uses of distraction, along with other methods of pain relief.

8. Teach a method of distraction during an acute pain (*e.g.,* painful procedure) that is not a burden (*e.g.,* count items in a picture, count anything in the room, such as patterns on wallpaper or count silently to self); breathe rhythmically; listen to music and increase the volume as the pain increases.

9. Teach noninvasive pain relief measures.

      a. Relaxation

         • Instruct on techniques to reduce skeletal muscle tension, which will reduce the intensity of the pain.

         • Promote relaxation with a back rub, massage, or warm bath.

         • Teach a specific relaxation strategy (*e.g.,* slow, rhythmic breathing or deep breath—clench fists—yawn).

      b. Cutaneous stimulation

         • Discuss with the person the various methods of skin stimulation and their effects on pain.

- Discuss each of the following methods and the precautions:
    Hot water bottle
    Electric heating pad
    Warm tub
    Moist heat pack
    Hot summer sun
    Thin plastic wrap over painful area to retain body heat (*e.g.,* knee, elbow)
- Discuss each of the following methods and the precautions of each:
    Cold towels (wrung out)
    Cold-water immersion for small body parts
    Ice bag
    Cold gel pack
    Ice massage
- Explain the therapeutic uses of menthol preparations and massage/back rub.

10. Provide the person with optimal pain relief with prescribed analgesics.
11. After administering a pain-relief medication, return in 30 minutes to assess effectiveness.
12. Give accurate information to correct family misconceptions (*e.g.,* addiction, doubts about pain).
13. Provide individuals with opportunities to discuss their fears, anger, and frustrations in private; acknowledge the difficulty of the situation.
14. Encourage individual to discuss his or her pain experience.
15. For children
    a. Assess the child's pain experience.
        - Determine the child's concept of the cause of pain, if feasible.
        - Ask child to point to the area that hurts.
        - For children under 4–5 use Oucher Scale of five faces from very happy (1) to crying (5).
        - For children over 4, ask child to rate the pain using a scale of 0–5 (0 = no pain and 5 = worst pain)
        - Ask the child what makes the pain better and what makes it worse.

- Assess if fear or loneliness is contributing to pain.
b. Promote security with honest explanations and opportunities for choice.
  - Tell the truth; explain
    How much it will hurt
    How long it will last
    What will help the pain
  - Do not threaten (*e.g., do not* tell the child, "If you don't hold still you won't go home.").
  - Explicitly explain and reinforce to the child that pain is not a means of punishment.
  - Explain to the parents that the child may cry more openly when they are present but that their presence is important for promoting trust.
  - Explain to the child that the procedure is necessary so he or she can get better, and it is important to hold still so it can be done quickly.
  - Discuss with the parents the importance of truth-telling; instruct parents to:
    Tell child when they are leaving and when they will return
    Relate to the child that they cannot take away the pain but that they will be there (except in circumstances when parents are not permitted to remain)
  - Allow the parents opportunities to share their feelings about witnessing their child's pain and their helplessness.
c. Prepare the child for a painful procedure.
  - Discuss the procedure with the parents; determine what they have told the child.
  - Explain the procedure in words suited to the child's age and developmental level.
  - Relate the discomforts that will be felt (*e.g.,* what the child will feel, taste, see, or smell).
  - Encourage the child to ask questions before and during the procedure; ask the child to share with you what he or she thinks is going to happen and why.

- Share with the child (who is old enough—over 3½) that

   You expect that the child will hold still and that such obedience will be pleasing to you.

   It is all right to cry or squeeze your hand if it hurts

   - Arrange to have parents present for procedures (especially for children 18 months to 5 years).

d. Explain to the child that he or she can be distracted from the procedure if that is the child's wish (the use of distraction without the child's knowledge of the impending discomfort is not advocated because the child will learn to mistrust).

   - Tell a story with a puppet.
   - Ask the child to name or count objects in a picture.
   - Ask the child to look at the picture and to locate certain objects ("Where is the dog?").
   - Ask child to tell you about a pet.
   - Ask child to count your blinks.

e. Provide the child with privacy during the painful procedure; use a treatment room rather than the child's bed.

f. Assist the child with the aftermath of pain.

   - Tell the child when the painful procedure is over.
   - Pick up the small child to indicate it is over.
   - Encourage the child to discuss the pain experience (draw or act out with dolls).
   - Encourage the child to perform the painful procedure using the same equipment on a doll under supervision.
   - Praise the child for endurance and convey that the pain was handled well regardless of the child's behavior (unless the child was violent to others).
   - Give the child a souvenir of the pain (Band-Aid, badge for bravery).
   - Teach the child to keep a record of painful experiences and to place a star next to those

he or she held still for (*e.g.,* gold stars on a
paper for each injection or venipuncture).

Chronic Pain

DEFINITION

Chronic Pain: The state in which an individual experiences
pain that is persistent or intermittent and lasts for more than
6 months.

DEFINING CHARACTERISTICS

Major (Must Be Present)

The person reports that pain has existed for more than 6 months
(may be the only assessment data present).

Minor (May Be Present)

Discomfort
Anger, frustration, depression because of situation
Facial mask of pain
Anorexia, weight loss
Insomnia
Guarded movement
Muscle spasms
Redness, swelling, heat
Color changes in affected area
Reflex abnormalities

OUTCOME CRITERIA

The person will

1. Relate that others validate that the pain exists
2. Practice selected noninvasive pain relief measures to
   manage the pain
3. Relate improvement of pain and an increase in daily
   activities as evident by (specify)

INTERVENTIONS

1. Assess the person's pain experience; determine the intensity of the pain at its worst and best.
2. Provide accurate information to reduce fear of addiction.
3. Relate your acceptance of the response to pain.
   a. Acknowledge the presence of the pain.
   b. Listen attentively to individual concerning the pain.
   c. Convey that you are assessing the pain because you want to better understand it (not determine if it is really present).
4. Assess the family for the presence of misconceptions about pain or its treatment.
5. Discuss the reasons why an individual may experience increased or decreased pain (*e.g.,* fatigue [increased] or presence of distractions [decreased]).
   a. Encourage family members to share their concerns privately (*e.g.,* fear that the person will use pain for secondary gains if they give the patient too much attention).
   b. Assess whether the family doubts the pain and discuss the effects of this on the person's pain and on the relationship.
   c. Encourage the family to give attention also when pain is not exhibited.
6. Provide person with opportunities to rest during the day and with periods of uninterrupted sleep at night (must rest when pain is ↓).
7. Discuss with the person and family the therapeutic uses of distraction, along with other methods of pain relief.
8. Teach a method of distraction during an acute pain (*e.g.,* painful procedure) that is not a burden (*e.g.,* count items in a picture, count anything in the room, such as patterns on wallpaper or count silently to self); breathe rhythmically; listen to music and increase the volume as the pain increases.
9. Teach noninvasive pain relief measures.
   a. Relaxation
      - Instruct on techniques to reduce skeletal muscle tension, which will reduce the intensity of the pain.

- Promote relaxation with a back rub, massage, or warm bath.
- Teach a specific relaxation strategy (*e.g.,* slow, rhythmic breathing or deep breath—clench fists—yawn).

b. Cutaneous stimulation

- Discuss with the person the various methods of skin stimulation and their effects on pain.
- Discuss each of the following methods and the precautions:

  Hot water bottle
  Electric heating pad
  Warm tub
  Moist heat pack
  Hot summer sun
  Thin plastic wrap over painful area to retain body heat (*e.g.,* knee, elbow)

- Discuss each of the following methods and the precautions of each:

  Cold towels (wrung out)
  Cold-water immersion for small body parts
  Ice bag
  Cold gel pack
  Ice massage

- Explain the therapeutic uses of menthol preparations and massage/back rub.

10. Provide the person with optimal pain relief with prescribed analgesics.
11. After administering a pain-relief medication, return in 30 minutes to assess effectiveness.
12. Give accurate information to correct family misconceptions (*e.g.,* addiction, doubts about pain).
13. Assess the effects of chronic pain on the individual's life, using the person and family.
    a. Performance (job, role responsibilities)
    b. Social interactions
    c. Finances
    d. Activities of daily living (sleep, eating, mobility, sexuality)
    e. Cognition/mood (concentration, depression)
    f. Family unit (response of members)

14. Explain the relationship between chronic pain and depression.
15. Discuss with the individual and family the various treatment modalities available (family therapy, group therapy, behavior modification, biofeedback, hypnosis, acupuncture, exercise program).

Communication, Impaired*

Communication, Impaired

DEFINITION

Impaired Communication: The state in which an individual experiences, or could experience, a decreased ability to send or receive messages (*i.e.,* has difficulty exchanging thoughts, ideas, or desires).

> **Author's Note:**
> Impaired Communication and Impaired Verbal Communication are diagnoses to describe individuals who desire to communicate but are encountering problems. Impaired Communication may not be useful to describe an individual in whom communication problems are a manifestation of a psychiatric illness or a coping problem. If nursing interventions are focusing on reducing hallucinations, fear, or anxiety the diagnosis of Fear or Anxiety is more appropriate.

DEFINING CHARACTERISTICS

Major (Must Be Present)

Inappropriate or absent speech or response

---

* This diagnostic category was developed by Rosalinda Alfaro–LeFevre and is not currently on the NANDA list but has been included for clarity or usefulness.

Minor (May Be Present)

Incongruence between verbal and nonverbal messages
Stuttering
Slurring
Problem in finding the correct word when speaking
Weak or absent voice
Decreased auditory comprehension
Confusion
Inability to speak the dominant language of the culture
Use of sign language

RELATED FACTORS
Pathophysiological

Cerebral impairment
  Expressive or receptive aphasia
  Cerebrovascular accident (CVA)
  Brain damage (*e.g.,* birth/head trauma)
  Central nervous system (CNS) depression/increased
    intracranial pressure
  Tumor (head, neck, or spinal cord)
  Mental retardation
  Chronic hypoxia/decreased cerebral blood flow
Neurological impairment
  Quadriplegia
  Nervous system diseases (*e.g.,* myasthenia gravis,
    multiple sclerosis)
  Vocal cord paralysis
  Auditory nerve damage
Respiratory impairment (*e.g.,* shortness of breath)
Auditory impairment (decreased hearing)
Laryngeal edema/infection
Oral deformities
  Cleft lip or palate
  Malocclusion or fractured jaw
  Missing teeth
  Dysarthria

Treatment-related

Surgery
  Endotracheal intubation
  Tracheostomy/tracheotomy/laryngectomy
  Surgery of the head, face, neck, or mouth

Pain (especially of the mouth or throat)
Drugs (*e.g.,* CNS depressants, anesthesia)

Situational (Personal, Environmental)

Fatigue (affecting ability to listen)
Anger, anxiety, pain
No access to hearing aid/malfunction of hearing aid
Speech pathology
   Stuttering
   Lisping
   Ankyloglossia ("tongue-tied")
   Voice problems
Language barrier (unfamiliar language or dialect)
Psychological barrier (*e.g.,* fear, shyness)
Lack of privacy
Lack of support system
Loss of recent memory recall

Maturational

Elderly (auditory losses)
Infant
Child

OUTCOME CRITERIA

The person will

1. Wear a hearing aid (if appropriate)
2. Receive messages through alternative methods (*e.g.,* written communication, sign language, speaking distinctly into "good" ear)
3. Relate/demonstrate an improved ability to communicate
4. Demonstrate increased ability to understand
5. Relate decreased frustration with communication

INTERVENTIONS

1. Use factors that promote hearing and understanding.
   a. Talk distinctly and clearly, facing the person.
   b. Minimize unnecessary sounds in the room.
      - Have only one person talk.
      - Be aware of background noises (*e.g.,* close the door, turn off the television or radio).

      c. Repeat, then rephrase a thought, if the person does not seem to understand the whole meaning.

      d. Use touch and gestures to enhance communication.

      e. If person can understand only sign language, have an interpreter present as often as possible.

      f. If the person is in a group (*e.g.,* diabetes class), place the individual in the front of the room near the teacher.

      g. Approach the person from the side on which hearing is best (*i.e.,* if hearing is better with left ear, approach the person from the left).

      h. If the person can lip read: look directly at the person and talk slowly and clearly.

      i. Assess functioning of hearing aids (*e.g.,* batteries).

2. Provide alternative methods of communication.

      a. Use pad and pencil, alphabet letters, hand signals, eye blinks, head nods, bell signals.

      b. Make flash cards with pictures or words depicting frequently used phrases (*e.g.,* "Wet my lips," "Move my foot," glass of water, bedpan).

      c. Encourage person to point, use gestures, and pantomime.

      d. Consult with speech pathologist for assistance in acquiring flash cards.

3. Provide a nonrushed environment.

      a. Use normal loudness level and speak unhurriedly, in short phrases.

      b. Encourage the person to take plenty of time talking and to enunciate words carefully with good lip movements.

      c. Decrease external distractions.

      d. Delay conversation when the person is tired.

4. Use techniques to increase understanding.

      a. Face the individual and establish eye contact if possible.

      b. Use uncomplicated one-step commands and directives.

      c. Have only one person talk.

      d. Encourage the use of gestures and pantomime.

      e. Match words with actions; use pictures.

      f. Terminate conversation on a note of success (*e.g.,* move back to an easier item).

      g. Use same words with same task.

5. Make a concerted effort to understand when the person is speaking.
   a. Allow enough time to listen if the person speaks slowly.
   b. Rephrase the person's message aloud to validate it.
   c. Respond to all attempts at speech even if they are unintelligible (*e.g.,* "I do not know what you are saying. Can you try to say it again?").
   d. Ignore mistakes and profanity.
   e. Don't pretend you understand if you don't.
   f. Allow the person time to respond; do not interrupt; supply words only occasionally.

6. Teach techniques to improve speech.
   a. Ask the person to slow down speech, and say each word clearly, while providing the example.
   b. Encourage the person to speak in short phrases.
   c. Suggest a slower rate of talking, or taking a breath prior to speech.
   d. Encourage the person to take time and concentrate on forming the words.
   e. Ask the person to write down the message or to draw a picture, if verbal communication is difficult.
   f. Encourage the person to speak in short phrases.
   g. Ask questions that can be answered with a yes or no.
   h. Focus on the present; avoid topics that are controversial, emotional, abstract, or lengthy.

7. Verbally address the problem of frustration over inability to communicate, and explain that patience is needed for both the nurse and the person who is trying to talk.

8. Give the person opportunities to make decisions about care (*e.g.,* "Do you want a drink? Would you rather have orange juice or prune juice?").

9. Teach techniques to significant others and repetitive approaches to improve communications.

10. If a translator is needed try to plan a daily visit from someone who has some knowledge of the person's language (many hospitals and social welfare offices keep a "language" bank with names and phone numbers of people who are willing to translate).

Communication, Impaired Verbal

DEFINITION

Impaired Verbal Communication: The state in which an individual experiences, or could experience, a decreased ability or inability to speak but can understand others.

DEFINING CHARACTERISTICS

Major (Must Be Present)

Inability to speak words but can understand others
or
Articulation or motor planning deficits

Minor (May Be Present)

Shortness of breath

RELATED FACTORS

See Impaired Communication.

OUTCOME CRITERIA

The person will

1. Demonstrate improved ability to express self
2. Relate decreased frustration with communication

INTERVENTIONS

1. Identify a method by which person can communicate basic needs.
2. Provide alternative methods of communication.
   a. Use pad and pencil, alphabet letters, hand signals, eye blinks, head nods, bell signals.
   b. Make flash cards with pictures or words depicting frequently used phrases (*e.g.,* "Wet my lips," "Move my foot," glass of water, bedpan).
   c. Encourage the person to point, use gestures, and pantomime.

    d. Consult with speech pathologist for assistance in acquiring flash cards.

3. For individuals with dysarthria:
   a. Reduce environmental noise.
   b. Encourage the person to make a conscious effort to slow down speech and to speak more loudly (*e.g.,* "Take a deep breath between sentences.").
   c. Ask person to repeat words that are unclear.
   d. If person is tired, ask questions that require only short answers.
   e. If speech is unintelligible, teach the person to use gestures, written messages, and communication cards.

4. Do not alter your speech, tone, or type of message, since the person's ability to understand is not affected; speak on an adult level.

5. Verbally address the problem of frustration over inability to communicate, and explain that patience is needed for both the nurse and the person who is trying to talk.

6. Write the method of communication that is used on care plan.

7. Teach significant others techniques and repetitive approaches to improve communications.

8. Encourage the family to share feelings concerning communication problems.

9. Seek consultation with a speech pathologist early in treatment regimen.

Coping, Ineffective Individual

Defensive Coping

Ineffective Denial

DEFINITION

Ineffective Individual Coping: The state in which an individual experiences or is at risk of experiencing an inability to manage internal or environmental stressors adequately because of inadequate resources (physical, psychological, behavioral, and/or cognitive).

Author's Note:
This diagnostic category can be used to describe a variety of situations in which an individual does not adapt effectively to stressors. Examples can be isolating behaviors, aggression, and destructive behavior. If the response is inappropriate use of the defense mechanisms of denial or defensiveness, the diagnosis Ineffective Denial or Defensive Coping can be used instead of Ineffective Individual Coping.

DEFINING CHARACTERISTICS*

Major (Must Be Present)

Change in usual communication patterns (if acute)
Verbalization of inability to cope
or
Inappropriate use of defense mechanisms
or
Inability to meet role expectations

Minor (May Be Present)

Anxiety
Reported life stress
Inability to problem-solve
Alteration in social participation
Destructive behavior toward self or others
High incidence of accidents
Frequent illnesses
Verbalization of inability to ask for help
Verbal manipulation
Inability to meet basic needs

* Adapted from Vincent KG: The validation of a nursing diagnosis. Nurs Clin North Am 20(4):631–639, 1985

RELATED FACTORS
Pathophysiological

Changes in body integrity
  Loss of body part
  Disfigurement secondary to trauma
Altered affect caused by changes in
  Body chemistry
  Tumor (brain)
  Intake of mood-altering substance
Physiological manifestations of persistent stress

Situational (Personal, Environmental)

Changes in physical environment
  War
  Natural disaster
  Relocation
  Seasonal work (migrant worker)
  Poverty
Disruption of emotional bonds due to
  Death
  Separation or divorce
  Desertion
  Relocation
  Incarceration
Unsatisfactory support system
Institutionalization
  Jail
  Foster home
  Orphanage
  Educational institution
  Maintenance institution for the disabled
Sensory overload
  Factory environment
  Urbanization: crowding, noise pollution, excessive activity
Inadequate psychological resources
  Poor self-esteem
  Excessive negative beliefs about self
  Helplessness
  Lack of motivation to respond
Culturally related conflicts with life experiences
  Premarital sex
  Abortion

Maturational

Child
  Developmental tasks (independence vs. dependence)
  Entry into school
  Competition among peers
  Peer relationships

Adolescent
  Physical and emotional changes
  Independence from family
  Heterosexual relationships
  Sexual awareness
  Educational demands
  Career choices

Young adult
  Career choices
  Educational demands
  Leaving home
  Marriage
  Parenthood

Middle adult
  Physical signs of aging
  Career pressures
  Child-rearing problems
  Problems with relatives
  Social status needs
  Aging parents

Elderly
  Physical changes
  Changes in financial status
  Changes in residence
  Retirement
  Response of others to older people

Treatment-related

Separation from family and home (*e.g.*, hospitalization, confinement to a nursing home)
Need for medical treatment conflicts with beliefs
Disfigurement due to surgery
Altered appearance due to drugs, radiation, or other treatment
Altered affect due to hormonal therapy
Sensory overload due to medical technology (*e.g.*, critical care units)

OUTCOME CRITERIA

The person will

1. Verbalize feelings related to emotional state
2. Identify personal coping patterns and the consequences of the behavior that results
3. Identify personal strengths and accept support through the nursing relationship
4. Make decisions and follow through with appropriate actions to change provocative situations in personal environment

INTERVENTIONS

1. Assess individual's present coping status.
    a. Determine onset of feelings and symptoms and their correlation with events and life changes.
    b. Assess ability to relate facts.
    c. Listen carefully and observe facial expressions, gestures, eye contact, body positioning, tone and intensity of voice.
    d. Determine risk of client's inflicting self-harm and intervene appropriately (Refer to High Risk for Self-Harm).
2. Offer support as person talks.
    a. Reassure that the feelings he or she has must be difficult.
    b. When person is pessimistic, attempt to provide a more hopeful, realistic perspective.

(See *High Risk for Self-Harm* for additional information on suicide prevention.)

3. Assist the person to problem-solve in a constructive manner.
    a. What is the problem?
    b. Who or what is responsible for the problem?
    c. What are the options? (Make a list.)
    d. What are the advantages and disadvantages of each option?
4. Discuss possible alternatives (*i.e.,* talk over the problem with those involved, try to change the situation, or do nothing and accept the consequences).
5. Assist the individual to identify problems that cannot be controlled directly and help individual to practice stress-reducing activities for control (*e.g.,* exercise program, yoga).
6. Instruct person in relaxation techniques; emphasize the importance of setting 15–20 minutes aside each day to practice relaxation.
7. Have person describe previous encounters with conflict and how he or she managed to resolve them.
8. Mobilize the person into a gradual increase in activity.
9. Find outlets that foster feelings of personal achievement and self-esteem.
10. Provide opportunities to learn and use stress management techniques (*e.g.,* jogging, yoga).
11. Establish a network of people who understand the situation.

12. Offer support to others when able.
13. For depression-related problems beyond the scope of nurse generalists, refer to appropriate professionals (marriage counselor, psychiatric nurse therapist, psychologist, psychiatrist).

Defensive Coping

DEFINITION

Defensive Coping: The state in which an individual repeatedly projects a falsely positive self-evaluation as a defense against underlying perceived threats to positive self-regard.

DEFINING CHARACTERISTICS*

Major (80%–100%)

Denial of obvious problems/weaknesses
Projection of blame/responsibility
Rationalizes failures
Hypersensitive to slight criticism
Grandiosity

Minor (50%–79%)

Superior attitude toward others
Difficulty in establishing/maintaining relationships
Hostile laughter or ridicule of others
Difficulty in testing perceptions against reality
Lack of follow through or participation in treatment or therapy

RELATED FACTORS

See Chronic Low Self-Esteem.

* Norris J, Kunes–Connell M: Self esteem disturbance: A clinical validation study. In McLane A (ed): Classification of Nursing Diagnoses: Proceedings of the Seventh Conference. St. Louis, CV Mosby, 1987.

OUTCOME CRITERIA

The person will:

1. Verbalize a realistic perception of self with strengths and limitations
2. Identify consequences of personal behavior

INTERVENTIONS

1. Be aware of how person is responding to stimuli (*e.g.,* increase in loudness, activity, irritability).
   a. Decrease noise, visitors and other persons in environment.
   b. Avoid group activities when individual is easily distractible.
2. Assist in appropriate expression of thoughts and feelings.
   a. Clarify what is being said.
   b. Refocus conversation so that only one topic at a time is discussed.
3. Assist individual to realistically evaluate personal behavior.
   a. Direct conversation from a delusional orientation to a reality-based one.
4. Encourage noncompetitive activities; avoid activities that require concentration and attention to rules.
   Use brief, one-to-one interactions during time when person is easily distracted; increase time as attention span increases.
5. Talk over with team members to prevent manipulation.
6. Define acceptable behavior.
7. Enforce established limits.
8. Maintain physical health (rest, nutrition, fluids, self-care).
9. Describe clues that will indicate the need for professional help (*e.g.,* promiscuity, alcohol/drug overuse, insomnia, euphoria, overspending).

Ineffective Denial

DEFINITION

Ineffective Denial: The state is which an individual minimizes or disavows symptoms or a situation to his or her detriment of health.

Author's Note:
This type of denial differs from the denial in response to a loss.
The denial in response to an illness or loss is necessary to maintain psychological equilibrium and is beneficial. Ineffective Denial is not beneficial when the individual will not participate in regimens to improve health or the situation, *e.g.,* denial of substance abuse. If the cause of the ineffective denial is not known, Ineffective Denial related to unknown etiology can be used; for example, Ineffective Denial related to unknown etiology as manifested by repetitive refusal to admit that barbiturate use is a problem.

DEFINING CHARACTERISTICS*

Major (80%–100%)

Delays seeking or refuses health care attention to the detriment of health
Does not perceive personal relevance of symptoms or danger

Minor (50%–79%)

Uses home remedies (self-treatment) to relieve symptoms
Does not admit fear of death or invalidism
Minimizes symptoms
Displaces source of symptoms to other areas of the body
Unable to admit impact of disease on life pattern
Makes dismissive gestures or comments when speaking of distressing events
Displaces fear of impact of the condition
Displays inappropriate affect

RELATED FACTORS
Pathophysiological

Any chronic and/or terminal illness

---

* Norris J, Kunes–Connell M: Self-esteem disturbance: A clinical validation study. In McLane A (ed): Classification of Nursing Diagnoses: Proceedings of the Seventh Conference. St. Louis, CV Mosby, 1987.

Treatment-related

Prolonged treatment with no positive results

Situational/Psychological

Loss of job
Loss of spouse/significant other
Financial crisis
Feelings of negative self-concept, inadequacy, guilt,
  loneliness, despair, failure
Feelings of increased anxiety/stress, need to escape
  personal problems, anger, and frustration
Feelings of omnipotence
Culturally permissive attitudes toward alcohol/drug use
Religious sanctions
Alcohol or drug abuse

Maturational

Adolescent
  Peer pressure
Adult
  Job stress
  Expectation of alcohol/drug use
  Losses (job, spouse, children)
Elderly
  Losses (spouse, function, financial)
  Retirement

Biological/Genetic

Family history of alcoholism

OUTCOME CRITERIA

The person will

1. Identify fears or anxieties
2. Express a sense of hope
3. Use alternative coping mechanisms

INTERVENTIONS

1. Provide opportunities to share fears and anxieties.
2. Focus on present response.

3. Assist in lowering anxiety level (see *Anxiety* for additional interventions).
4. Avoid confronting person on use of denial.
5. Carefully explore with person his or her interpretation of the situation.
    a. Reflect back self-reported cues used to minimize the situation (*e.g.,* "a little," "only").
6. Emphasize strengths and past successful coping.

Coping: Potential for Growth, Family

DEFINITION

Family Coping: Potential for Growth. Effective management of adaptive tasks by a family member involved with the individual's health challenge, who now is exhibiting the desire and readiness for enhanced health and growth in regard to self and in relation to the client.

Author's Note:
This diagnostic category describes components that are found in Altered Family Processes and Health-Seeking Behaviors. Until clinical research differentiates the category from the preceding ones, use Altered Family Processes or Health-Seeking Behaviors, depending on the data presented.

DEFINING CHARACTERISTICS

Family member attempts to describe the growth impact of a crisis on his or her own values, priorities, goals, or relationships

Family member moves in the direction of a health-promoting and enriching life-style that supports and monitors maturational processes, audits and negotiates

treatment programs, and generally chooses experiences
that optimize wellness
Individual expresses interest in making contact on a one-
to-one basis or in a mutual-aid group with another
person who has experienced a similar situation

RELATED FACTORS

See *Health Seeking Behaviors* and *Altered Family Processes.*

Coping: Compromised, Ineffective Family

DEFINITION

Ineffective Family Coping: Compromised: The state in which
a usually supportive primary person (family member or close
friend) is providing insufficient, ineffective, or compromised
support, comfort, assistance, or encouragement that may be
needed by the client to manage or master adaptive tasks related
to his or her health challenge.

Author's Note:

This diagnostic category describes situations that are similar to
the diagnostic categories Impaired Adjustment and Altered
Family Processes. Until clinical research differentiates this category from the preceding ones, use Impaired Adjustment and/
or Altered Family Processes.

DEFINING CHARACTERISTICS
Subjective

Client expresses or confirms a concern or complaint about
a significant other's response to his or her health problem
Significant person describes preoccupation with personal
reactions, *e.g.,* fear, anticipatory grief, guilt, anxiety, to

client's illness, disability, or other situational or
developmental crises

Significant person describes or confirms an inadequate
understanding or knowledge base that interferes with
effective assistive or supportive behaviors

Objective

Significant person attempts assistive or supportive
behaviors with less than satisfactory results

Significant person withdraws or enters into limited or
temporary personal communication with the client at
times of need

Significant person displays protective behavior
disproportionate (too little or too much) to the client's
abilities or need for autonomy

RELATED FACTORS

See *Altered Family Processes.*

Coping: Disabling, Ineffective Family

DEFINITION

Ineffective Family Coping: Disabling The state in which a family demonstrates destructive behavior in response to an inability to manage internal or external stressors due to inadequate resources (physical, psychological, cognitive, and/or behavioral).

Author's Note:

The diagnostic category Ineffective Family Coping: Disabling describes a family that has a history of demonstrating destructive
(Continued)

> **Author's Note** (*Continued*)
> overt or covert behavior or has adapted detrimentally to a
> stressor. This category differs from Altered Family Processes,
> which describes a family that usually functions constructively
> but is challenged by a stressor that has altered or may alter its
> functioning. Sustained Altered Family Processes may progress
> to Ineffective Family Coping.

DEFINING CHARACTERISTICS

Major (Must Be Present)

Neglectful care of the client
Decisions/actions that are detrimental to economic and/or
  social well-being
Neglectful relationships with other family members

Minor (May Be Present)

Distortion of reality regarding the client's health problem
Intolerance
Rejection
Abandonment
Desertion
Psychosomaticism
Taking on illness signs of client
Agitation
Depression
Aggression
Hostility
Impaired restructuring of a meaningful life for self
Prolonged overconcerns for client
Client's development of helpless inactive dependence

RELATED FACTORS

The following describes those individuals or families who are
at high risk for contributing to a family's destructive coping
behavior.

Parent(s)
  Single   Drug addicted
  Adolescent   Terminally ill

71

Abusive	Acutely disabled/
Emotionally disturbed	accident victim
Alcoholic	Elderly dependent

Child

Of unwanted pregnancy	Physically handicapped
Of undesired gender or	Mentally handicapped
of forced intercourse	Hyperactive
With undesired	Terminally ill
characteristics	Adolescent rebellion

Pathophysiological

Any condition that challenges one's ability for self-care, for fulfilling role responsibilities, and for financial independence can contribute to Ineffective Family Coping. See Altered Family Process for specific situations.

Other

History of ineffective relationship with own parents
History of abusive relationships with parents
Unrealistic expectations of child by parent
Unrealistic expectations of self by parent
Unrealistic expectations of parent by child
Unmet psychosocial needs of child by parent
Unmet psychosocial needs of parent by child

OUTCOME CRITERIA

The person will

1. Identify responses that are neglectful or harmful
2. Verbalize the need for assistance with situation
3. Relate community resources available

INTERVENTIONS

1. Assist family to evaluate past and present family functioning.
2. Provide all family members an opportunity to discuss their appraisal of the situation.
3. Discourage blaming but allow ventilation of anger.
4. Clarify feelings of members.
5. Assist family with appraisal of the situation.
   a. What is wrong?
   b. What are the causes?
   c. Who has contributed to the problem?
   d. What are the options?

      e. What are the advantages/disadvantages of each option?

6. If indicated, ask members to consider the problem from the perspective of another family member.

7. If a member is ill, assist family to have more realistic expectations.

8. If domestic abuse is present:

      a. Provide an opportunity to validate abuse and talk about feelings.

      b. Be direct and nonjudgmental (Blair).*
   - How do you handle stress?
   - How does your partner or caregiver handle stress?
   - How do you and your partner argue?
   - Are you afraid of your partner?
   - Have you ever been hit, pushed, or injured by your partner?

      c. Provide options but allow them to make a decision at their own pace.

      d. Encourage a realistic appraisal of the situation; dispel guilt and myths.
   - Violence is not normal for most families.
   - Violence may stop but it usually becomes increasingly worse.
   - The victim is not responsible for the violence.

      e. Provide a list of community agencies available to victim and abuser (emergency and long-term):
   - Hotlines
   - Legal services
   - Shelters
   - Counseling agencies

      f. Discuss the availability of the social service department for assistance.

      g. Consult with the legal resources in the community and familiarize the victim with the state laws regarding:
   - Eviction of abuser
   - Counseling
   - Temporary support
   - Protection orders

---

* Blair K. The battered woman: Is she a silent partner? Nurse Pract 11(6):38, 1986

- Criminal law
- Types of police interventions

    h. Document findings and dialogue for possible future court use.

9. If child abuse or neglect is suspected:

    a. Report suspected cases of child abuse.

- Know your state's child abuse laws and procedures for reporting child abuse (*e.g.*, Bureau of Child Welfare, Department of Social Services, Child Protective Services).
- Maintain an objective record:

    Description of injuries

    Conversations with parents and child in quotes

    Description of behaviors, not interpretation (*e.g.*, avoid "angry father;" instead, "Father screamed at child, 'If you weren't so bad this wouldn't have happened.' ")

    Description of parent–child interactions (*e.g.*, shies away from mother's touch)

    Nutritional status

    Growth and development compared to age-related norms

    b. Provide the child with acceptance and affection.

    c. Assist child with grieving if foster home placement is necessary.

    d. Allow opportunities for child to ventilate feelings.

    e. Provide interventions that promote parents' self-esteem and sense of trust.

- Tell them it was good that they brought the child to the hospital.
- Promote their confidence by presenting a warm, helpful attitude and acknowledging any competent parenting activities.
- Provide opportunities for parents to participate in their child's care (*e.g.*, feeding, bathing).

    f. Refer abusive parents to community agencies and professionals for counseling.

    g. Disseminate information to the community about the problem of child abuse (*e.g.*, parent–school organizations, radio, television, newspaper).

Decisional Conflict

DEFINITION

Decisional Conflict: The state in which an individual/group experiences uncertainty about course of action when the choice involves risk, loss, or challenge.

DEFINING CHARACTERISTICS*

Major (80%–100%)

Verbalized uncertainty about choices
Verbalization of undesired consequences of alternative actions being considered
Vacillation between alternative choices
Delayed decision making

Minor (50%–79%)

Verbalized feeling of distress while attempting a decision
Self-focusing
Physical signs of distress or tension (increased heart rate, increased muscle tension, restlessness, etc.) whenever the decision comes within focus of attention
Questioning personal values and beliefs while attempting to make a decision

RELATED FACTORS

Many situations can contribute to decisional conflict, particularly those that involve complex medical interventions of great risk. Any decisional situation can precipitate conflict for an individual; thus, the examples listed below are not exhaustive but reflective of situations that may be problematic and possess factors that increase the difficulty.

Treatment-related

Surgery
Tumor removal   Cosmetic
Cataract   Joint replacement

---

* Hiltunen E: Diagnostic content validity of the nursing diagnosis: Decisional Conflict. Unpublished raw data, 1987

    Laminectomy   Hysterectomy
    Orchiectomy   Transplant
Diagnostics
    Amniocentesis   X-rays
    Ultrasound
Chemotherapy
Radiation
Dialysis
Mechanical ventilation
Enteral feedings
Intravenous hydration

Situational

Personal
    Marriage   Institutionalization
    Separation   (child, parent)
    Divorce   Breast vs bottle feeding
    Parenthood   Abortion
    Birth control   Sterilization
    Artificial insemination   Nursing home placement
    Adoption
    Foster home placement
Work/Task
    Career change   Business investments
    Relocation   Professional ethics
Lack of relevant information
Confusing information
Disagreement within support systems
Inexperience with decision making
Unclear personal values/beliefs
Conflict with personal values/beliefs
Resignation
Family history of poor prognosis
Hospital environment—loss of control
Ethical dilemmas
    Quality of life
    Cessation of life-support systems
    "Do not resuscitate" orders

Maturational

Adolescent
    Peer pressure   Whether to continue a
    Sexual activity   relationship

Alcohol/drug use	College
Illegal/dangerous situations	Career choice
Use of birth control	
Adult	
Career change	Parenthood
Marriage	
Older adult	
Retirement	Nursing home placement

OUTCOME CRITERIA

The individual/group will

1. Relate the advantages and disadvantages of choices
2. Share fears and concerns regarding choices and responses of others
3. Make an informed choice

INTERVENTIONS

1. Establish a trusting and meaningful relationship that promotes mutual understanding and caring.
2. Facilitate a logical decision-making process.
   a. Assist the person in recognizing what the problem is and clearly identify the decision that needs to be made.
   b. Have person make a list of all the possible alternatives or options.
   c. Help identify the probable outcomes of the various alternatives.
   d. Aid in evaluating the alternatives based on actual or potential threats to beliefs/values.
   e. Encourage the person to make a decision.
3. Encourage the person's significant others to be involved in the entire decision-making process.
4. Assist the individual in exploring personal values and relationships that may have an impact on the decision.
5. Support individual making informed decision—even if decision conflicts with own values.
   a. Consult own spiritual leader.
6. Actively reassure the person that the decision is his or hers to make and that he or she has the right to do so.
7. Do not allow others to undermine the person's confidence in making own decision.

77

8. Explore with individual and family if they have discussed and recorded their end-of-life decisions.
9. Discuss the purpose of a living will. Provide information when requested. To obtain a copy of your state's living will, write to the Society for the Right to Die, 250 West 57th Street, New York, NY 10107.

Disuse Syndrome: High Risk for

DEFINITION

High Risk for Disuse Syndrome: The state in which an individual is at risk for deterioration of body systems as a result of musculoskeletal inactivity.

Author's Note:

High Risk for Disuse Syndrome represents an individual at risk for the adverse effects of immobility. As a syndrome diagnosis, the etiology of the diagnosis is in the diagnostic label, *i.e.,* Disuse, thus no related to's are used. The same is true for Rape Trauma Syndrome.

High Risk for Disuse Syndrome has 11 "high risk for" or actual nursing diagnoses clustered under it: (NANDA-adapted)

High Risk for Impaired Skin Integrity
High Risk for Constipation
High Risk for Altered Respiratory Function
High Risk for Altered Peripheral Tissue Perfusion
High Risk for Infection
High Risk for Activity Intolerance
High Risk for Impaired Physical Mobility
High Risk for Injury
High Risk for Sensory–Perceptual Alterations
Powerlessness
Body Image Disturbance

It is no longer necessary to use separate categories as High Risk for Altered Respiratory Function or High Risk for Impaired
(*Continued*)

RISK FACTORS

Presence of risk factors (see Related Factors)

RELATED FACTORS

Pathophysiological

Decreased sensorium
Unconsciousness
Neuromuscular impairment
    Multiple sclerosis   Muscular dystrophy
    Parkinsonism   Partial or total paralysis
    Guillain-Barré syndrome   Spinal cord injury
Musculoskeletal conditions
    Fractures   Rheumatic diseases
End-stage disease
    Acquired immuno-   Renal disease
      deficiency syndrome   Cardiac disease
      (AIDS)   Cancer
Psychiatric/mental health disorders
    Major depression   Severe phobias
    Catatonic state

Treatment-related

Surgery (amputation, skeletal)
Traction/casts/splints
Prescribed immobility
Mechanical ventilation
Invasive vascular lines

Situational

Depression
Fatigue

Debilitated state
Pain

Maturational

Newborn/infant/child/adolescent
    Down Syndrome
    Legg–Calvé–Perthes
     Disease
    Osteogenesis imperfecta
    Cerebral palsy
    Spina bifida
Elderly
    Decreased motor agility
    Muscle weakness
    Presenile dementia

Risser turnbuckle jacket
Juvenile arthritis
Autism
Mental/physical
  disability

OUTCOME CRITERIA

The person will demonstrate continued

1. Intact skin/tissue integrity
2. Maximum pulmonary function
3. Maximum peripheral blood flow
4. Full range of motion
5. Bowel, bladder, and renal functioning
6. Use of social contacts and activities when possible

The person will

1. Explain rationale for treatments
2. Make decisions regarding care when possible
3. Share feelings regarding immobile state

INTERVENTIONS

1. Promote optimal respiratory function.
   a. Vary the position of the bed.
2. Assist to reposition, turning frequently from side to side (hourly if possible).
3. Encourage deep breathing and controlled coughing exercises 5 times every hour.
4. Auscultate lung fields every 8 hours.
5. Maintain usual pattern of bowel elimination. Refer to Constipation for specific interventions.
6. Prevent pressure ulcers.

   a. Use repositioning schedule that relieves vulnerable area most often.
   b. Turn person or instruct person to turn or shift weight every 30 minutes to 2 hours.
   c. Keep bed as flat as possible to reduce shearing forces; limit Fowler's position to only 30 minutes at a time.
   d. Use foam blocks or pillows to provide a bridging effect.
   e. Use enough personnel to lift person up in bed or chair.

7. Observe for erythema and blanching and palpate for warmth and tissue sponginess with each position change.
8. Massage vulnerable areas with each position change.
9. Refer to *Impaired Skin Integrity* for additional interventions.
10. Elevate extremity above the level of the heart (may be contraindicated if severe cardiac or respiratory disease is present).
11. Perform range of motion exercises (frequency to be determined by condition of the individual).
12. Position the person in alignment to prevent complications.
13. Provide a daily intake of fluid of 2000 ml or greater a day (unless contraindicated); refer to *Fluid Volume Deficit* for specific interventions.
14. Provide weight-bearing when possible.
15. Encourage the person to share feelings and fears regarding restricted movement.
16. Encourage the person to wear own clothes rather than pajamas.
17. Include the individual in planning schedule for daily routine.
18. Be creative; vary the physical environment and daily routine when possible.
19. Provide opportunities for individual to control decisions.

Diversional Activity Deficit

DEFINITION

Diversional Activity Deficit: The state in which an individual or group experiences or is at risk of experiencing decreased stimulation from or interest in leisure activities.

DEFINING CHARACTERISTICS

Major (Must Be Present)

Observed on statements of boredom/depression from inactivity

Minor (May Be Present)

Constant expression of unpleasant thoughts or feelings
Yawning or inattentiveness
Flat facial expression
Body language (shifting of body away from speaker)
Restlessness/fidgeting
Immobile (on bed rest or confined)
Weight loss or gain
Hostility

RELATED FACTORS

Pathophysiological

Communicable disease
Pain

Treatment-related

Long or frequent treatments

Situational (Personal, Environmental)

No peers or friends
Monotonous environment
Long-term hospitalization or confinement
Lack of motivation
Loss of ability to perform usual or favorite activities

Excessive long hours of stressful work
No time for leisure activities
Career changes (*e.g.,* teacher to homemaker, retirement)
Children leaving home ("empty nest")
Immobility
Decreased sensory perception (*e.g.,* blindness, hearing
loss)

Maturational

Infant/child
   Lack of appropriate toys/peers
Elderly
   Sensory-motor deficits

OUTCOME CRITERIA

The person will

1. Relate feelings of boredom and discuss methods of finding diversional activities
2. Related methods of coping with feelings of anger or
   depression caused by boredom
3. Engage in a diversional activity

INTERVENTIONS

1. Stimulate motivation by showing interest and encour-
   aging sharing of feelings and experiences.
2. Help the person to work through feelings of anger and
   grief.
3. Vary daily routine when possible (*e.g.,* give bath in the
   afternoon, so that the person can watch a special show
   or talk with a visitor who drops in).
4. Include the individual in planning schedule for daily
   routine.
5. Plan time for visitors.
6. Be creative, vary the physical environment and daily
   routine when possible.
7. Place the person near a window, if possible.
8. Provide reading material, radio, television "books on
   tape" (if person is visually impaired).
9. Plan an activity daily to give person something to look
   forward to and always keep your promises.

10. Discourage the use of television as the primary source of recreation unless it is highly desired.
11. Consider using a volunteer to spend time reading to the person or helping with an activity.
12. Provide an environment with accessible playthings that suit the child's developmental age and see that they are well within reach.
13. Encourage family to bring in child's favorite playthings, including items from nature that will help to keep the real world alive (*e.g.,* goldfish, leaves in fall).

Dysreflexia

DEFINITION

Dysreflexia: The state in which an individual with a spinal cord injury at T7 or above experiences or is at risk for experiencing uninhibited sympathetic response of the nervous system to a noxious stimulus.

> **Author's Note:**
> This is a situation that the nurse and/or client can prevent or treat. If the nurse's initial treatment does not abate the symptoms, medical treatment is imperative. An individual does not experience dysreflexia as a continued state but rather is at risk for it, so if it is experienced, it is abated. Thus High Risk for Dysreflexia better describes the clinical situation than does Dysreflexia.

DEFINING CHARACTERISTICS

Major (Must Be Present)

Individual with spinal cord injury T7 or above with
Paroxysmal hypertension (sudden periodic elevated blood pressure in which systolic pressure is over 140 mm Hg and diastolic is above 90 mm Hg)

Bradycardia or tachycardia (pulse rate of less than 60 or more than 100 beats/min)
Diaphoresis (above the injury)
Red splotches on the skin (above the injury)
Pallor (below the injury)
Headache (a diffuse pain in different portions of the head and not confined to any nerve distribution area)

Minor (May Be Present)

Chilling
Conjunctival congestion
Horner's syndrome (contraction of the pupil, partial ptosis of the eyelid, enophthalmos and sometimes loss of sweating over the affected side of the face)
Paresthesia
Pilomotor reflex
Blurred vision
Chest pain
Metallic taste in the mouth
Nasal congestion

RELATED FACTORS
Pathophysiological

Visceral stretching and irritation
  Bowel
    Constipation   Fecal impaction
  Bladder
    Distended bladder   Infection
    Urinary calculi
Stimulation of skin (abdominal, thigh)
Acute abdominal condition
Spastic sphincter

Treatment-related

Removal of fecal impaction
Clogged or nonpatent catheter
Surgical incision

Situational (Personal, Environmental)

Lack of knowledge

OUTCOME CRITERIA

The individual/family will

1. State factors that cause dysreflexia
2. Describe the treatment for dysreflexia
3. Relate when emergency treatment is indicated

INTERVENTIONS

1. If signs of dysreflexia occur, *raise the head of the bed* and remove the noxious stimuli.
2. Check for distended bladder.
3. If catheterized:
   a. Check catheter for kinks or compression.
   b. Irrigate with only 30 ml saline very slowly.
   c. Replace catheter if it will not drain.
4. If not catheterized, insert catheter using Nupercaine ointment and remove 500 ml, then clamp for 15 minutes; repeat cycle until bladder is drained.
5. For fecal impaction:
   a. First apply dibucaine hydrochloride ointment (Nupercaine) to the anus and into the rectum for 1 inch (2.54 cm).
   b. Gently check rectum with a well-lubricated glove.
   c. Insert rectal suppository or gently remove impaction.
6. Continue to monitor blood pressure every 3–5 minutes.
7. Immediately consult physician for pharmacological treatment if symptoms or noxious stimuli are not eliminated.
8. Teach signs and symptoms and treatment of dysreflexia to person and family.
9. Teach when immediate medical intervention is warranted.
10. Explain what situations can trigger dysreflexia (menstrual cycle, sexual activity, bladder or bowel routines).
11. Advise consultation with physician for long-term pharmacological management if individual is very vulnerable.

Family Processes, Altered

DEFINITION

Altered Family Processes: The state in which a normally supportive family experiences a stressor that challenges its previously effective functioning ability.

Author's Note:

The nursing diagnosis Altered Family Processes describes a family that usually functions optimally but is challenged by a stressor that has altered or may alter the family's function. This diagnosis differs from Ineffective Family Coping: Disabling, which describes a family that has a pattern of destructive behavioral responses. Unsuccessful resolution of a problem can change Altered Family Processes to Ineffective Family Coping: Disabling.

DEFINING CHARACTERISTICS

Major (Must Be Present)

Family system cannot or does not
  Adapt constructively to crisis
  Communicate openly and effectively among family
    members

Minor (May Be Present)

Family system cannot or does not
  Meet physical needs of all its members
  Meet emotional needs of all its members
  Meet spiritual needs of all its members
  Express or accept a wide range of feelings
  Seek or accept help appropriately

RELATED FACTORS

Any factor can contribute to Altered Family Processes. Some common factors are listed below.

Pathophysiological

Illness of family member
    Discomforts related to
      the symptoms of the
      illness
    Change in the family
      member's ability to
      function
    Time-consuming
      treatments
Trauma
    Surgery

Disabling treatments
Expensive treatments

Loss of body part or
    function

Treatment-related

Disruption of family routines due to time-consuming
    treatments (*e.g.,* home dialysis)
Physical changes due to treatments of ill family member
Emotional changes in all family members due to
    treatments of ill family member
Financial burden of treatments for ill family member
Hospitalization of ill family member

Situational (Personal, Environmental)

Loss of family member
    Death
    Going away to school
    Separation
    Divorce
Gain of family member
    Birth
    Adoption
Poverty
Disaster
Relocation
Economic crisis
    Unemployment
Change in family roles
    Working mother
Birth of child with defect

Incarceration
Desertion
Hospitalization

Marriage
Elderly relative

Financial loss

Retirement

Conflict
  Goal conflicts
  Moral conflict with
    reality

Cultural conflict with
  reality
Personality conflict in
  family

Breach of trust among members
  Dishonesty
  Adultery
History of psychiatric illness in family
Social deviance by family member (including crime)

OUTCOME CRITERIA

The person (family members) will

1. Frequently verbalize feelings to professional nurse and each other
2. Participate in care of ill family member
3. Facilitate return of ill family member from sick role to well role
4. Maintain functional system of mutual support for each member
5. Seek appropriate external resources when needed

INTERVENTIONS

1. Assist family with appraisal of the situation.
   a. What is at stake? Encourage family to have a realistic perspective by providing accurate information and answers to questions.
   b. What are the choices? Assist family to reorganize roles at home and set priorities to maintain family integrity and reduce stress.
   c. Where is there help? Direct family to community agencies, home health care organizations, and sources of financial assistance as needed (see *Impaired Home Maintenance Management* for additional interventions).
2. Create a private and supportive hospital environment for family.
3. Acknowledge strengths to family when appropriate.
   a. "I can tell you are a very close family."
   b. "You know just how to get your mother to eat."
   c. "Your brother means a great deal to you."

4. Involve family members in care of ill member when possible (feeding, bathing, dressing, ambulating).
5. Involve family members in patient care conferences when appropriate.
6. Encourage family to acquire substitutes to care for the ill person, to provide the family with time away.
7. Encourage verbalization of guilt, anger, blame, hostility, and subsequent recognition of own feelings in family members.
8. Aid family members to change their expectations of the ill member in a realistic manner.
9. Provide the family with anticipatory guidance as illness continues.
    a. Inform parents of the effects of prolonged hospitalization on children (appropriate to developmental age).
    b. Prepare family members for signs of depression, anxiety, and dependency, which are a natural part of the illness experience.
10. Enlist help of other professionals when problems extend beyond realm of nursing (*e.g.,* social worker, clinical psychologist, nurse therapist, clinical specialist, psychiatrist, child care specialist).

Fatigue

DEFINITION

Fatigue: The self-recognized state in which an individual experiences an overwhelming sustained sense of exhaustion and decreased capacity for physical and mental work that is not relieved by rest.

Author's Note:
Fatigue is different from tiredness. Tiredness is a transient, temporary state from lack of sleep, improper nutrition, sedentary
(*Continued*)

DEFINING CHARACTERISTICS*

Major (80%–100%)

Verbalization of an unremitting and overwhelming lack of energy
Inability to maintain usual routines

Minor (50%–79%)

Perceived need for additional energy to accomplish routine tasks
Increase in physical complaints
Emotionally labile or irritable
Impaired ability to concentrate
Decreased performance
Lethargic or listless
Lack of interest in surroundings/introspection
Decreased libido
Accident prone

RELATED FACTORS

Many factors can cause fatigue; some common factors are the following:

* Voith AM, Frank AM, Pigg JS: Validations of fatigue as a nursing diagnosis. In McLane A (ed): Classification of Nursing Diagnoses: Proceedings of the Seventh National Conference, p. 280. St Louis, CV Mosby, 1987

Pathophysiological

Acute infections
    Mononucleosis   Viruses
    Hepatitis
Fever
Chronic infection
    Hepatitis   Endocarditis
Impaired oxygen transport system (chronic)
    Congestive heart failure   Anemia
    Chronic obstructive lung   Peripheral vascular
      disease   disease
Endocrine/metabolic disorders
    Diabetus Mellitus   Pituitary disorders
    Hypothyroidism   Addison's disease
Chronic diseases (*e.g.,* renal failure, cirrhosis)
Neuromuscular disorders
    Parkinson's disease   Myasthenia gravis
    Arthritis   Multiple sclerosis
Obesity
Electrolyte imbalances
Cancer
Nutritional disorders
Gait disorders
Acquired immunodeficiency syndrome (AIDS)

Treatment-related

Chemotherapy
Radiation therapy
Antidepressants
Drug withdrawal

Situational

Excessive role demands
Overwhelming emotional demands
Depression
Extreme stress

Maturational

Adult
    Pregnancy (first trimester)
    Caregiver (ill child, aging parent)

OUTCOME CRITERIA

The person will:

1. Discuss the causes of fatigue
2. Share feelings regarding the effects of fatigue on his or her life
3. Establish priorities for daily and weekly activities
4. Participate in activities that stimulate and balance physical, cognitive, affective, and social domains

INTERVENTIONS

1. Explain the causes of the person's fatigue.
2. Allow expression of feelings regarding the effects of fatigue on person's life.
3. Assist the individual to identify strengths, abilities, interests.
4. Instruct individual to record fatigue levels each hour during a 24-hour period (select a usual day).
   a. Ask to rate fatigue 0–10 using the Rhoten fatigue scale
      (0 = not tired, peppy; 10 – total exhaustion).*
   b. Record the activities at the time of each rating.
5. Analyze together the 24-hour fatigue levels.
   a. Times of peak energy
   b. Times of exhaustion
   c. Activities associated with increasing fatigue
6. Assist individual to identify what tasks can be delegated.
7. Plan the important tasks during periods of high energy.
8. Assist individual to identify priorities and to eliminate nonessential activities.
9. Distribute difficult tasks throughout the week.
10. Rest before difficult tasks and stop before fatigue ensues.
11. Teach energy conservation technique (*e.g.,* organize kitchen or work areas, reduce trips up and down stairs).
12. Explain the psychological and physiological benefits of exercise and discuss what is realistic.
13. Provide significant others with opportunities to discuss their feelings in private.

* Rhoten D: Fatigue and the postsurgical patient. In Norris C (ed): Concept Clarification in Nursing. Rockville, MD, Aspen Systems, 1982

14. Refer to community services (Meals on Wheels, housekeeper).

Fear

DEFINITION

Fear: The state in which an individual or group experiences a feeling of physiological or emotional disruption related to an identifiable source that is perceived as dangerous.

> **Author's Note**
> See *Author's Note, Anxiety,* page 10.

DEFINING CHARACTERISTICS

Major (Must Be Present)

Feelings of: dread, fright, apprehension
and/or
Behaviors of: avoidance, narrowing of focus on danger, and deficits in attention, performance, and control

Minor (May Be Present)

Verbal reports of: panic, obsessions
Behavioral acts of
 Aggression
 Escape
 Hypervigilance
 Dysfunctional immobility
 Compulsive mannerisms
 Increased questioning/verbalization
Visceral–somatic activity
 Musculoskeletal
  Muscle tightness
  Fatigue

Cardiovascular
  Palpitations
  Rapid pulse
  Increased blood pressure
Respiratory
  Shortness of breath
  Increased rate
Gastrointestinal
  Anorexia
  Nausea/vomiting
  Diarrhea
Genitourinary
  Urinary frequency
Skin
  Flush/pallor
  Sweating
  Paresthesia
Central nervous system/perceptual
  Syncope
  Insomnia
  Lack of concentration
  Irritability
  Absentmindedness
  Nightmares
  Dilated pupils

RELATED FACTORS

Fear can occur as a response to a variety of health problems, situations, or conflicts. Some common sources are indicated below.

Pathophysiological

Loss of body part
Loss of body function
Disabling illness

Long-term disability
Terminal disease

Treatment-related

Hospitalization
Surgery and its outcome
Anesthesia

Invasive procedures
Radiation

Situational (Personal, Environmental)

Influences of others
Pain
New environment
New people
Lack of knowledge

Change or loss of
  significant other
Divorce
Success
Failure

Maturational

Child
    Age-related fears (dark, strangers)
    Influence of others
Adolescent
    School adjustments
    Social and intellectual competitiveness
    Independence
    Authorities
Adult
    Marriage
    Pregnancy
    Parenthood
Elderly
    Retirement
    Relinquishing roles
    Functional losses

OUTCOME CRITERIA

The adult will

1. Relate increase in psychological and physiological comfort
2. Differentiate real from imagined situations
3. Describe effective and ineffective coping patterns
4. Identify own coping responses

The child will

1. Discuss fears
2. Relate an increase in psychological comfort

INTERVENTIONS

1. Orient to environment using simple explanations.
2. Speak slowly and calmly.
3. Allow personal space.

4. Use simple direct statements (avoid detail).
5. Encourage expression of feelings (helplessness, anger).
6. Encourage responses that reflect reality.
7. Provide an emotionally nonthreatening atmosphere.
8. Accept the child's fear and provide an explanation, if possible, or some form of control; share with child that these fears are okay.
   a. Fear of imaginary animals, intruders ("I don't see a lion in your room, but I will leave the light on for you, and if you need me again, please call.").
   b. Fear of parent being late (establish a contingency plan, *e.g.,* "If you come home from school and Mommy is not here, go to Mrs. S. next door.").
   c. Fear of vanishing down a toilet or bathtub drain. Wait until child is out of tub before releasing drain.
      Wait until child is off the toilet before flushing.
      Leave toys in bathtub and demonstrate how they do not go down the drain.
      • Fear of dark: give child a nightlight.
      • Fear of dogs, cats:
           Allow child to watch a child and a dog playing from a distance.
           Do not force child to touch the animal.
9. Discuss with parents the normalcy of fears in children; explain the necessity of acceptance and the negative outcomes of punishment or of forcing the child to overcome the fear.
10. Provide child with opportunity to observe how other children cope successfully with feared object.
11. When intensity of feelings has decreased, bring behavioral cues into the person's awareness.

Fluid Volume Deficit

DEFINITION

Fluid Volume Deficit: The state in which an individual who is not NPO experiences or is at risk of experiencing vascular, interstitial, or intracellular dehydration.

Author's Note:
This diagnostic category represents situations in which nurses can prescribe definitive treatment to prevent fluid depletion or to reduce or eliminate related factors such as insufficient oral intake. Situations that represent hypovolemia caused by hemorrhage or NPO states should be considered collaborative problems, not nursing diagnoses. Nursing monitors to detect these situations and collaborates with medicine for treatment. These situations can be labeled Potential Complication: Hemorrhage, or Potential Complication: Hypovolemia.

DEFINING CHARACTERISTICS

Major (Must Be Present)

Output greater than intake
Dry skin/mucous membranes

Minor (May Be Present)

Increased serum sodium
Increased pulse rate (from baseline)
Decreased urine output or excessive urine output
Concentrated urine or urinary frequency
Decreased fluid intake
Decreased skin turgor
Thirst/nausea/anorexia

RELATED FACTORS

Pathophysiological

Excessive urinary output
 Uncontrolled diabetes
 Diabetes insipidus (inappropriate antidiuretic hormone)
Burns (postacute)
Fever or increased metabolic rate
Infection
Abnormal drainage
 Wound
 Excessive menses
 Other

Peritonitis
Diarrhea

Situational (Personal, Environmental)

Vomiting/nausea
Decreased motivation to drink liquids
    Depression
    Fatigue
Dietary problems
    Fad diets/fasting
    Anorexia
    High-solute tube feedings
Difficulty swallowing or feeding self
    Oral pain
    Fatigue
Climate exposure
    Extreme heat/sun
    Extreme dryness
Hyperpnea
Extreme exercise effort/diaphoresis
Excessive use of
    Laxatives or enemas
    Diuretics or alcohol

Maturational

Infant/child
    Decreased fluid reserve
    Decreased ability to concentrate urine
Elderly
    Decreased fluid reserve
    Decreased sensation of thirst

OUTCOME CRITERIA

The person will

1. Increase intake of fluids to a minimum of 2000 ml (unless contraindicated)
2. Relate the need for increased fluid intake during stress or heat
3. Maintain a urine specific gravity within a normal range
4. Demonstrate no signs and symptoms of dehydration

INTERVENTIONS

1. Assess likes and dislikes; provide favorite fluids within dietary restrictions.
2. Plan an intake goal for each shift (*e.g.,* 1000 ml during day; 800 ml during evening; 300 ml at night).
3. Assess the person's understanding of the reasons for maintaining adequate hydration and methods for reaching goal of fluid intake.
4. For children, offer:
   a. Appealing forms of fluids (popsicles, frozen juice bars, snow cones, water, milk, Jell-O with vegetable coloring added; let child help make it)
   b. Unusual containers (colorful cups, straws)
   c. A game or activity (have child take a drink when it is child's turn in a game)
5. Have person maintain a written record (log) of fluid intake and urinary output (if necessary).
6. Monitor intake; assure at least 1500 ml of oral fluids every 24 hours.
7. Monitor output; assure at least 1000–1500 ml/24 hours.
8. Weigh daily in same type of clothing, at same time. A 2%–4% weight loss indicates mild dehydration; 5%–9% weight loss indicates moderate dehydration.
9. Monitor serum electrolytes, blood urea nitrogen, urine and serum, osmolality, creatinine, hematocrit, and hemoglobin.
10. Teach that coffee, tea, and grapefruit juice are diuretics and can contribute to fluid loss.
11. Consider the additional fluid losses associated with vomiting, diarrhea, fever.
12. For wound drainage:
    a. Keep careful records of the amount and type of drainage.
    b. Weigh dressings, if necessary, to estimate fluid loss.

Fluid Volume Excess

DEFINITION

Fluid Volume Excess: The state in which an individual experiences or is at risk of experiencing intracellular or interstitial fluid overload.

Author's Note:
This diagnostic category represents situations in which nursing can prescribe definitive treatment to reduce or eliminate factors that contribute to edema or can teach preventive actions. Situations that represent vascular fluid overload should be considered collaborative problems, not nursing diagnoses. They can be labeled Potential Complication: Congestive heart failure, or Potential Complication: Hypervolemia.

DEFINING CHARACTERISTICS

Major (Must Be Present)

Edema
Taut, shiny skin

RELATED FACTORS
Pathophysiological

Renal failure, acute or chronic
Decreased cardiac output
    Myocardial infarction   Valvular disease
    Congestive heart failure   Tachycardia/arrhythmias
    Left ventricular failure
Varicosities of the legs
Liver disease
    Cirrhosis   Cancer
    Ascites
Tissue insult
    Injury to the cell wall   Hypoxia of the cell
Inflammatory process

Hormonal disturbances
Pituitary   Estrogen
Adrenal

Treatment-related

Corticosteroid therapy

Situational (Personal, Environmental)

Excessive sodium intake/fluid intake
Low protein intake
Fad diets   Malnutrition
Dependent venous pooling/venostasis
Immobility   Standing or sitting for
long periods

Venous pressure point
Tight cast or bandage
Pregnancy
Inadequate lymphatic drainage

Maturational

Elderly (decreased cardiac output)

OUTCOME CRITERIA

The person will

1. Relate causative factors and methods of preventing edema
2. Exhibit decreased peripheral edema

INTERVENTIONS

1. Assess dietary intake and habits that may contribute to fluid retention.
2. Encourage the person to decrease salt intake.
3. Teach the person to:
    a. Read labels for sodium content.
    b. Avoid convenience foods, canned foods, and frozen foods.
    c. Cook without salt and use spices to add flavor (lemon, basil, tarragon, mint).
    d. Use vinegar in place of salt to flavor soups, stews,

etc. (*e.g.,* 2–3 teaspoons of vinegar to 4–6 quarts, according to taste).

4. Assess for evidence of dependent venous pooling or venostasis.

5. Keep edematous extremity elevated above the level of the heart whenever possible (unless contraindicated by heart failure).

6. Instruct person to avoid panty girdles/garters, knee-highs, and leg crossing and to practice keeping legs elevated when possible.

7. For inadequate lymphatic drainage:
   a. Keep extremity elevated on pillows.
   b. Take blood pressures in unaffected arm.
   c. Do not give injections or start intravenous fluids in affected arm.
   d. Protect the affected arm from injury.
   e. Teach the person to avoid strong detergents, carrying heavy bags, holding a cigarette, injuring cuticles or hangnails, reaching into a hot oven, wearing jewelry or a wristwatch, or using Ace bandages.
   f. Caution the person to see a physician if the arm becomes red, swollen or unusually hard.

8. Protect edematous skin from injury.

Grieving*

Grieving, Anticipatory

Grieving, Dysfunctional

DEFINITION

Grieving: The state in which an individual or group experiences an actual or perceived loss (person, object, function, status, relationship) or the state in which an individual or group responds to the realization of a future loss (anticipatory grieving).

* This diagnostic category is not currently on the NANDA list but has been included for clarity or usefulness.

> **Author's Note:**
> Grieving, Anticipatory Grieving, and Dysfunctional Grieving
> represent three types of responses of individuals or families ex-
> periencing a loss. Grieving describes normal grieving after a loss
> and participation in grief work.
>
> Anticipatory Grieving describes someone engaged in grief
> work prior to an expected loss. Dysfunctional Grieving is a
> maladaptive process that occurs when grief work is suppressed
> or absent or when there is prolonged exaggerated responses. For
> all three diagnoses, the goal of nursing is to promote grief work.
> In addition, for Dysfunctional Grieving, the nurse will direct
> interventions to reduce excessive, prolonged problematic re-
> sponses.

DEFINING CHARACTERISTICS

Major (Must Be Present)

The person
Reports an actual or perceived loss (person, object,
function, status, relationship)
or
Anticipates a loss

Minor (May Be Present)

Denial
Guilt
Anger
Despair
Feelings of worthlessness
Suicidal thoughts
Crying
Sorrow
Hallucinations

Delusions
Phobias
Anergia
Inability to concentrate
Visual, auditory, and
tactile hallucinations
about the object or person

RELATED FACTORS

Many situations can contribute to feelings of loss. Some common situations are listed below.

Pathophysiological

Loss of function (actual or potential) related to a disorder

Neurological	Digestive
Cardiovascular	Respiratory
Sensory	Renal
Musculoskeletal	

Loss of function or body part related to
Trauma

Treatment-related

Dialysis
Surgery (mastectomy, colostomy, hysterectomy)

Situational (Personal, Environmental)

Chronic pain
Terminal illness
Death
Changes in life-style

Childbirth	Child leaving home (*e.g.,*
Marriage	college or marriage)
Separation	Loss of career
Divorce	

Type of relationship (with the person who is leaving or is gone)
Multiple losses or crises
Lack of social support system

Maturational

Loss associated with aging

Friends	Function
Occupation	Home

OUTCOME CRITERIA

The individual will

1. Express grief
2. Describe the meaning of the death or loss
3. Share grief with significant others (children, spouses)

INTERVENTIONS

1. Promote a trust relationship.
2. Support the person and the family's grief reactions.
3. Explain grief reactions:
   a. Shock and disbelief
   b. Developing awareness
   c. Restitution
   d. Somatic manifestations
4. Assess for past experiences with loss.
5. Recognize and reinforce the strengths of each family member.
6. Encourage the family to evaluate their feelings and support one another.
7. Promote grief work with each response.
   a. Denial
      - Explain the use of denial by one family member to the other members.
      - Do not push client to move past denial without emotional readiness.
   b. Isolation
      - Reinforce the person's self-worth by allowing privacy.
      - Encourage client/family to gradually increase social activities (support groups, church groups, etc.).
   c. Depression
      - Identify the level of depression and develop the approach accordingly.
      - Use empathic sharing; acknowledge grief ("It must be very difficult.").
   d. Anger
      - Explain to family that anger serves to try to control one's environment more closely because of inability to control loss.
      - Encourage verbalization of the anger.
   e. Guilt
      - Encourage client to identify positive contributions/aspects of the relationship.
      - Avoid arguing and participating in the person's system of shoulds and should nots.
   f. Fear
      - Focus on the present and maintain a safe and secure environment.

g. Rejection
  - Explain this response to family members.
h. Hysteria
  - Reduce environmental stresses (*e.g.,* limit personnel).
  - Provide person with a safe, private area to display grief.

8. Promote grief work in children.
   a. Encourage parents and staff to be truthful and offer explanations that can be understood.
   b. Encourage parents and/or significant others to nurture children during the grieving process.
   c. Explore with child his or her concept of death in the context of maturational level.
   d. Correct misconceptions about death, illness, and rituals (funerals).
   e. Prepare the child for grief responses of others.
   f. If the child plans to attend the funeral or visit the funeral home, a thorough explanation of the setting, rituals, and expected behaviors of mourners is necessary beforehand (the family can plan the visit of the child to be short and also before the other mourners arrive).
   g. Allow child to share fears.
   h. Allow child to remain with significant others while they grieve at home.
   i. Provide accurate explanations for sibling illness or death.

9. Identify persons who are at high risk for potential pathological grieving reactions.
   a. Absence of any emotion
   b. Previous conflict with deceased person
   c. History of ineffective coping patterns

10. Teach the person and the family signs of resolution.

11. Identify agencies that may be helpful.

Grieving, Anticipatory

DEFINITION

Anticipatory Grieving: The state in which an individual/group experiences feelings in response to an expected significant loss.

DEFINING CHARACTERISTICS

Major (Must Be Present)

Expressed distress at potential loss

Minor (May Be Present)

Denial
Guilt
Anger
Sorrow
Change in eating habits
Change in sleep patterns
Change in social patterns
Change in communication patterns
Decreased libido

RELATED FACTORS

See *Grieving.*

OUTCOME CRITERIA

The person will

1. Express grief
2. Participate in decision-making for the future
3. Share concerns with significant others

INTERVENTIONS

1. Encourage the person to share concerns.
2. Promote the integrity of the person and the family by acknowledging strengths.
3. Prepare person and family for grief reactions.
4. Promote family cohesiveness.
5. Provide for the concept of hope by:
   a. Supplying accurate information
   b. Resisting the temptation to give false hope
   c. Discussing concerns willingly
6. Promote grief work with each response.
   a. Denial
      • Initially support and then strive to increase the development of awareness (when individual indicates readiness for awareness).

b. Isolation
  - Listen and spend designated time consistently with person and family.
  - Offer the person and the family opportunity to explore their emotions.
c. Depression
  - Begin with simple problem-solving and move toward acceptance.
  - Enhance self-worth through positive reinforcement.
d. Anger
  - Allow for crying to release this energy.
  - Encourage concerned support from significant others as well as professional support.
e. Guilt
  - Allow for crying.
  - Promote more direct expression of feelings.
  - Explore methods to resolve guilt.
f. Fear
  - Help person and family recognize the feeling.
  - Explore person's and family's attitudes about loss, death, etc.
  - Explore person's and family's methods of coping.
g. Rejection
  - Allow for verbal expression of this feeling state to diminish the emotional strain.
  - Recognize that expression of anger may create a rejection of self to significant others.

7. Caution against the use of sedatives and tranquilizers, which may prevent and/or delay emotional expressions of loss.
8. Teach signs of pathological responses and referrals needed.
9. Encourage person and family to engage in life review.
   a. Focus on and support the social network relationships.
   b. Reevaluate past life experiences and integrate them into a new meaning.

Grieving, Dysfunctional

DEFINITION

Dysfunctional Grieving: The state in which an individual or group experiences prolonged unresolved grief and engages in detrimental activities.

> **Author's Note:**
> How one responds to loss is highly individual. Responses to acute loss should not be labeled Dysfunctional regardless of the severity. Dysfunctional grieving is characterized by its sustained or prolonged detrimental response. The validation of dysfunctional grieving cannot occur until several months to a year after the loss. In many clinical settings, the diagnosis of High Risk for Dysfunctional Grieving for individuals at high risk for unsuccessful reintegration after a loss may be more useful.

DEFINING CHARACTERISTICS

Major (Must Be Present)

Unsuccessful adaptation to loss
Prolonged denial, depression
Delayed emotional reaction

Minor (May Be Present)

Social isolation or withdrawal
Failure to develop new relationships/interests
Failure to restructure life after loss

RELATED FACTORS

See *Grieving.*

OUTCOME CRITERIA

The person will

1. Acknowledge the loss

2. Demonstrate a lessening response of the pain of grief
3. Identify treatments available

INTERVENTIONS

1. Identify which tasks of mourning must be accomplished (Worden).*
   a. Acknowledgment of the loss
   b. Experiencing the pain
   c. Adjusting to the loss
   d. Reinvesting and goal-setting
2. Encourage persons to share perceptions of the situation and their response.
3. If denial persists, see *Ineffective Denial.*
4. Discuss the reality of the loss.
5. Explore the positive and negative aspects of the loss.
6. Assess risk for suicide (See *High Risk for Self-Harm*).
7. Encourage sharing of guilt and ambivalent feelings. Validate that they are normal.
8. Correct misinformation.
9. Emphasize past successful coping.
10. Share community resources available for sharing experiences with others.
11. Refer for counseling, if indicated.

Growth and Development, Altered

DEFINITION

Altered Growth and Development: The state in which an individual has or is at risk for an impaired ability to perform tasks of his or her age group or impaired growth.

---

* Worden J: Grief Counseling and Grief Therapy: A Handbook for the Mental Health Practitioner, New York, Springer, 1982

Author's Note:
The focus of this category will be children and adolescents. When an adult has not accomplished a developmental task, the nurse should assess for the altered functioning that has resulted from the failure to meet a developmental task; for example, Impaired Social Interactions or Ineffective Individual Coping.

DEFINING CHARACTERISTICS

Major (Must Be Present)

Inability to perform or difficulty performing skills or behaviors typical of his or her age group; for example, motor, personal/social, language/cognition
and/or
Altered physical growth: Weight lagging behind height by two standard deviations; pattern of height and weight percentiles indicating a drop in pattern

Minor (May Be Present)

Inability to perform self-care or self-control activities appropriate for age
Flat affect, listlessness, decreased responses, slow in social responses, shows limited signs of satisfaction to caregiver, shows limited eye contact, difficulty feeding, decreased appetite, lethargic, irritable, negative mood, regression in self-toileting, regression in self-feeding
Infants: watchfulness, interrupted sleep pattern

RELATED FACTORS

Pathophysiological

Circulatory impairment
    Congenital heart defects
    Congestive heart failure
Neurological impairment
    Cerebral damage
    Congenital defects
    Cerebral palsy
    Microcephaly

Gastrointestinal impairment
   Malabsorption syndrome
   Gastroesophageal reflux
   Cystic fibrosis
Endocrine or renal impairment
   Hormonal disturbance
Musculoskeletal impairments
   Congenital anomalies of extremities
   Muscular dystrophy
Acute illness
Prolonged pain
Repeated acute illness, chronic illness
Inadequate caloric, nutritional intake

Treatment-related

Prolonged, painful treatments
Repeated or prolonged hospitalization
Traction or casts that alter locomotion
Prolonged bed rest
Isolation due to disease processes
Confinement for ongoing treatment

Situational (Personal, Environmental)

Parental lack of knowledge
Stress (acute, transient, or chronic)
Hospitalization or change in usual environment
Separation from significant others (parents, primary
  caregiver)
Inadequate, inappropriate parental support (neglect,
  abuse)
Inadequate sensory stimulation (neglect, isolation)
Parent–child conflict
School-related stressors
Maternal or parental anxiety
Loss of significant other
Loss of control over environment (established rituals,
  activities, established hours of contact with family)
Multiple caregivers

Maturational

Infant–toddler (birth to 3 years)
   Lack of stimulation
   Separation from parents/significant others

Change in environment
Restriction of activity
Inadequate parental support
Inability to trust significant other
Inability to communicate (deafness)
Pre-school age (4-6 years)
Restriction of activity
Loss of ability to communicate
Lack of stimulation
Lack of significant other
Loss of significant other (death, divorce)
Loss of peer group
Loss of independence
Fear of mutilation/pain/abandonment
Removal from home environment
School age (6-11 years)
Loss of individual control
Loss of significant other
Loss of peer group
Fear of immobility, mutilation, death
Fear of intrusive procedures
Strange environment
Adolescent (12-18 years)
Loss of independence and autonomy
Disruption of peer relationships
Disruption in body image
Interruption of intellectual achievement
Loss of significant other

OUTCOME CRITERIA

The child will

1. Demonstrate an increase in behaviors in personal/social, language, cognition, motor activities appropriate to age group (specify the behaviors)

INTERVENTIONS

1. Teach parents the age-related developmental tasks (see Table I-1).
2. Carefully assess child's level of development in all areas of functioning by using specific assessment tools, (*e.g.,*

Brazelton Assessment Table, Denver Developmental Screening Tool).
3. Provide opportunities for an ill child to meet age-related developmental tasks.
   a. Birth to 1 year
      - Provide increased stimulation using variety of colored toys in crib (*i.e.,* mobiles, musical toys, stuffed toys of varied textures, frequent periods of holding and speaking to infant).
      - Hold while feeding; feed slowly and in relaxed environment.
      - Provide periods of rest prior to feeding.
      - Observe mother and child during interaction, especially during feeding.
      - Investigate crying promptly and consistently.
      - Assign consistent caregiver.
      - Encourage parental visits/calls and involvement in care, if possible.
      - Provide buccal experience if infant desires (*i.e.,* thumb, pacifier).
      - Allow hands and feet to be free, if possible.
   b. 1–3½ years
      - Assign consistent caregiver.
      - Encourage self-care activities (*i.e.,* self-feeding, self-dressing, bathing).
      - Reinforce word development by repeating words child uses, naming objects by saying words, and speaking to child often.
      - Provide frequent periods of play with peers present and with a variety of toys (puzzles, books with pictures, manipulative toys, trucks, cars, blocks, bright colors).
      - Explain all procedures as you do them.
      - Provide safe area where the child can locomote, use walker, creeping area, hold hand while taking steps.
      - Encourage parental visits/calls and involvement in care, if possible.
      - Provide comfort measures after painful procedures.
   c. 3½–5 years
      - Encourage self-care: self-grooming, self-dressing, mouth care, hair care.

(Text continues on p. 120)

TABLE I-1.
Age-related Developmental Needs

Developmental Tasks/Needs

BIRTH TO 1 YEAR	3½–5 YEARS	11–15 YEARS
PERSONAL/SOCIAL	PERSONAL/SOCIAL	PERSONAL/SOCIAL
Learns to trust and anticipate satisfaction	Attempts to establish self as like parents, but independent	Family values continue to be significant influence
Sends cues to mother/caretaker	Explores environment on own initiative	Peer group values have increasing significance
Begins understanding self as separate from others (body image)	Boasts, brags, has feelings of indestructibility	Early adolescence: outgoing and enthusiastic
MOTOR	Family is primary group	Emotions are extreme, mood swings, introspection
Responds to sound	Peers increasingly important	Sexual identity full mature
Social smile	Assumes sex roles	Wants privacy/independence
Reaches for objects	Aggressive	

Begins to sit, creep, pull up, and stand with support
Attempts to walk

LANGUAGE/COGNITION
Learns to signal wants/needs with sounds, crying
Begins to vocalize with meaning (two-syllable words: Dada, Mama)
Comprehends some verbal/nonverbal messages (no, yes, bye-bye)
Learns about words through senses

FEARS
Loud noises
Falling

MOTOR
Locomotion skills increase, and coordinates easier
Rides tricycle/bicycle
Throws ball, but has difficulty catching

LANGUAGE/COGNITION
Egocentric
Language skills flourish
Generates many questions, how, why, what?
Simple problem-solving; uses fantasy to understand, problem-solve

FEARS
Mutilation
Castration

Develops interests not shared with family
Concern with physical self
Explores adult roles

MOTOR
Well-developed
Rapid physical growth
Secondary sex characteristics

LANGUAGE/COGNITION
Plans for future career
Able to abstract solutions and problem-solve in future tense

FEARS
Mutilation

(Continued)

TABLE I-1. (Continued)

Developmental Tasks/Needs

1–3½ YEARS

PERSONAL/SOCIAL

Establishes self-control, decision-making, self-independence (autonomy)

Extremely curious, prefers to do things independently

Demonstrates independence through negativism

Very egocentric: believes he or she controls the world

Learns about words through senses

Dark

Unknown

Inanimate, unfamiliar objects

5–11 YEARS

PERSONAL/SOCIAL

Learns to include values and skills of school, neighborhood, peers

Peer relationships important

Focuses more on reality, less on fantasy

Family is main base of security and identity

Disruption in body image

Rejection from peers

MOTOR
Begins to walk and run well
Drinks from cup, feeds self
Develops fine-motor control
Climbs
Begins self-toileting

LANGUAGE/COGNITION
Has poor time sense
Increasingly verbal (4–5 word
    sentences by age 3½)
Talks to self/others
Misconceptions about cause/effect

FEARS
Loss/separation from parents
Darkness
Machines/equipment
Intrusive procedures

Sensitive to reactions of others
Seeks approval, recognition
Enthusiastic, noisy, imaginative,
    desires to explore
Likes to complete a task
Enjoys helping

MOTOR
Moves constantly
Physical play prevalent (sports,
    swimming, skating, etc.)

LANGUAGE/COGNITION
Organized, stable thought
Concepts more complicated
Focuses on concrete understanding

FEARS
Rejections, failure
Immobility
Mutilation
Death

- Provide frequent play time with others and with variety of toys (*i.e.,* models, musical toys, dolls, puppets, books, mini-slide, wagon, tricycle, etc.).
- Read stories aloud.
- Ask for verbal responses and requests.
- Say words for equipment, objects, and people and ask the child to repeat.
- Allow time for individual play and exploration of play environment.
- Encourage parental visits/calls and involvement in care, if possible.
- Monitor television and utilize television as means to help child understand time ("After Sesame Street, your mother will come.").

d. 5–11 years
- Talk with child about care provided.
- Request input from child (*i.e.,* diet, clothes, routine, etc.).
- Allow child to dress in clothes instead of pajamas.
- Provide periods of interaction with other children on unit.
- Provide craft project that can be completed each day or week.
- Continue school work at intervals each day.
- Praise positive behaviors.
- Read stories, and provide variety of independent games, puzzles, books, video games, painting, etc.
- Introduce child by name to persons on unit.
- Encourage visits with and/or telephone calls from parents, sibling, and peers.

e. 11–15 years
- Speak frequently with child about feelings, ideas, concerns over condition or care.
- Provide opportunity for interaction with others of the same age on unit.
- Identify interest or hobby that can be supported on unit in some manner and support it daily.
- Allow hospital routine to be altered to suit child's schedule.
- Dress in child's own clothes if possible.

- Involve in decisions about care.
- Provide opportunity for involvement in variety of activities (*i.e.,* reading, video games, movies, board games, art, trips outside or to other areas).
- Encourage visits and/or telephone calls from parents, siblings, and peers.
4. Refer to community programs specific to contributing factors (*e.g.,* WIC, social services, family services, counseling).

Health Maintenance, Altered

DEFINITION

Altered Health Maintenance: The state in which an individual or group experiences or is at risk of experiencing a disruption in health because of an unhealthy life-style or lack of knowledge to manage a condition.

Author's Note:
Altered Health Maintenance is a diagnostic category that can be used to describe a person or persons who desire to change an unhealthy life-style (obesity, tobacco use) or who need teaching for self-management of a disease or condition.

DEFINING CHARACTERISTICS (in the Absence of Disease)

Major (Must Be Present)

Reports or demonstrates an unhealthy practice or life-style
Reckless driving of vehicle
Substance abuse

Participation in high-risk activities (*e.g.,* recreational: skydiving/scuba diving, hang gliding; occupational: police, firefighting, mining, etc.)

Presence of obvious behavior disorders (compulsiveness, belligerence)

Overeating

Reports or demonstrates

Skin and nails

Malodorous

Unclean

Skin lesions (pustules, rashes, dry or scaly skin)

Sunburn

Unusual color, pallor

Unexplained scars

Respiratory system

Frequent infections

Chronic cough

Dyspnea with exertion

Oral cavity

Frequent sores (on tongue, buccal mucosa)

Loss of teeth at early age

Lesions associated with lack of oral care or substance abuse (leukoplakia, fistulas)

Gastrointestinal system and nutrition

Obesity

Anorexia

Cachexia

Chronic anemia

Chronic bowel irregularity

Chronic dyspepsia

Musculoskeletal system

Frequent muscle strain, backaches, neck pain

Diminished flexibility and muscle strength

Genitourinary system

Frequent venereal lesions and infections

Frequent use of potentially unhealthful over-the-counter products (chemical douches, perfumed vaginal products, nasal sprays, etc.)

Constitutional

Chronic fatigue, malaise, apathy

Neurosensory

Presence of facial tics (nonconvulsant)

Headaches

Psychoemotional

Emotional fragility

Behavior disorders (compulsiveness, belligerence)

Frequent feelings of being overwhelmed

RELATED FACTORS

A variety of factors can produce altered health maintenance. Some common causes are listed below.

Pathophysiological

Any new medical condition, regardless of the severity of illness

Treatment-related

Lack of previous exposure
New or complex treatment

Situational (Personal, Environmental)

Lack of exposure to the experience
Language differences
Information misinterpretation
Personal characteristics
Lack of motivation
Lack of education or readiness

Ineffective coping patterns (*e.g.,* anxiety, depression, nonproductive denial of situation, avoidance coping)

Changes in finances
Lack of access to adequate health care services
Inadequate health practice
External locus of control
Religious beliefs
Cultural beliefs

Maturational

Lack of education of age-related factors. Examples include
Child
Sexuality and sexual development
Safety hazards

Substance abuse
Nutrition

Adolescent
Same as child
Automobile safety practices

Substance abuse (alcohol, other drugs, tobacco)
Health maintenance practices

Adult
    Parenthood   Safety practices
    Sexual function   Health maintenance
                           practices

Elderly
    Effects of aging   Sensory deficits

See Table I-2 for age-related conditions.

OUTCOME CRITERIA

The person will

1. Describe life-styles that promote health
2. Describe/demonstrate health behaviors needed to manage condition
3. Describe signs and symptoms that need reporting

INTERVENTIONS

1. Assess knowledge of primary prevention.
   a. Safety–accident prevention (*e.g.,* car, machinery, outdoor safety)
   b. Healthful diet (*e.g.,* "basic four," low fat and salt, sufficient intake of vitamins, minerals, 2–3 quarts of water daily)
   c. Weight control
   d. Avoidance of substance abuse (*e.g.,* alcohol, drugs, tobacco)
   e. Avoidance of sexually transmitted diseases
   f. Dental/oral hygiene (*e.g.,* daily, dentist)
   g. Immunizations
   h. Regular exercise pattern
   i. Stress management
   j. Life-style counseling (*e.g.,* family planning, parenting skills)
2. Teach importance of secondary prevention.
   a. Physical exams (age-related)
   b. Monthly self-breast or testicular exams
   c. Annual mammography at 35 and after
   d. Glaucoma testing every 3–5 years after 30
3. Determine knowledge needed to manage condition.
   a. Causes
   b. Treatments
   c. Medications

    d. Diet
    e. Activity
    f. Risk factors
    g. Signs/symptoms of complications
    h. Restrictions
    i. Follow-up care
4. Assess if needed at-home resources are available.
    a. Caregiver
    b. Finances
    c. Equipment
5. Determine if referrals are indicated (*e.g.,* social services, housekeeping, home health).

Health-Seeking Behaviors:
(Specify)

DEFINITION

Health-Seeking Behaviors: The state in which an individual in stable health actively seeks ways to alter personal health habits and/or the environment to move toward a higher level of wellness.*

Author's Note:

This diagnostic category can be used to describe the individual/family that desires health teaching related to the promotion and maintenance of health (preventive behavior, age-related screening, optimal nutrition, etc.). This diagnostic category should be used to describe an asymptomatic person. However, it can be used for a person with a chronic disease to help that person attain a higher level of wellness. For example, a woman with lupus erythematosus can have the diagnosis Health-Seeking Behaviors: regular exercise program.

---

* Stable health status is defined as follows: age-appropriate illness prevention measures are achieved; client reports good or excellent health; signs and symptoms of disease, if present, are controlled.

(Text continues on p. 134)

TABLE I-2.
Primary and Secondary Prevention for Age-related Conditions

Developmental Level	Primary Prevention	Secondary Prevention
Infancy (0–1 year)	Parent education	Complete physical examination every 2–3 months
	Infant safety	Screening at birth
	Nutrition	Congenital hip
	Breastfeeding	Phenylketonuria (PKU)
	Sensory stimulation	Sickle cell disease
	Infant massage and touch	Cystic fibrosis
	Visual stimulation	Vision (startle reflex)
	Activity	Hearing (response to and localization of sounds)
	Colors	Tuberculin test at 12 months
	Auditory stimulation	Developmental assessments
	Verbal	Screen and intervene for high risk
	Music	Low birth weight
	Immunizations	Maternal substance abuse during pregnancy
	DPT ⎫ at 2, 4, and 6 months	Alcohol: fetal alcohol syndrome
	TOPV ⎭	Cigarettes: sudden infant death syndrome (SIDS)
	Oral hygiene	Drugs: addicted neonate
	Teething biscuits	Maternal infections during pregnancy

Prescool
(1–5 years)

Fluoride
Avoid sugared food and drink
Parent education
 Teething
 Discipline
 Nutrition
 Accident prevention
 Normal growth and development
Child education
 Dental self-care
 Dressing
 Bathing with assistance
 Feeding self-care
Immunizations
 DPT ⎫ at 18 months
 TOPV ⎭
MMR at 15 months
Dental/oral hygiene
 Fluoride treatments
 Fluoridated water
 Dietary counsel

Complete physical examination between 2 and 3 years
 and preschool (urinalysis, CBC)
Tuberculin test at 3 years
Developmental assessments (annual)
 Speech development
 Hearing
 Vision
Screen and intervene
 Plumbism
 Developmental lag
 Neglect or abuse
 Strabismus
 Hearing deficit
 Vision deficit

(Continued)

127

TABLE I-2. (Continued)

Developmental Level	Primary Prevention	Secondary Prevention
School age (6–11 years)	Health education of child "Basic 4" nutrition Accident prevention Outdoor safety Substance abuse counsel Anticipatory guidance for physical changes at puberty Immunizations Tetanus, at 10 years DPT } Boosters between TOPV } 4 and 6 years Professional dental hygiene every 6–12 months Continue fluoridation Complete physical examination	Complete physical examination Tuberculin test every 3 years (at ages 6 and 9) Developmental measurements Language Vision: Snellen charts at school 6–8 years, use "E" chart Over 8 years, use alphabet chart Hearing: audiogram
Adolescence (12–19 years)	Health education Proper nutrition and healthful diets	Complete physical examination (prepuberty or age 13) Blood pressure

	Sex education with family planning, male/female	Cholesterol
	Safe driving skills	Tuberculin test at 12 years
	Adult challenges	VDRL, CBC, urinalysis
	Seeking employment and career choices	Female: breast self-examination
	Dating and marriage	Male: testicular self-examination
	Confrontation with substance abuse	Female, if sexually active: Papanicolaou test and pelvic examination twice, one year apart (cervical gonorrhea culture with pelvic examination), then every 3 years if both are negative
	Safety in athletics	Screening and interventions if high risk
	Skin care	Depression
	Professional dental hygiene every 6–12 months	Suicide
	Immunization	Substance abuse
	Tetanus without trauma	Pregnancy
	TOPV booster at 12–14 years	Family history of alcoholism or domestic violence
Young adult (20–39 years)	Health education	Complete physical examination at about 20 years, then every 5–6 years
	Weight management with good nutrition as basal metabolic rate changes	Cancer checkup every 3 years
	Life-style counseling	Female: breast self-examination monthly
	Stress management skills	Male: testicular self-examination monthly

(Continued)

TABLE I-2. *(Continued)*

Developmental Level	Primary Prevention	Secondary Prevention
	Safe driving	All females: baseline mammography between ages 35 and 40
	Family planning	Parents-to-be: high-risk screening for Down syndrome, Tay-Sachs disease
	Parenting skills	Pregnant female: screen for sexually transmitted disease, rubella titer, Rh factor
	Regular exercise	Screening and interventions if high risk
	Environmental health choices	Female with previous breast cancer: annual mammography at 35 years and after
	Professional dental hygiene every 6–12 months	Female with mother or sister who has had breast cancer, same as above
	Immunization	Family history of colorectal cancer or high risk: annual stool guaiac, digital rectal examination, and sigmoidoscopy
	Tetanus at 20 years and every 10 years	PPD if exposed to tuberculosis
	Female: rubella, if zero negative for antibodies	

Middle-aged adult (40–59 years)	Health education: continue with young adult	Complete physical examination every 5–6 years with complete laboratory evaluation (serum/urine tests, x-ray, ECG)
	Midlife changes, male and female counseling	Cancer checkup every year
	"Empty-nest syndrome"	Female: breast self-examination monthly
	Anticipatory guidance for retirement	Male: testicular self-examination monthly
	Grandparenting	All females: annual mammography 50 years and over
	Professional dental hygiene every 6–12 months	Schiøtz tonometry (glaucoma) every 3–5 years
	Immunizations	Pregnant female: perinatal screening by amniocentesis if desired
	Tetanus every 10 years	Sigmoidoscopy at 50 and 51, then every 4 years if negative
	Pneumococcal influenza } Annual if high risk; *i.e.*, major chronic disease (COPD, CAD)	Stool guaiac annually at 50 and thereafter
		Screening and intervention if high risk
		Endometrial cancer: have endometrial sampling at menopause
		Oral cancer: screen more often if substance abuser
Elderly adult (60–74 years)	Health education: continue with previous counseling	Complete physical examination every 2 years with laboratory assessments

(Continued)

131

TABLE I-2. (Continued)

Developmental Level	Primary Prevention	Secondary Prevention
	Home safety	Annual cancer checkup
	Retirement	Blood pressure annually
	Loss of spouse	Female: breast self-examination monthly
	Special health needs	Male: testicular self-examination monthly
	Nutritional changes	Female: annual mammogram
	Changes in hearing or vision	Annual stool guaiac
	Alterations in bowel or bladder habits	Sigmoidoscopy every 4 years
	Professional dental/oral hygiene every 6–12 months	Schiøtz tonometry every 3–5 years
		Podiatric evaluation with foot care PRN

	Immunizations
	  Tetanus every 10 years
	  Pneumococcal ⎫ Annual if high risk
	  influenza ⎭
	Health education: continue counsel
	Anticipatory guidance
	  Dying and death
	  Loss of spouse
	  Increasing dependency on others
	Professional dental/oral hygiene every 6–12 months
		Screen for high risk
		  Depression
		  Suicide
		Complete physical examination annually
		Laboratory assessments
		Cancer checkup
		Blood pressure
		Stool guaiac
		Female: mammogram, sigmoidoscopy every 4 years
		Schiøtz tonometry every 3–5 years
		Podiatrist PRN

Old-age adult (75 years and over)	Immunizations Tetanus every 10 years Pneumococcal ⎫ Annual influenza ⎭	

DEFINING CHARACTERISTICS

Major (Must Be Present)

Expressed or observed desire to seek information for health promotion

Minor (May Be Present)

Expressed or observed desire for increased control of health practice

Expression of concern about current environmental conditions on health status

Stated or observed unfamiliarity with community wellness resources

Demonstrated or observed lack of knowledge in health promotion behaviors

RELATED FACTORS

Situational (Personal, Environmental)

Role changes
   Marriage
   Parenthood
   "Empty-nest syndrome"
   Retirement
Lack of knowledge of need for
   Preventive behavior (disease)
   Screening practices for age and risk
   Optimal nutrition and weight control
   Regular exercise program
   Constructive stress management
   Supportive social networks
   Responsible role participation

Maturational

See Table I-2 (Primary and Secondary Prevention for Age-related Conditions).

OUTCOME CRITERIA

The person will

1. Describe screening that is appropriate for age and risk factors

2. Perform self-screening for cancer
3. Participate in a regular physical exercise program
4. State an intent to use positive coping mechanisms and constructive stress management
5. Agree with self-responsibility for wellness (physical, dental, safety, nutritional, family)

INTERVENTIONS

1. Determine the person's or family's knowledge or perception of:
   a. Specific diseases (*e.g.,* heart disease, cancer, respiratory disease, childhood diseases, infections, dental disease)
   b. Susceptibility (*e.g.,* presence of risk factors, family history)
   c. Seriousness
   d. Value of early detection
2. Determine the person's or family's past patterns of health care.
   a. Expectations
   b. Interactions with health care system or providers
   c. Influences of family, cultural group, peer group, mass media
3. Provide specific information concerning screening for age-related conditions (refer to Table I-2).
4. Discuss the role of nutrition in health maintenance and the prevention of illness.
5. Discuss the benefits of a regular exercise program.
6. Discuss the elements of constructive stress management.
   a. Assertiveness training
   b. Problem-solving
   c. Relaxation techniques
7. Discuss strategies for developing positive social networks.
8. Review the daily health practices of the individual (adults, children).
   a. Dental care
   b. Food intake
   c. Fluid intake
   d. Exercise regimen
   e. Leisure activities
   f. Responsibilities in the family
      Use of:
   g. Tobacco
   h. Salt, sugar, fat products

    i. Alcohol
    j. Drugs (over-the-counter, prescribed)
        Knowledge of safety practices:
    k. Fire prevention
    l. Water safety
    m. Automobile (maintenance, seat belts)
    n. Bicycle
    o. Poison control

Home Maintenance Management, Impaired

DEFINITION

Impaired Home Maintenance Management: The state in which an individual or family experiences or is at risk of experiencing a difficulty in maintaining self or family in a home environment.

> **Author's Note:**
> This diagnostic category can describe situations in which the individual and/or family needs specific instruction to manage home care of a family member and/or activities of daily living.

DEFINING CHARACTERISTICS

Major (Must Be Present)

Outward expressions by individual or family of difficulty in maintaining the home (cleaning, repairs, financial needs)
or
In caring for self or family member at home

Minor (May Be Present)

Poor hygienic practices
    Infections
    Accumulated wastes

    Infestations
    Unwashed cooking and
      eating equipment
    Offensive odors

Impaired caregiver
    Overtaxed
    Anxious

    Lack of knowledge
    Negative response to ill
      member

Unavailable support system

RELATED FACTORS

Pathophysiological

Chronic debilitating disease
    Diabetes mellitus
    Chronic obstructive
      pulmonary disease
    Congestive heart failure
    Cancer

    Arthritis
    Multiple sclerosis
    Muscular dystrophy
    Parkinsonian syndrome
    Cerebrovascular accident

Situational (Personal, Environmental)

Injury to individual or family member (fractured limb,
spinal cord injury)
    Surgery (amputation, ostomy)
    Impaired mental status (memory lapses, depression,
      anxiety—severe, panic)
    Substance abuse (alcohol, other drugs)
    Unavailable support system
    Loss of family member
    Addition of family member (newborn, aged parent)
    Lack of knowledge
    Insufficient finances

Maturational

Infant
    Newborn care
    High risk for sudden infant death syndrome
Elderly
    Family member with deficits (cognitive, motor, sensory)

OUTCOME CRITERIA

The person or caretaker will

1. Identify factors that restrict self-care and home management
2. Demonstrate the ability to perform skills necessary for the care of the individual or home
3. Express satisfaction with home situation

INTERVENTIONS

1. Determine with the person and family the information needed to be taught and learned.
2. Determine the type of equipment needed, considering availability, cost, and durability.
3. Determine the type of assistance needed (*e.g.,* meals, housework, transportation) and assist the individual to obtain them.
4. Discuss the implications of caring for a chronically ill family member.
   a. Amount of time
   b. Effects on other role responsibilities (spouse, children, job)
   c. Physical requirements (lifting)
5. Stress to maintain contacts with friends and relatives even if only by phone; let friends know that you do use sitters so they can include you in some social activities.
6. Allow the caretaker opportunities to share problems and feelings.
7. Refer to community agencies as indicated (*e.g.,* nursing, social service, meals).

Hopelessness

DEFINITION

Hopelessness: A sustained subjective emotional state in which an individual sees no alternatives or personal choices available to solve problems or to achieve what is desired and cannot mobilize energy on own behalf to establish goals.

Author's Note:
Hopelessness differs from powerlessness in that a hopeless person sees no solution to the problem and/or way to achieve what is desired, even if he or she has control of his or her life. A powerless person may see an alternative or answer to the problem yet be unable to do anything about it because of perceived lack of control and resources.

DEFINING CHARACTERISTICS

Major (Must Be Present)

Expresses profound, overwhelming apathy in response to a situation perceived as impossible with no solutions (overt or covert)

Examples of expressions are:
"I might as well give up because I can't make things better."
"My future seems awful to me."
"I can't imagine what my life will be like in 10 years."
"I've never been given a break, so why should I in the future?"
"Life looks unpleasant when I think ahead."
"I know I'll never get what I really want."
"Things never work out how I want them to."
"It's foolish to want to get anything because I never do."
"It's unlikely that I'll get satisfaction in the future."
"The future seems vague and uncertain."

Physiological
Slowed responses to stimuli

Emotional
The hopeless person often has difficulty experiencing feelings, but may feel
Unable to seek good fortune, luck, or God's favor
That he or she has no meaning or purpose in life
"Empty or drained"
A sense of loss and deprivation

Person exhibits
Passiveness
Decreased verbalization
Lack of ambition, initiative, and interest

Cognitive
  Decreased problem-solving and decision-making
    capabilities
  Deals with past and future, not the here and now
  Decreased flexibility in thought processes
  Lacks imagination and wishing capabilities
  Unable to identify and/or accomplish desired objectives
    and goals
  Unable to plan, organize, or make decisions
  Unable to recognize sources of hope

Minor (May Be Present)

Physiological
  Anorexia
  Weight loss
  Decreased exercise
  Increased sleep
Emotional
  Patient feels
    Incompetent
    "A lump in the throat"
    Discouraged with self and others
    "At the end of his or her rope"
    Tense
    Helpless
    Overwhelmed ("I just can't . . .")
    Loss of gratification from roles and relationships
    Vulnerable
Person exhibits
  Poor eye contact; turns away from speaker; shrugs in
    response to speaker
  Apathy (decreased response to internal and external
    stimuli)
  Decreased affect
  Decreased motivation
  Despondency
  Sighing
  Social withdrawal
  Lack of involvement in self-care (may be cooperative in
    nursing care but offers little help to self)
  Passively *allows* care
  Regression
  Resignation

Depression
Anger
Destructiveness
Cognitive
  Conveys negative and/or slowed thought processes
  Decreased ability to integrate information received
  Loss of time perception for past, present, and future
  Decreased ability to recall from the past
  Confusion
  Inability to communicate effectively
  Distorted thought perceptions and associations
  Unreasonable judgment
  Suicidal thoughts
  Unrealistic perceptions in relation to hope

RELATED FACTORS

Pathophysiological

Any chronic and/or terminal illness can cause or
  contribute to hopelessness (heart disease, kidney disease,
  cancer, acquired immunodeficiency syndrome).
Associated factors include
  Failing or deteriorating physiological condition
  Impaired body image
  New and unexpected signs or symptoms of previous
    disease process
  Prolonged pain, discomfort, weakness
  Impaired functional abilities (walking, elimination,
    eating)

Treatment-related

Prolonged treatments (*e.g.,* chemotherapy, radiation) that
  cause discomfort
Prolonged treatments with no positive results
Treatments that alter body image (*e.g.,* surgery,
  chemotherapy)
Prolonged diagnostic studies with no results
Prolonged dependence on equipment for life support
  (dialysis, ventilator)
Prolonged dependence on equipment for monitoring
  bodily functions (telemetry)

Situational (Personal, Environmental)

Prolonged activity restriction (*e.g.,* fractures, spinal cord injury)

Prolonged isolation for disease processes (*e.g.,* infectious diseases, reverse isolation for compromised immune system)

Separation from significant others (parents, spouse, children, others)

Inability to achieve goals that one values in life (marriage, education, children)

Inability to participate in activities one desires (walking, sports)

Loss of something or someone valued (spouse, children, friend, financial resources)

Prolonged caretaking responsibilities (spouse, child, parent)

Exposure to long-term physiological or psychological stress

Loss of belief in transcendent values/God

Maturational

Child
　Loss of caregivers
　Loss of trust in significant other (parents, sibling)
　Abandonment by caregivers
　Loss of autonomy related to illness (*e.g.,* fracture)
　Loss of bodily functions
　Inability to achieve developmental tasks (trust, autonomy, initiative, industry)
Adolescent
　Loss of significant other (peer, family)
　Loss of bodily functions
　Change in body image
　Inability to achieve developmental task (role identity)
Adult
　Impaired bodily functions, loss of body part
　Impaired relationships (separation, divorce)
　Loss of job, career
　Loss of significant others (death of children, spouse)
　Inability to achieve developmental tasks (intimacy, commitment, productivity)

Elderly
   Sensory deficits
   Motor deficits
   Loss of independence
   Loss of significant others, things
   Inability to achieve developmental tasks (integrity)

OUTCOME CRITERIA

Short-Term

The person will

1. Share suffering openly and constructively with others
2. Reminisce and review life positively
3. Consider values and the meaning of life
4. Express feelings of optimism about the present
5. Express feelings of positive relationships with significant others
6. Express confidence in a desired outcome
7. Express confidence in self and others
8. Verbalize realistic goals

Long-Term

The person will

1. Demonstrate an increase in energy level as evidenced by activities (*i.e.,* self-care, exercise, hobbies, etc.)
2. Express positive expectations about the future
3. Demonstrate initiative, self-direction, and autonomy in decision-making and activities
4. Make statements similar to the following:
   a. "I am looking forward to . . ."
   b. "When things are not so good, it helps me to think of . . ."
   c. "I have enough time to do what I want."
   d. "There are more good times ahead."
   e. "I expect to succeed in . . ."
   f. "I expect to get more out of the good things in life."
   g. "My past experiences have helped me be prepared for my future."
   h. "In the future, I'll be happier."
   i. "I have faith in the future."

INTERVENTIONS

1. Convey empathy to promote verbalization of doubts, fears, and concerns.
2. Encourage the person to verbalize why and how hope is significant in his or her life.
3. Encourage expressions of how hope is uncertain and areas in which hope has failed.
4. Assist the person to understand that he or she can deal with the hopeless aspects by separating them from the hopeful aspects.
5. Assess and mobilize the person's internal resources (autonomy, independence, rationale, cognitive thinking, flexibility, spirituality).
6. Assist the client to identify sources of hope (*i.e.,* relationships, faith, things to accomplish).
7. Assist the client to develop realistic short-term and long-term goals (progress from simple to more complex; may use a "goals poster" to indicate type and time for achieving specific goals).
8. Teach the client to anticipate experiences he or she takes delight in each day (*e.g.,* walking, reading favorite book, writing letter).
9. Assess and mobilize person's external resources (significant others, health care team, support groups, God and/or higher powers).
10. Help the client to recognize that he or she is loved, cared about, and important to the lives of others regardless of failing health.
11. Encourage person to share concerns with others who have had similar problem and/or disease and have had positive experiences from coping effectively with it.
12. Assess belief support system (value, past experiences with, religious activities, relationship with God, meaning and purpose of prayer; refer to *Spiritual Distress*).
13. Allow the client time and opportunities to reflect on the meaning of suffering, death, and dying.
14. Initiate referrals as indicated (*e.g.,* counseling, spiritual leader).

Infection, High Risk for

Infection Transmission, High Risk for

DEFINITION

High Risk for Infection: The state in which an individual is at risk of being invaded by an opportunistic or pathogenic agent (virus, fungus, bacterium, protozoan, or other parasite) from external sources.

> **Author's Note:**
> High Risk for Infection describes a situation when host defenses are compromised, making the host more susceptible to environmental pathogens.

RISK FACTORS

Evidence of risk factors, such as
    Altered production of leukocytes
    Altered immune response
    Altered circulation (lymph, blood)
    Presence of favorable conditions for infection (see
      Related Factors)
History of infection

RELATED FACTORS

A variety of health problems and situations can create conditions that would encourage the development of infections. Some common factors are listed below.

Pathophysiological

Chronic diseases
    Cancer   Hepatic disorders
    Renal failure   Respiratory disorders

Arthritis
Hematological disorders
Diabetes mellitus
Collagen diseases
Heritable disorders
Alcoholism
Immunosuppression
Immunodeficiency
Altered or insufficient leukocytes
Blood dyscrasias
Impaired oxygen transport
Altered integumentary system
Periodontal disease
Obesity
Loss of consciousness
Hormonal factors

Treatment-related

Medications
Antibiotics
Corticosteroids
Antiviral agents
Insulin
Antifungal agents
Tranquilizers
Immuno-
suppressants
Surgery
Radiation therapy
Dialysis
Total parenteral nutrition
Tracheostomy
Chemotherapy
Lack of immunizations
Presence of invasive lines
(*e.g.,* IVs, Foley catheter,
enteral feedings)

Situational (Personal, Environmental)

Prolonged immobility
Trauma (accidental, intentional)
Postpartum period
Contact with contagious agents (nosocomial or
community acquired)
Postoperative period
Increased length of hospital stay
Malnutrition
Stress
Bites (animal, insect, human)
Thermal injuries
Warm, moist, dark environment (skinfolds, casts)
Inadequate personal hygiene
Lack of immunizations
Smoking

Maturational

Newborn
Lack of maternal antibodies (dependent on maternal exposure)
Lack of normal flora
Open wounds (umbilical, circumcision)
Immature immune system
Infant/child
Lack of immunization
Elderly
Debilitated
Decreased immune response
Chronic diseases

OUTCOME CRITERIA

The person will

1. Demonstrate meticulous handwashing technique by the time of discharge
2. Be free from nosocomial infectious processes during hospitalization
3. Demonstrate knowledge of risk factors associated with potential for infection and will practice appropriate precautions to prevent infection

INTERVENTIONS

1. Identify individuals at high risk for nosocomial infections.
   a. Assess for predictors.
      - Infection (preoperatively)
      - Abdominal or thoracic surgery
      - Surgery longer than 2 hours
      - Genitourinary procedure
      - Instrumentation (ventilator, suction, catheters, nebulizers, tracheostomy, invasive monitoring)
      - Anesthesia
   b. Assess for confounding factors.
      - Age less than 1 year or greater than 65 years
      - Obesity
      - Underlying disease conditions (chronic obstructive pulmonary disease, diabetes, cardiovascular blood dyscrasias)

- Substance abuse
- Medications (steroids, chemotherapy, antibiotic therapy)
- Nutritional status (intake less than minimum daily requirements)
- Smoker

2. Reduce the entry of organisms into individuals.
   a. Meticulous handwashing
   b. Aseptic technique
   c. Isolation measures
   d. Unnecessary diagnostic or therapeutic procedures
   e. Reduction of airborne microorganisms
3. Protect the immune-deficient individual from infection.
   a. Instruct individual to ask all visitors and personnel to wash their hands before approaching individual.
   b. Limit visitors when appropriate.
   c. Restrict invasive devices (IV, lab specimens) to those that are absolutely necessary.
   d. Teach individual and family members signs and symptoms of infection.
4. Reduce individual's susceptibility to infection.
   a. Encourage and maintain caloric and protein intake in diet (see *Altered Nutrition*).
   b. Monitor use or overuse of antimicrobial therapy.
   c. Administer prescribed antimicrobial therapy within 15 minutes of scheduled time.
   d. Minimize length of stay in hospital.
5. Instruct individual and family regarding the causes, risks, and communicability of the infection.
6. Report communicable diseases as appropriate to public health department.

Infection Transmission, High Risk for*

DEFINITION

High Risk for Infection Transmission: The state in which an individual is at risk for transferring an opportunistic or pathogenic agent to others.

---

* This diagnostic category is not currently on the NANDA list but has been included for clarity or usefulness.

RISK FACTORS

Presence of risk factors (see Related Factors)

RELATED FACTORS

Pathophysiological

Colonization with highly antibiotic-resistant organism
Airborne transmission exposure
Contact transmission exposure (direct, indirect, contact
droplet)
Vehicle transmission exposure
Vector-borne transmission exposure

Treatment-related

Contaminated or dirty surgical procedures (incision and
drainage, traumatic wound)
Drainage devices (urinary, chest tubes)
Suction equipment
Invasive devices (endotracheal tubes)

Situational (Personal, Environmental)

Disaster with hazardous infectious material
Unsanitary living conditions (sewage, personal hygiene)
Areas considered high risk for vector-borne diseases
(malaria, rabies, bubonic plague)
Areas considered high risk for vehicle-borne diseases
(hepatitis A, shigella, salmonella)
Lack of knowledge
Intravenous drug use
Multiple sexual partners

Maturational

Newborn
Birth outside a hospital setting in an uncontrolled
environment
Exposure during prenatal or perinatal period to
communicable disease via mother

OUTCOME CRITERIA

The person will

1. Relate the need to be isolated until noninfectious

149

2. Describe the mode of transmission of disease by the time of discharge
3. Demonstrate meticulous handwashing during hospitalization

INTERVENTIONS

1. Identify susceptible host individuals based on focus assessment for potential for infection and history of exposure.
2. Identify the mode of transmission based on infecting agent.
   a. Airborne
   b. Contact
      - Direct
      - Indirect
      - Contact droplet
   c. Vehicle-borne
   d. Vector-borne
3. Initiate appropriate isolation precautions.
4. Secure appropriate room assignment, dependent on the type of infection and hygienic practices of the infected person.
5. Adhere to the Universal Infection Precautions.
6. Referral to infection control practitioner for follow-up with the health department regarding family exposure and cause of exposure and to assist in appropriate isolation of the patient.
7. Teach patient regarding the chain of infection and patient responsibility in both the hospital and at home.

Injury, High Risk for

Aspiration, High Risk for

Poisoning, High Risk for

Suffocation, High Risk for

Trauma, High Risk for

DEFINITION

High Risk for Injury: The state in which an individual is at risk for harm because of a perceptual or physiological deficit, a lack of awareness of hazards, or maturational age.

Author's Note:

This diagnostic category has four subcategories: High Risk for Aspiration, Poisoning, Suffocation, and Trauma. Should the nurse choose to isolate interventions only for prevention of poisoning, then the diagnostic category High Risk for Poisoning would be useful.

RISK FACTORS

Presence of risk factors such as (see Related Factors for specific factors)
Evidence of environmental hazards
Lack of knowledge of environmental hazards
Lack of knowledge of safety precautions
History of accidents
Impaired mobility
Sensory deficits

RELATED FACTORS

Pathophysiological

Altered cerebral function
    Tissue hypoxia   Syncope
    Post-trauma   Confusion
    Vertigo
Altered mobility
    Unsteady gait   Loss of limb
Impaired sensory function
    Vision   Thermal/touch
    Hearing   Smell
Pain
Fatigue
Orthostatic hypotension

Vertebrobasilar insufficiency
Cervical spondylosis
Subclavian steal
Vestibular disorders
Carotid sinus syncope
Seizures
Hypoglycemia
Electrolyte imbalance
Amputation
Arthritis
Cerebrovascular accident
Parkinsonism
Congestive heart failure
Dysrhythmias
Depression

Treatment-related

Medications
  Sedatives   Hypoglycemics
  Vasodilators   Diuretics
  Antihypertensives   Phenothiazines
Casts/crutches, canes, walkers

Situational (Personal, Environmental)

Decrease in or loss of short-term memory
Dehydration (*e.g.,* summer)
Prolonged bed rest
Stress
Vasovagal reflex
Faulty judgment
Alcohol
Poisons (plants, toxic chemicals)
Household hazards
  Unsafe walkways   Faulty electric wires
  Unsafe toys   Improperly stored
                      poisons
Automotive hazards
  Lack of use of seatbelts   Mechanically unsafe
    or child seats   vehicle
Fire hazards
  Smoking in bed   Improperly stored
  Gas leaks   petroleum products

Unfamiliar setting (hospital, nursing home)
Improper footwear
Inattentive caretaker
Improper use of aids (crutches, canes, walkers,
   wheelchairs)
Environmental hazards (home, school, hospital)
History of accidents

Maturational

Infant/child
   High risk for maturational age
      Suffocation hazards (improper crib, pillow in crib,
         plastic bags, unattended in water —bath, pool,
         choking on such things as toys or food)
      Improper use of bicycles, kitchen utensils/appliances,
         sports equipment, lawn equipment
      Poison (plants, cleaning agents, medications)
      Fire (matches, fireplace, stove)
      Falls
Adolescent
   Automobile
   Bicycle
   Alcohol
   Drugs
Adult
   Drugs
   Automobile
   Alcohol
Elderly
   Motor and sensory deficits
   Medication (accidental overdose, sedation)
   Cognitive deficits

OUTCOME CRITERIA

The person will

1. Identify factors that increase the potential for injury
2. Relate an intent to use safety measures to prevent injury
   (*e.g.,* remove throw rugs or anchor them)
3. Relate an intent to practice selected prevention measures
   (*e.g.,* wear sunglasses to reduce glare)

INTERVENTIONS

1. Orient each new admission to surroundings, explain the call system, and assess the person's ability to use it.
2. Closely supervise the person during the first few nights to assess safety.
3. Use night light.
4. Encourage the person to request assistance during the night.
5. Keep bed at lowest level during the night.
6. Teach proper use of crutches, canes, walkers, prosthesis.
7. Instruct person to wear shoes that fit properly and have nonskid soles.
8. Assess for the presence of side effects of drugs that may cause vertigo.
9. Teach person to:
    a. Eliminate throw rugs, litter, and highly polished floors
    b. Provide nonslip surfaces in bathtub or shower by applying commercially available traction tapes
    c. Provide hand grips in bathroom
    d. Provide railings in hallways and on stairs
    e. Remove protruding objects (*e.g.,* coat hooks, shelves, light fixtures) from stairway walls
10. Protect infant/child from injury by controlling age-related hazards.

Aspiration, High Risk for

DEFINITION

High Risk for Aspiration: The state in which an individual is at risk for entry of secretions, solids, or fluids into the tracheobronchial passages.

RISK FACTORS

Presence of risk factors (see Related Factors)

RELATED FACTORS
Pathophysiological

Reduced level of consciousness
- Anesthesia
- Head injury
- Seizures
- Intoxicated
- Drug overdose
- Cerebrovascular accident (CVA)
- Coma
- Presenile dementia

Depressed cough and gag reflexes

Increased intragastric pressure
- Lithotomy position
- Enlarged uterus
- Obesity
- Ascites

Hiatal hernia

Delayed gastric emptying
- Intestinal obstruction
- Ileus
- Gastric outlet syndrome

Impaired swallowing
- Achalasia
- Scleroderma
- Hiatal hernia
- Esophageal strictures
- Myasthenia gravis
- Guillain–Barré syndrome
- Multiple sclerosis
- Muscular dystrophy

Impaired ability to chew

Facial/oral/neck surgery or trauma

Paraplegia or hemiplegia

CVA

Parkinsonism

Debilitating conditions

Catatonia

Tracheoesophageal fistula

Treatment-related

Presence of tracheostomy/endotracheal tube

Gastrointestinal tubes

Tube feedings

Medication administration

Wired jaws

Imposed prone position

Situational (Personal, Environmental)

Impaired ability to elevate upper body

Eating when intoxicated

Maturational

Premature
  Impaired sucking/swallowing reflexes
Neonate
  Decreased muscle tone of inferior esophageal sphincter
Elderly
  Poor dentition

OUTCOME CRITERIA

The person will

1. Not experience aspiration
2. Relate measures to prevent aspiration

INTERVENTIONS

1. Reduce the risk of aspiration in:
   a. Individuals with decreased strength, decreased sensorium, or autonomic disorders
      - Maintain a side-lying position if not contraindicated by injury.
      - Assess for position of the tongue, assuring that it has not dropped backward, occluding the airway.
      - Keep the head of the bed elevated, if not contraindicated by hypertension or injury.
      - Clear secretions from mouth and throat with a tissue or gentle suction.
      - Reassess frequently for presence of obstructive material in mouth and throat.
   b. Persons with tracheostomies or endotracheal tubes
      - Inflate cuff (during continuous mechanical ventilation, during and after eating, during and 1 hour after tube feeding, during intermittent positive-pressure breathing treatments).
      - Suction q1–2 hours and PRN.
   c. Persons with gastrointestinal tubes and feedings
      - Verify placement of feeding tube with air auscultation for tubes positioned via the nasogastric or nasojejunal route.

- Aspirate for residual contents before each feeding for tubes positioned gastrically.
- Elevate head of bed 30–45 minutes during feeding periods, and 1 hour after to prevent reflux by use of reverse gravity.
- Administer feeding if residual contents are less than 150 ml (intermittent) or
- Administer feeding if residual is not greater than 150 ml at 10%–20% of hourly rate (continuous).
- Regulate gastric feedings using an intermittent schedule allowing periods for stomach emptying between feeding intervals.

Poisoning, High Risk for

DEFINITION

High Risk for Poisoning: The state in which an individual is at high risk of accidental exposure to or ingestion of drugs or dangerous substances.

RISK FACTORS

Presence of risk factors (see Related Factors under High Risk for Injury)

Suffocation, High Risk for

DEFINITION

High Risk for Suffocation: The state in which an individual is at risk for smothering and asphyxiation.

RISK FACTORS

Presence of risk factors (see Related Factors under High Risk for Injury)

Trauma, High Risk for

DEFINITION

High Risk for Trauma: The state in which an individual is at high risk of accidental tissue injury (*e.g.,* wound, burns, fracture)

RISK FACTORS

Presence of risk factors (see Related Factors under High Risk for Injury)

Knowledge Deficit

DEFINITION

Knowledge Deficit: The state in which an individual or group experiences a deficiency in cognitive knowledge or psychomotor skills regarding the condition or treatment plan.

Author's Note:

Knowledge Deficit does not represent a human response, alteration, or pattern of dysfunction but rather an etiological or contributing factor.* Lack of knowledge can contribute to a variety of responses, *e.g.,* anxiety, self-care deficits. All nursing diagnostic categories have related patient/family teaching as a part of nursing interventions, *e.g.,* Altered Bowel Elimination, Impaired Verbal Communication. When the teaching directly relates to a specific nursing diagnosis, incorporate the teaching into the plan. When specific teaching is indicated prior to a procedure, the diagnosis Anxiety related to unfamiliar environment or procedure can be used. When information-giving is directed to assist a person or family with a decision, the diagnosis Decisional Conflict may be indicated.

---

* Jenny J: Knowledge Deficit: Not a Nursing Diagnosis. Image 19(4): 184–185, 1987

DEFINING CHARACTERISTICS

Major (Must Be Present)

Verbalizes a deficiency in knowledge or skill/request for
information
Expresses an inaccurate perception of health status
Does not correctly perform a desired or prescribed health
behavior

Minor (May Be Present)

Lack of integration of treatment plan into daily activities
Exhibits or expresses psychological alteration (*e.g.*,
anxiety, depression) resulting from misinformation or
lack of information

Mobility, Impaired Physical

DEFINITION

Impaired Physical Mobility: The state in which an individual
experiences or is at risk of experiencing limitation of purpose-
ful/independent physical movement.

Author's Note:

Impaired Physical Mobility describes an individual with limited
use of arm(s) or leg(s) or limited muscle strength. Impaired
Physical Mobility should not be used to describe complete immobility; instead, Potential for Disuse Syndrome is more applicable. Limitation of physical movement can also be the etiology of other nursing diagnoses such as Self Care Deficit or High
Risk for Injury.

Nursing Interventions for Impaired Physical Mobility would
focus on strengthening and restoring function and preventing
deterioration.

DEFINING CHARACTERISTICS

Major (Must Be Present)

Inability to move purposefully within the environment, including bed mobility, transfers, ambulation

Minor (May Be Present)

Range of motion limitations
Limited muscle strength or control
Impaired coordination

RELATED FACTORS
Pathophysiological

Neuromuscular impairment
Autoimmune alterations (multiple sclerosis, arthritis)
Nervous system diseases (parkinsonism, myasthenia gravis)
Muscular dystrophy
Partial or total paralysis (spinal cord injury, stroke)
Central nervous system tumor
Increased intracranial pressure
Sensory deficits
Musculoskeletal impairment
Spasms
Flaccidity, atrophy, weakness
Connective tissue disease (systemic lupus erythematosus)
Edema (increased synovial fluid)

Treatment-related

External devices (casts or splints, braces, IV tubing)
Surgical procedures (amputation)

Situational (Personal, Environmental)

Trauma or surgical procedures
Nonfunctioning or missing limbs (fractures)
Pain

Maturational

Elderly
  Decreased motor agility
  Muscle weakness

OUTCOME CRITERIA

The person will

1. Demonstrate the use of adaptive devices to increase mobility
2. Use safety measures to minimize potential for injury
3. Demonstrate measures to increase mobility
4. Report an increase in mobility

INTERVENTIONS

1. Refer to *High Risk for Disuse* syndrome for interventions to prevent the complications of immobility.
2. Teach to perform active range of motion on unaffected limbs at least four times a day.
    a. Perform passive range of motion on affected limbs.
        *   Perform slowly.
        *   Support the extremity above and below the joint.
    b. Gradually progress active range of motion to functional activities.
3. Provide progressive mobilization.*
    a. Assist the person slowly to sitting position.
    b. Allow the person to dangle legs over the side of the bed for a few minutes before standing.
    c. Limit time to 15 minutes, three times a day, the first few times out of bed.
    d. Increase the person's time out of bed, as tolerated, by 15-minute increments.
    e. Progress to ambulation with or without assistive devices.
    f. If unable to walk, assist the person out of bed to a wheelchair or chair.

---

* May require a physician's order.

      g. Encourage ambulating for short frequent walks (at least three times daily), with assistance if unsteady.

      h. Increase lengths of walks progressively each day.

4. Observe and teach the use of:

      a. Crutches

- No pressure should be exerted on axilla; hand strength should be used.
- Type of gait varies with individual's diagnosis.
- Measure crutches 2 to 3 inches below axilla, and tips 6 inches away from feet.

      b. Walkers

- Use arm strength to support weakness in lower limbs.
- Gait varies with individual's problems.

      c. Wheelchairs

- Practice transfers.
- Practice maneuvering around barriers.

      d. Prostheses (teach about the following)

- Stump wrapping prior to application of the prosthesis.
- Application of the prosthesis.
- Principles of stump care.
- Importance of cleaning the stump, keeping it dry, and applying the prosthesis only when the stump is dry.

      e. Slings

- Assess for correct application; sling should be loose around neck and should support elbow and wrist above level of the heart.
- Remove slings for range of motion.*

      f. Ace bandages

- Observe for correct position.
- Apply with even pressure, wrapping distally to proximally.
- Observe for "bunching."
- Observe for signs of skin irritation (redness, ulceration) or tightness (compression).
- Rewrap Ace bandages b.i.d. or as needed, unless contraindicated (*e.g.,* if bandage is postoperative compression dressing, check physician's orders).

---

* May require a physician's order.

5. Teach the individual safety precautions.
   a. Protect areas of decreased sensation from extremes of heat and cold.
   b. Practice falling and how to recover from falls while transferring or ambulating.
   c. For decreased perception of lower extremity (post-cerebrovascular accident [CVA] "neglect"), instruct the individual to check where limb is placed when changing positions or going through doorways; and check to make sure both shoes are tied, that affected leg is dressed with trousers, and that pants are not dragging.
   d. Instruct individuals who are confined to wheelchair to shift position and lift up buttocks every 15 minutes to relieve pressure; maneuver curbs, ramps, inclines, and around obstacles; and lock wheelchairs prior to transferring.
6. Encourage use of affected arm when possible.
   a. Encourage the person to use affected arm for self-care activities (*e.g.,* feeding himself, dressing, brushing hair).
   b. For post-CVA neglect of upper limb (see also *Unilateral Neglect*).
   c. Instruct the person to use unaffected arm to exercise the affected arm.
   d. Use appropriate adaptive equipment to enhance the use of arms.
      • Universal cuff for feeding in individuals who have poor control in both arms, hands
      • Large-handled or padded silverware to assist individuals with poor fine motor skills
      • Dishware with high edges to prevent food from slipping
      • Suction-cup aids to hold dishes in place to prevent sliding of plate
   e. Use a warm bath to alleviate early morning stiffness and improve mobility.
7. Proceed with health teaching, as indicated.

Noncompliance

DEFINITION

Noncompliance: The state in which an individual or group desires to comply, but factors are present that deter adherence to health-related advice given by health professionals.

> **Author's Note:**
> Noncompliance describes the individual who desires to comply, but the presence of certain factors prevents him or her from doing so. The nurse must attempt to reduce or eliminate these factors for the interventions to be successful. However, the nurse is cautioned against using the diagnosis of Noncompliance to describe an individual who has made an informed, autonomous decision not to comply.

DEFINING CHARACTERISTICS

Major (Must Be Present)

Verbalization of noncompliance or nonparticipation or confusion about therapy
and/or
Direct observation of behavior indicating noncompliance

Minor (May Be Present)

Missed appointments
Partially used or unused medications
Persistence of symptoms
Progression of disease process
Occurrence of undesired outcomes (postoperative morbidity, pregnancy, obesity, addiction, regression during rehabilitation)

RELATED FACTORS

Pathophysiological

Impaired ability to perform tasks because of disability
(*e.g.,* poor memory, motor and sensory deficits)
Chronic nature of illness
Increasing amount of disease-related symptoms despite
adherence to advised regimen

Treatment-related

Side effects of therapy
Previous unsuccessful experiences with advised regimen
Impersonal aspects of referral process
Nontherapeutic environment
Complex, unsupervised, or prolonged therapy
Financial cost of therapy
Nontherapeutic relationship between client and nurse

Situational (Personal, Environmental)

Concurrent illness of family member
Inclement weather keeping client from keeping
appointment
Nonsupportive family, peers, community
Knowledge deficit
Lack of autonomy in health-seeking behavior
Health beliefs run counter to professional advice
Poor self-esteem
Disturbance in body image

Maturational

Developmental maturity of the client is incompatible with the
individual's age.

OUTCOME CRITERIA

The person will

1. Verbalize fears related to health needs
2. Identify factors that are contributing to anxiety
3. Identify alternatives to present coping patterns

INTERVENTIONS

1. Using open-ended questions, encourage person to talk about previous experiences with health care (*e.g.,* hospitalizations, family deaths, diagnostic tests, blood tests, x-rays).
2. Ask client directly, "What are your concerns about
   a. taking this drug?"
   b. following this diet?"
   c. having a blood test?"
   d. going through the cystoscopy?"
   e. having your gallbladder removed?"
   f. using a diaphragm?"
   g. paying for the operation?"
3. Assess person for recent changes in life-style (personal, work, family, health, financial).
4. Assess for problems with present medication therapy (*e.g.,* side effects, finances).
5. Assist to reduce side effects, if possible.
   a. For gastric irritation, suggest that drug be taken with milk or food; may be advisable to eat yogurt (unless contraindicated).
   b. For drowsiness, take medication at bedtime or late in afternoon; consult physician for dose reduction.
6. Teach importance of adhering to prescribed regimen.

Nutrition, Altered: Less Than Body Requirements

Impaired Swallowing

DEFINITION

Altered Nutrition: Less Than Body Requirements: The state in which an individual who is not NPO experiences or is at risk of experiencing reduced weight related to inadequate intake or metabolism of nutrients.

> **Author's Note:**
> This diagnostic category describes individuals who can ingest food but only in less-than-adequate amounts. This category should not be used to describe individuals who are NPO or cannot ingest food. These situations should be described by the collaborative problem of
>
>   Potential Complication:
>   Electrolyte imbalances
>   Negative nitrogen balance
>
> Nurses monitor to detect complications of an NPO state and confer with physicians for parenteral therapy. Some nursing diagnoses that may relate to an individual who is NPO are High Risk for Altered Oral Mucous Membrane and Altered Comfort.

DEFINING CHARACTERISTICS

Major (Must Be Present)

Reported inadequate food intake less than recommended daily allowance (RDA) with or without weight loss
and/or
Actual or potential metabolic needs in excess of intake

Minor (May Be Present)

Weight 10%–20% or more below ideal for height and frame
Triceps skin fold, mid-arm circumference, and mid-arm muscle circumference less than 60% standard measurement
Tachycardia on minimal exercise and bradycardia at rest
Muscle weakness and tenderness
Mental irritability or confusion
Decreased serum albumin
Decreased serum transferrin or iron-binding capacity
Decreased lymphocyte count

RELATED FACTORS
Pathophysiological

Hyperanabolic/catabolic states
    Burns (postacute phase)   Cancer
    Infection   Trauma

Chemical dependence
Faulty metabolism
    Cirrhosis
    Gastric resection
Dysphagia
    Cerebrovascular accident   Parkinson's disease
    Amyotrophic lateral   Neuromuscular disorders
     sclerosis   Muscular dystrophy
    Cerebral palsy
Absorptive disorders
    Crohn's disease
    Cystic fibrosis
Diverticulosis
Stomatitis
Trauma
Altered level of consciousness
Fear of choking

Treatment-related

Surgery
Medications (cancer chemotherapy)
Surgical reconstruction of the mouth
Wired jaw
Radiation therapy
Inadequate absorption as a side effect
    Colchicine
    Pyrimethamine
    Antacid
    Neomycin
    Para-aminosalicylic acid

Situational (Personal, Environmental)

Anorexia
Depression
Stress
Social isolation
Nausea and vomiting
Allergies
Parasites
Inability to procure food (physical limitations, financial or
    transportation problems)
Lack of knowledge of adequate nutrition
Crash or fad diet

Inability to chew (wired jaw, damaged or missing teeth,
  ill-fitting dentures)
Diarrhea
Lactose intolerance
Ethnic/religious eating patterns

Maturational

Infant/child
    Congenital anomalies
    Growth spurts
    Developmental eating disorders
Adolescent
    Anorexia nervosa (postacute phase)
Elderly
    Altered sense of taste

OUTCOME CRITERIA

The person will

1. Increase oral intake as evidenced by (specify)
2. Describe causative factors when known
3. Describe rationale and procedure for treatments

INTERVENTIONS

1. Explain to person the importance of consuming adequate amounts of nutrients.
2. Teach person to use spices to help improve the taste and aroma of food (lemon juice, mint, cloves, basil, thyme, cinnamon, rosemary, bacon bits).
3. Encourage individual to eat with others (meals served in dining room or group area, at local meeting place such as community center, by church groups).
4. Plan care so that unpleasant or painful procedures do not take place before meals.
5. Provide pleasant, relaxed atmosphere for eating (no bedpans in sight; don't rush); try a "surprise" (*e.g.*, flowers with meal).
6. Arrange plan of care to decrease or eliminate nauseating odors or procedures near mealtimes.
7. Teach or assist individual to rest before meals.
8. Teach person to avoid cooking odors—frying foods, brewing coffee—if possible (take a walk; select foods that can be eaten cold).

169

9.   Maintain good oral hygiene (brush teeth, rinse mouth) before and after ingestion of food.
10. Offer frequent small feedings (6/day plus snacks) to reduce the feeling of a distended stomach.
11. Arrange to have highest protein/calorie nutrients served at the time individual feels most like eating (*e.g.,* if chemotherapy is in early morning, serve in late afternoon).
12. Instruct person to:
     a. Eat dry foods (toast, crackers) on arising.
     b. Eat salty foods if permissible.
     c. Avoid overly sweet, rich, greasy, or fried foods.
     d. Try clear cool beverages.
     e. Sip slowly through straw.
     f. Take whatever can be tolerated.
     g. Eat small portions low in fat and eat more frequently.
13. Try commercial supplements available in many forms (liquids, powder, pudding); keep switching brands until some are found that are acceptable to individual in taste and consistency.

Impaired Swallowing

DEFINITION

Impaired Swallowing: The state in which an individual has decreased ability to voluntarily pass fluids and/or solid foods from the mouth to the stomach.

DEFINING CHARACTERISTICS

Major (Must Be Present)

Observed evidence of difficulty in swallowing
and/or
Stasis of food in oral cavity
Evidence of aspiration

Minor (May Be Present)

Coughing
Choking
Apraxia (ideational, constructional, or visual)

RELATED FACTORS
Pathophysiological

Cleft lip/palate

Neuromuscular disorders (*e.g.,* cerebral palsy, muscular dystrophy, amyotrophic lateral sclerosis, myasthenia gravis, Guillain-Barré syndrome, botulism, poliomyelitis, parkinsonism)

Neoplastic disease (disease affecting brain and/or brain stem)

Cerebrovascular accident

Right or left hemispheric damage to the brain

Damage to the 5th, 7th, 9th, 10th, or 11th cranial nerves

Tracheoesophageal fistula

Tracheoesophageal tumors, edema

Treatment-related

Surgical reconstruction of the mouth and/or throat

Anesthesia

Mechanical obstruction (tracheostomy tube)

Situational (Personal, Environmental)

Altered level of consciousness

Fatigue

Limited awareness

Altered sense of taste

Irritated oropharyngeal cavity

Maturational

Infant/child
  Congenital anomalies
  Developmental disorders

OUTCOME CRITERIA

The person will

1.   Report improved ability to swallow

The person and/or family will

1.   Describe causative factors when known
2.   Describe rationale and procedures for treatment

INTERVENTIONS

1. Assist the individual with moving the bolus of food from the anterior to the posterior of mouth.
   a. Place food in the posterior mouth where swallowing can be assured.
2. Prevent/decrease thick secretions.
3. Progress to ice chips, water, and then food when danger of aspiration is decreased.
4. For individuals with impaired cognition or awareness:
   a. Concentrate on solids rather than liquids, since liquids are generally less well tolerated.
   b. Keep extraneous stimuli at minimum while eating (*e.g.,* no television or radio, no verbal stimuli unless directed at task).
   c. Have person concentrate on task of swallowing.
   d. Have person sit up in chair with neck slightly flexed.
   e. Instruct person to hold breath while swallowing.
   f. Observe for swallowing and check mouth for emptying.
   g. Avoid overloading mouth, because this decreases swallowing effectiveness.
   h. Give solids and liquids separately.
   i. Reinforce behaviors with simple one-word commands.
5. Reduce the possibility of aspiration.
   a. Before beginning feeding, assess that person is adequately alert and responsive, is able to control mouth, has cough/gag reflex, and can swallow own saliva.
   b. Have suction equipment available and functioning properly.
   c. Position correctly.
      - Sit upright (60°–90°) in chair or dangle feet at side of bed if possible (prop pillows if necessary).
      - Assume position 10–15 minutes before eating and maintain position for 10–15 minutes after finishing eating.
      - Flex head forward on the midline about 45° to keep esophagus patent.
   d. Keep individual focused on task by giving directions until he or she has finished swallowing each mouthful.

e. Start with small amounts and progress slowly as person learns to handle each step.
- Ice chips
- Part of eyedropper filled with water
- Use juice in place of water
- ¼, ½, 1 teaspoon semisolid
- Pureed food or commercial baby foods
- One-half cracker
- Soft diet—regular diet

6. Feed slowly, making certain previous bite has been swallowed.
7. Consult with speech pathologist.

Nutrition, Altered: More Than Body Requirements

DEFINITION

Altered Nutrition: More Than Body Requirements: The state in which an individual experiences or is at risk of experiencing weight gain related to an intake in excess of metabolic requirements.

Author's Note:

Obesity is a complex condition with sociocultural, psychological, and metabolic implications. This diagnostic category, when used to describe obesity or overweight conditions, focuses on them as nutritional problems. The focus of treatment is behavioral modification and life-style changes. It is recommended that Altered Health Maintenance related to intake in excess of metabolic requirements be used in place of this diagnostic category. When weight gain is the result of physiological conditions, *e.g.,* altered taste or pharmacological interventions such as corticosteroid therapy, this diagnostic category can be clinically useful.

173

DEFINING CHARACTERISTICS

Major (Must Be Present)

Overweight (weight 10% over ideal for height and frame)
or
Obese (weight 20% or more over ideal for height and
frame)
Triceps skin fold greater than 15 mm in men and 25 mm
in women

Minor (May Be Present)

Reported undesirable eating patterns
Intake in excess of metabolic requirements
Sedentary activity patterns

RELATED FACTORS
Pathophysiological

Altered satiety patterns
Decreased sense of taste and smell

Treatment-related

Medications (corticosteroids)
Radiation (decreased sense of taste and smell)

Situational (Personal, Environmental)

Pregnancy (at risk to gain more than 25–30 pounds)
Lack of basic nutritional knowledge

Maturational

Adult/elderly
Decreased activity patterns
Decreased metabolic needs

OUTCOME CRITERIA

The person will

1. Experience increased activity expenditure with weight
loss
2. Describe relationship between activity level and weight
3. Identify eating patterns that contribute to weight gain
4. Lose weight

INTERVENTIONS

1. Increase individual's awareness of amount/type of food consumed.
   a. Instruct person to keep a diet diary for 1 week.
      - What, when, where, and why eaten?
      - Whether doing anything else (*e.g.,* watching television, preparing dinner)
      - Emotions just before eating
      - Others present (snacking with spouse, children)
   b. Review diet diary with individual to point out patterns (*i.e.,* time, place, persons, emotions, foods) that affect intake.
   c. Review high- and low-calorie food items.
2. Assist person to set realistic goals (*i.e.,* decreasing oral intake by 500 calories will result in a 1-to-2-pound loss each week)
3. Teach behavior modification techniques.
   a. Eat only at a specific spot at home (*i.e.,* kitchen table).
   b. Do not eat while doing other activities such as reading or watching television; eat only when sitting.
   c. Drink 8-oz glass of water immediately before eating.
   d. Use small plates (portions look bigger).
   e. Prepare small portions, just enough for a meal, and discard leftovers.
   f. Never eat from another person's plate.
   g. Eat slowly and chew thoroughly.
   h. Put down utensils and wait 15 seconds between bites.
   i. Eat low-calorie snacks that need to be chewed to satisfy oral need (carrots, celery, apples).
   j. Decrease liquid calories; drink diet sodas or water.
4. Plan a daily walking program and gradually increase rate and length of walk.
   a. Start out at 5–10 blocks for 0.5–1.0 mile/day; increase 1 block or 0.1 mile/week
   b. Progress slowly.
   c. Avoid straining or pushing too hard and becoming overly fatigued.
   d. Stop immediately if any of the following signs occur:

- Lightness or pain in chest
- Severe breathlessness
- Lightheadedness
- Dizziness
- Loss of muscle control
- Nausea

e. Establish a regular time of day to exercise, with the goal of 3–5 times/week for a duration of 15–45 minutes and with a heart rate of 80% of stress test or gross calculation (170 beats/min for 20–29 age group; decrease 10 beats/min for each additional decade of life—*e.g.,* 160 beats/min for ages 30–39, 150 beats/min for ages 40–49, etc.)

5. Refer to support groups (*e.g.,* Weight Watchers, Overeaters Anonymous, TOPS, trim clubs, The Diet Workshop, Inc.).

Nutrition, Altered: Potential for More Than Body Requirements

DEFINITION

Altered Nutrition: Potential for More Than Body Requirements: The state in which an individual is at risk of experiencing an intake of nutrients that exceeds metabolic needs.

Author's Note:

This diagnostic category is similar to High Risk for Altered Nutrition: More Than Body Requirements. It describes an individual who has a family history of obesity, who is demonstrating a pattern of higher weight, and/or who has had a history of excessive weight gain (*e.g.,* previous pregnancy). Until clinical
(*Continued*)

DEFINING CHARACTERISTICS

Reported or observed obesity in one or both parents
Rapid transition across growth percentiles in infants or
  children
Reported use of solid food as major food source before 5
  months of age
Observed use of food as a reward or comfort measure
Reported or observed higher baseline weight at beginning
  of each pregnancy
Dysfunctional eating patterns

Parenting, Altered

Parental Role Conflict

DEFINITION

Altered Parenting: The state in which one or more caregivers
experiences a real or potential inability to provide a constructive
environment that nurtures the growth and development of his/
her/their child (children).

DEFINING CHARACTERISTICS

Major (Must Be Present)

Inappropriate parenting behaviors and/or lack of parental attachment behavior

Minor (May Be Present)

Frequent verbalization of dissatisfaction or disappointment with infant/child
Verbalization of frustration of role
Verbalization of perceived or actual inadequacy
Diminished or inappropriate visual, tactile, or auditory stimulation of infant
Evidence of abuse or neglect of child
Growth and development lag in infant/child

RELATED FACTORS

Individuals or families who may be at high risk for developing or experiencing parenting difficulties
Parent(s)

Single	Alcoholic
Adolescent	Addicted to drugs
Abusive	Terminally ill
Emotionally disturbed	Acutely disabled
	Accident victim

Child

Of unwanted pregnancy	Physically handicapped
Of undesired gender	Mentally handicapped
With undesired characteristics	Hyperactive
	Terminally ill
	Rebellious

Situational (Personal, Environmental)

Separation from nuclear family
Lack of extended family
Lack of knowledge
Economic problems

Inflation	Unemployment
Relationship problems	
Marital discord	Live-in sexual partner
Divorce	Relocation

Separation
Step-parents
Change in family unit
    New child   Relative moves in

Other

History of ineffective relationships with own parents
Parental history of abusive relationship with parents
Unrealistic expectations of child by parent
Unrealistic expectations of self by parent
Unrealistic expectations of parent by child
Unmet psychosocial needs of child by parent
Unmet psychosocial needs of parent by child

OUTCOME CRITERIA

The person will

1. Share feelings regarding parenting
2. Identify factors that interfere with effective parenting
3. Describe appropriate disciplinary measures
4. Share feelings regarding parenting
5. Identify resources available for assistance with parenting

INTERVENTIONS

1. Assess parenting behaviors and determine the level of impairment.
2. Encourage to share parenting difficulties and usual and/ or recent stressors.
3. If abuse is suspected, notify appropriate authorities (see *Ineffective Family Coping: Disabling*).
4. Provide with information on:
    a. Age-related development needs
    b. Age-related problematic behavior
5. Observe the parent interacting with child.
    a. Support strengths.
    b. Role model in areas that are uncomfortable or problematic.
    c. Emphasize the child's strengths or unique characteristics.
6. Encourage parent to participate in care.
7. Explain all procedures and the associated discomforts.

8. Encourage parents to be present for procedures when possible and to comfort the child.
9. Explore parent(s) expectations of child and to differentiate realistic from unrealistic.
10. Assess usual discipline methods for appropriateness and follow-through.
11. Discuss discipline methods:
    a. For small child—sit in chair 2 minutes (if child gets up, put back in chair and reset timer).
    b. For older child—deprive of favorite pastime (*e.g.,* bicycle, TV show).
    c. Avoid hitting except one hand slap for a small child for dangerous touching (*e.g.,* stove, electric plug).
    d. Don't threaten. Clarify punishment and follow through with it.
    e. Expect child to obey.
    f. Parents should jointly agree and follow through with consistency.
12. Discuss resources available (*e.g.,* counseling, community, social service, parenting classes).

Parental Role Conflict

DEFINITION

Parental Role Conflict: The state in which a parent experiences or perceives a change in role in response to external factors (*e.g.,* illness, hospitalization, divorce, separation).

Author's Note:
This diagnostic category describes a parent or parents whose previously effective functioning ability is challenged by external factors. In certain situations, such as illness, role confusion and conflict are expected. This category differs from Altered Parenting, which describes a parent (or parents) who demonstrates or is at high risk of demonstrating inappropriate parenting behaviors and/or lack of parental attachment. If parents are not assisted in adapting their role to external factors, Parental Role
(*Continued*)

> *Author's Note (Continued)*
> Conflict can lead to Altered Parenting. The term *parent* refers
> to any individual(s) defined as the primary caregiver(s) for a
> child.
>   This diagnostic category was developed by the Nursing Di-
> agnosis Discussion Group, Rainbow Babies' and Children's
> Hospital, University Hospitals of Cleveland.

DEFINING CHARACTERISTICS

Major (Must Be Present)

Parent(s) expresses concerns about changes in parental
role
and/or
Demonstrates disruption in caregiving routines

Minor (May Be Present)

Parent(s) expresses concerns/feelings of inadequacy to
provide for child's physical and emotional needs during
hospitalization or in the home.
Parent(s) expresses concern about effect of child's illness
on family.
Parent(s) expresses concerns about care of siblings at
home.
Parent(s) expresses guilt about contributing to the child's
illness through lack of knowledge, judgment, and so
forth.
Parent(s) expresses concern about perceived loss of control
over decisions relating to the child.
Parent(s) reluctant, unable, or unwilling to participate in
normal caregiving activities even with encouragement
and support.
Parent(s) verbalizes/demonstrates feelings of guilt, anger,
fear, anxiety, and/or frustration.

RELATED FACTORS

Situational (Personal, Environmental)

Illness of child
  Birth of a child with a congenital defect and/or chronic
  illness

Hospitalization of a child with an acute or chronic illness

Change in acuity, prognosis, or environment of care (*e.g.,* transfer to or from an ICU)

Invasive or restrictive treatment modalities (*e.g.,* isolation, intubation)

Home care of a child with special needs (*e.g.,* apnea monitoring, postural drainage, hyperalimentation)

Interruptions of family life due to treatment regimen

Separation

Divorce

Remarriage

Death

Illness of caregiver

Change in family membership

Birth, adoption

Addition of relatives (*e.g.,* grandparent, siblings)

OUTCOME CRITERIA

The person will

1. Identify source of role conflict
2. Define the parental role desired
3. Participate in decision-making regarding health/illness care of child
4. Participate in care of child at level desired

INTERVENTIONS

1. Discuss what has influenced a change in role, *e.g.,* divorce, remarriage, illness (child, parent), boarding away, family additions (newborn, aging parent).
2. Allow person to share frustrations.
3. Assist person to determine the type of role desired and if realistic.
4. If indicated, refer for counseling for management of stressors and role changes.
5. For ill or hospitalized child:
   a. Help parent(s) adapt parenting behaviors to allow for continuation of parenting role during hospitalization and/or illness.
   b. Provide information about hospital routines and policies such as visiting hours, mealtimes, division

routines, medical and nursing routines, rooming-in, etc.

c. Explain procedures and tests to parent(s); help them interpret these activities to the child; discuss child's age-appropriate range of responses.

d. Instruct parents to continue limit-setting strategies and demonstrations of caring behaviors (*e.g.,* touching, hugging despite hospitalization and equipment).

e. Provide information to empower parent(s) to adapt parenting role to the situation of hospitalization and/or the event of chronic illness of the child.

f. Foster open communication between self and parent(s), allowing time for questions, frequent repetition of information; provide direct and honest answers.

g. Approach parents with new information; do not make them assume the responsibility for seeking out the information.

h. When parents cannot be with their child, facilitate information-sharing through telephone calls; allow parents to call primary nurse or nurse caring for child.

i. Support continued decision-making of parent(s) regarding the child's care.
   • Provide parent(s) opportunity to help formulate plan of care for their child.
   • Use parent(s) as source of information about the child, child's usual behaviors, reactions, and preferences.
   • Recognize parent(s) as "expert(s)" about their child.
   • Allow parent(s) the choice to be present during treatments and procedures.

j. Allow parents to participate in caring for their child to the degree they desire.
   • Provide for 24-hour rooming-in for at least one parent and extended visiting for other family members.
   • Collaborate and negotiate with parent(s) about parental tasks they wish to continue to do, tasks they wish others to assume, tasks they wish to share, and tasks they want to

learn to do; continually assess changes in their desired involvement in care.
- Allow parent(s) to have uninterrupted time with the child.

k. Explore with parent(s) their personal responsibilities (*i.e.,* work schedule, sibling care, household responsibilities, responsibilities to extended family); assist them in establishing a schedule that allows for sufficient caretaking time for the child and/or visiting time with the hospitalized child without frustration in meeting other role responsibilities (*e.g.,* if visiting is not possible until evening hours, delay child's bath time and allow parent to bathe child then).

l. Support parental ability to normalize the hospital/home environment for themselves and the child.
- Encourage parent(s) to bring clothing and toys from home.
- Allow parent(s) to prepare home-cooked food or bring food from home if desired.
- Encourage opportunities for families to eat meals together.
- Encourage opportunities for parent(s) to take the child on leaves from the hospital, including visits home, as possible.

m. Help parent(s) verbalize feelings about the child's illness and/or hospitalization and adaptation of the parenting role to the situation.

n. Provide for physical and emotional needs of parent(s).
- Assess and facilitate parental ability to meet self-care needs (*i.e.,* rest, nutrition, activity, privacy, etc.).
- Allow parent(s) an opportunity to determine the caregiving schedule to correspond with a schedule to meet their own needs.
- Assess support systems: parent to parent, family, friends, minister, etc.

o. Initiate referrals if indicated: chaplain, social service, community agencies (respite care), parent self-help groups.

Post-Trauma Response

Rape Trauma Syndrome

DEFINITION

Post-Trauma Response: The state in which an individual experiences a sustained painful response to (an) overwhelming traumatic event(s) that has (have) not been assimilated.

DEFINING CHARACTERISTICS

Major (Must Be Present)

Reexperience of the traumatic event, which may be identified in cognitive, affective, and/or sensory-motor activities such as
  Flashbacks, intrusive thoughts
  Repetitive dreams/nightmares
  Excessive verbalization of the traumatic events
  Survival guilt or guilt about behavior required for survival
  Painful emotion, self-blame, shame, or sadness
  Vulnerability or helplessness, anxiety, or panic
  Fear of
      Repetition
      Death
      Loss of bodily control
  Anger outburst/rage, startle reaction
  Hyperalertness or hypervigilance

Minor (May Be Present)

Psychic/emotional numbness
  Impaired interpretation of reality, impaired memory
  Confusion, dissociation, or amnesia
  Vagueness about traumatic event
  Narrowed attention, or inattention/daze
  Feeling of numbness, constricted affect
  Feeling detached/alienated
  Reduced interest in significant activities
  Rigid role-adherence or stereotyped behavior

Altered life-style
    Submissiveness, passiveness, or dependency
    Self-destructiveness (alcohol/drug abuse, suicide
        attempts, reckless driving, illegal activities, etc.)
    Difficulty with interpersonal relationships
    Development of phobia regarding trauma
    Avoidance of situations or activities that arouse
        recollection of the trauma
    Social isolation/withdrawal, negative self-concept
    Sleep disturbances, emotional disturbances
    Irritability, poor impulse control, or explosiveness
    Loss of faith in people or the world/feeling of
        meaninglessness in life
Chronic anxiety or/and chronic depression
Somatic preoccupation/multiple physiological symptoms

RELATED FACTORS

Situational (Personal, Environmental)

Traumatic events of natural origin, including
    Floods
    Earthquakes
    Volcanic eruptions
    Storms
    Avalanches
    Epidemics (may be of human origin)
    Other natural disasters, which are overwhelming to
        most people
Traumatic events of human origin, such as
    Wars
    Airplane crashes
    Serious car accidents
    Large fires
    Bombing
    Concentration camp confinement
    Torture
    Assault
    Rape
    Industrial disasters (nuclear, chemical, or other life-
        threatening accidents)
    Other traumatic events of human origin that involve
        death and destruction or the threat of them

OUTCOME CRITERIA

Short-term goals
The person will

1. Report a lessening of reexperiencing of numbing symptoms
2. Acknowledge the traumatic event and begin to work with the trauma by talking over the experience and expressing feelings such as fear, anger, and guilt
3. Identify and make connection with support persons/resources

Long-term goals
The person will

1. Assimilate the experience into a meaningful whole and go on to pursue his or her life as evidenced by goal setting

INTERVENTIONS

1. Determine if the person has experienced (a) traumatic event(s).
2. Evaluate the severity of the responses and the effects on current functioning level.
3. Assist the person to decrease extremes of reexperiencing or numbing symptoms.
   a. Provide a safe, therapeutic environment where the person can regain control.
   b. Stay with the person and offer support during an episode of high anxiety.
   c. Assist the person to control impulsive acting-out behavior by setting limits, promoting ventilation, and redirecting excess energy into physical exercise activity (gym, walking, jogging, etc.).
4. Reassure the person that these feelings/symptoms are often experienced by the individuals who underwent such traumatic events.
5. Assist person to acknowledge the traumatic event and begin to work through the trauma by talking over the experience and expressing feelings such as fear, anger, and guilt.
6. Assist individual to make connections with support and resources according to his or her needs.

7. Encourage to resume old activities and begin some new ones.
8. Assist child to describe the experience and to express feelings (fear, guilt, rage, etc.) in safe, supportive places, such as play therapy sessions.
9. Assist family/significant others to understand what is happening to the victim.
   a. Encourage ventilation of their feelings.
   b. Provide counseling sessions and/or link them with appropriate community resources as necessary.
10. Provide or arrange follow-up treatment where person/family can continue to work through the trauma and to integrate the experience into new ego synthesis.

Rape Trauma Syndrome

DEFINITION

Rape Trauma Syndrome: The state in which an individual experiences a forced, violent sexual assault (vaginal or anal penetration) against his or her will and without his or her consent. The trauma syndrome that develops from this attack or attempted attack includes an acute phase of disorganization of the victim and family's life-style and a long-term process of reorganization of life-style.*

DEFINING CHARACTERISTICS

Major (Must Be Present)

Reports or evidence of sexual assault

Minor (May Be Present)

If the victim is a child, parent(s) may experience similar responses.

Acute phase
Somatic responses

---

* Holmstrom L, Burgess AW: Development of diagnostic categories: Sexual traumas. Am J Nurs 75:1288–1291, 1975

Gastrointestinal irritability (nausea, vomiting, anorexia)
Genitourinary discomfort (pain, pruritus)
Skeletal muscle tension (spasms, pain)
Psychological responses
    Denial
    Emotional shock
    Anger
    Fear—of being alone or that the rapist will return (a
        child victim will fear punishment, repercussions,
        abandonment, rejection)
    Guilt
    Panic on seeing assailant or scene of attack
Sexual responses
    Mistrust of men (if victim is a woman)
    Change in sexual behavior
Long-term phase

Any response of the acute phase may continue if resolution
does not occur.

Psychological responses
    Phobias
    Nightmares or sleep disturbances
    Anxiety
    Depression

OUTCOME CRITERIA

Short-term goals
The person will

1. Share feelings
2. Describe rationale and treatment procedures
3. Identify members of support system and use them appropriately

Long-term goals
The person will

1. Return to precrisis level of functioning

The child will:

1. Discuss the assault
2. Express feelings concerning the assault and the treatment

The parent(s), spouse, or significant other will

1. Discuss their response to the assault
2. Return to precrisis level of functioning

INTERVENTIONS

1. Promote trusting relationship and stay with person during acute stage or arrange for other support.
2. Explain the care and examination she or he will experience.
   a. Conduct the exams in an unhurried manner.
   b. Explain every detail prior to action.
   c. If this is the person's first pelvic exam, explain the position and the instruments.
   d. Discuss the possibility of pregnancy and a sexually transmitted disease and treatments available.
3. Explain the legal issues and police investigation (Heinrich).*
   a. Explain the need to collect specimens for future possible court use.
   b. Explain that the choice to report the rape is the victim's.
   c. If the police interview is permitted:
      • Negotiate with victim and police for an advantageous time.
      • Explain to victim what kind of questions will be asked.
      • Remain with the victim during the interview; do not ask questions or offer answers.
4. Whenever possible, provide crisis counseling within 1 hour of rape trauma event.
5. Before person leaves hospital, provide card with information about follow-up appointments and names and telephone numbers of local crisis and counseling centers.
6. Encourage person to recognize positive responses or support from sexual partner or members of opposite sex.
7. Record presence and location of bruises, lacerations, edema, or abrasion.

* Heinrich L: Care of the female rape victim. Nurse Pract 12(11):9, 1987

Powerlessness

DEFINITION

Powerlessness: The state in which an individual or group perceives a lack of personal control over certain events or situations.

> **Author's Note:**
> Most individuals are subject to feelings of powerlessness in varying degrees in various situations. This diagnostic category can be used to describe individuals who respond to loss of control with apathy, anger, or depression. Prolonged states of powerlessness may lead to hopelessness.

DEFINING CHARACTERISTICS

Major (Must Be Present)

Overt or covert expressions of dissatisfaction over inability to control situation (*e.g.,* illness, prognosis, care, recovery rate)

Minor (May Be Present)

Refuses or is reluctant to participate in decision-making

Apathy	Uneasiness
Aggressive behavior	Resignation
Violent behavior	Acting-out behavior
Anxiety	Depression

RELATED FACTORS
Pathophysiological

Any disease process—acute or chronic—can contribute to powerlessness. Some common sources are the following:

Inability to communicate (cerebrovascular accident [CVA], Guillain-Barré syndrome, intubation)

Inability to perform activities of daily living (CVA, cervical trauma, myocardial infarction, pain)

Inability to perform role responsibilities (surgery, trauma, arthritis)

Progressive debilitating disease (multiple sclerosis, terminal cancer)

Mental illness

Substance abuse

Obesity

Disfigurement

Situational (Personal, Environmental)

Lack of knowledge

Personal characteristics that highly value control (*e.g.,* internal locus of control)

Hospital or institutional limitations

Some control relinquished to others

No privacy

Altered personal territory

Social isolation

Lack of explanations from caregivers

Lack of consultation regarding decisions

Social displacement

Relocation

Insufficient finances

Sexual harassment

Maturational

Adolescent
  Dependence on peer group
  Independence from family
Young adult
  Marriage
  Pregnancy
  Parenthood
Adult
  Adolescent children
  Physical signs of aging
  Career pressures
  Divorce
Elderly
  Sensory deficits
  Motor deficits
  Losses (money, significant others)

OUTCOME CRITERIA

The person will

1. Identify factors that can be controlled by self
2. Make decisions regarding own care, treatment, and future when possible

INTERVENTIONS

1. Explain all procedures, rules, and options to person.
2. Allow time to answer questions; ask person to write questions down so as not to forget them.
3. Keep person informed about condition, treatments, and results.
4. Anticipate questions/interest and offer information.
5. While being realistic, point out positive changes in person's condition.
6. Provide opportunities for individual to control decisions.
7. Allow person to manipulate surroundings, such as deciding what is to be kept where (shoes under bed, picture on window).
8. Record person's specific choices on care plan to ensure that others on staff acknowledge preferences ("Dislikes orange juice," "Takes showers," "Plan dressing change at 7:30 prior to shower.").
9. Provide daily recognition of progress.

Protection, Altered

DEFINITION

Altered Protection: The state in which an individual experiences a decrease in the ability to guard the self from internal or external threats such as illness or injury.

Author's Note:
Altered Protection represents a broad diagnostic category under which several specific nursing diagnoses are clustered: Impaired Tissue Integrity, Altered Oral Mucous Membrane, and Impaired Skin Integrity. As a diagnostic category, Altered Protection serves to classify the above nursing diagnoses, which are more clinically useful because of their specificity.

The nurse should be cautioned regarding the substitution of Altered Protection as a new name for compromised immune system, AIDS, disseminated intravascular coagulation, diabetes mellitus, etc. The nurse should focus on the functional abilities of the individual that are or may be compromised because of altered protection such as Fatigue, High Risk for Infection, Potential Social Isolation. The nurse should also focus on the physiological complications of altered protection that require nursing and medical interventions for management, *i.e.*, collaborative problems such as Potential Complication: Thrombocytopenia or Potential Complication: Septicemia.

DEFINING CHARACTERISTICS

Major

Deficient immunity
Impaired healing
Altered clotting
Maladaptive stress response
Neurosensory alterations

Minor

Chilling
Perspiring
Dyspnea
Cough
Itching
Restlessness
Insomnia
Fatigue
Anorexia
Weakness
Immobility
Disorientation
Pressure sores

194

Tissue Integrity, Impaired

Skin Integrity, Impaired

Oral Mucous Membrane, Altered

DEFINITION

Impaired Tissue Integrity: The state in which an individual experiences or is at risk for damage to the integumentary, corneal, or mucous membranous tissues.

Author's Note:

Impaired Tissue Integrity is the broad category under which the more specific nursing diagnoses of Impaired Skin Integrity and Altered Oral Mucous Membranes fall. Since tissue is composed of epithelium and connective muscle, and nervous tissue, Impaired Tissue Integrity correctly describes some pressure ulcers that are deeper than dermal. Impaired Skin Integrity should be used to describe potential or actual disruptions of epidermal and dermal tissue only. When a pressure ulcer is stage IV, necrotic or infected, it may be more appropriate to label the diagnosis a collaborative problem as Potential Complication: Stage IV pressure ulcer. This would represent a situation a nurse manages with physician- and nurse-prescribed interventions. When a stage II or III pressure ulcer needs a dressing that requires a physician's order in an acute care setting, the nurse should continue to label the situation a nursing diagnosis because other than hospital regulation it would be appropriate and legal for a nurse to treat the ulcer independently, e.g., in the community. If an individual is at risk for damage to corneal tissue, the nurse can use the diagnosis High Risk for Impaired Corneal Tissue Integrity related to; for example: to corneal drying and reduced lacrimal production secondary to unconscious state. If an individual is immobile and multiple systems—respiratory, circulatory, musculoskeletal, and integumentary—are threatened, the nurse can use High Risk for Disuse Syndrome to describe the entire situation.

DEFINING CHARACTERISTICS

Major (Must Be Present)

Disruptions of corneal, integumentary, or mucous membranous tissue or invasion of body structure (incision, dermal ulcer, corneal ulcer, oral lesion)

Minor (May Be Present)

Lesions (primary, secondary)
Edema
Erythema
Dry mucous membrane
Leukoplakia
Coated tongue

RELATED FACTORS

Pathophysiological

Autoimmune alterations
  Lupus erythematosus   Scleroderma
Metabolic and endocrine alterations
  Diabetes mellitus   Jaundice
  Hepatitis   Cancer
  Cirrhosis   Thyroid dysfunction
  Renal failure
Nutritional alterations
  Obesity   Emaciation
  Dehydration   Malnutrition
  Edema
Impaired oxygen transport
  Peripheral vascular   Anemia
    alterations   Cardiopulmonary
  Venous stasis   disorders
  Arteriosclerosis
Medications (corticosteroid therapy)
Psoriasis
Eczema
Infections
  Bacterial (impetigo, folliculitis, cellulitis)
  Viral (herpes zoster [shingles], herpes simplex, gingivitis, acquired immunodeficiency syndrome [AIDS])

Fungal (ringworm [dermatophytosis], athlete's foot, vaginitis)
Dental caries/periodontal disease

Treatment-related

NPO status
Therapeutic extremes in body temperature
Therapeutic irradiation
Surgery
Drug therapy (local and systemic)
    Corticosteroids
Imposed immobility related to sedation
Mechanical trauma
    Therapeutic fixation devices
        Wired jaw
        Traction
        Casts
        Orthopedic devices/braces
    Inflatable or foam "donuts"
    Tourniquets
    Footboards
    Restraints
    Dressings, tape, solutions
    External urinary catheters
    Nasogastric tubes
    Endotracheal tubes
    Oral prostheses/braces
    Contact lenses

Situational (Personal, Environmental)

Chemical trauma
    Excretions   Noxious agents/
    Secretions   substances
Environmental
    Radiation—sunburn   Bites (insect, animal)
    Temperature   Inhalants
    Humidity   Poison plants
    Parasites
Immobility
    Related to pain; fatigue; motivation; cognitive, sensory, or motor deficits
Personal
    Allergies

Inadequate personal habits (hygiene/dental/dietary/
sleep)
Body build/weight distribution/bony prominences/
muscle mass/range of motion/joint mobility
Stress
Occupation
Pregnancy

Maturational

Infants/children
  Diaper rash
  Childhood diseases (chickenpox)
Elderly
  Dry skin
  Thin skin
  Loss of skin elasticity
  Loss of subcutaneous tissue

OUTCOME CRITERIA

The person will

1. Identify cause of mechanical tissue destruction
2. Participate in plan to promote wound healing
3. Demonstrate progressive healing of tissue

INTERVENTIONS

1. Encourage highest degree of mobility to avoid prolonged periods of pressure.
2. For neuromuscular impairment:
   a. Teach patient/significant other appropriate mea-
      sures to prevent pressure, shear, friction, mac-
      eration.
   b. Teach to recognize early signs of tissue damage.
   c. Change position at least every 2 hours around
      the clock.
   d. Frequently supplement full body turns with mi-
      nor shifts in body weight.
3. Keep patient clean and dry.
4. Avoid stripping of epidermis when removing adhesives.
5. Use pressure-dispersing devices as appropriate.
6. Limit Fowler's position in high-risk patients. Avoid
   use of knee gatch on bed.

7. Devise method to contain bowel or bladder incontinence. See *Altered Patterns of Urinary Elimination* and *Altered Bowel Elimination* for specific interventions.
8. Teach correct application of stoma pouch.
9. Use stoma pouching techniques to contain drainage from fistulas/ulcers.
10. Recommend mild soaps that do not alter skin pH.
11. Teach use of protective gloves/clothing when using chemical products in occupational setting.

Skin Integrity, Impaired

DEFINITION

Impaired Skin Integrity: The state in which an individual experiences or is at risk for damage to the epidermal and dermal tissue.

DEFINING CHARACTERISTICS

Major (Must Be Present)

Disruptions of epidermal and dermal tissue

Minor (May Be Present)

Denuded skin
Erythema
Lesions (primary, secondary)
Pruritus

RELATED FACTORS

See *Impaired Tissue Integrity*

OUTCOME CRITERIA (For *Impaired Skin Integrity*)

The person will

1. Identify causative factors for pressure ulcers
2. Identify rationale for prevention and treatment
3. Participate in the prescribed treatment plan to promote wound healing
4. Demonstrate progressive healing of dermal ulcer

199

INTERVENTIONS (For *Impaired Skin Integrity*)

1. Identify the stage of pressure ulcer development.
   a. Stage I: Nonblanchable erythema or ulceration limited to epidermis
   b. Stage II: Ulceration of dermis not involving underlying subcutaneous fat
   c. Stage III: Ulceration involving subcutaneous fat
   d. Stage IV: Extensive ulceration penetrating muscle and bone
2. Wash reddened area gently with a mild soap, rinse area thoroughly to remove soap, and pat dry.
3. Gently massage healthy skin around the affected area to stimulate circulation; do not massage reddened area.
4. Protect the healthy skin surface with one or a combination of the following:
   a. Apply a thin coat of liquid copolymer skin sealant.
   b. Cover area with moisture-permeable film dressing.
   c. Cover area with a hydroactive wafer barrier and secure with strips of 1-inch microscope tape; leave in place for 4–5 days.
5. Increase protein and carbohydrate intake to maintain a positive nitrogen balance: weigh the person daily and determine serum albumin level weekly to monitor status.
6. Devise plan for pressure ulcer management using principles of moist wound healing.
   a. Assess status of pressure ulcer (color, odor, amount of drainage from wound and surrounding skin).
   b. Debride necrotic tissue (collaborate with physician).
   c. Flush ulcer base with sterile saline solution.
   d. Protect granulating wound bed.
   e. Cover pressure ulcer with a sterile dressing that maintains a moist environment over the ulcer base (*e.g.,* film dressing, hydroactive wafer dressing, moist gauze dressing).
   f. Avoid the use of drying agents (heat lamps, Maalox, Milk of Magnesia).
   g. Monitor for clinical signs of wound infection.
7. Consult with nurse specialist or physician for treatment of stage IV pressure ulcers.
8. Refer to community nursing agency if additional assistance at home is needed.

OUTCOME CRITERIA (For *High Risk for Impaired Skin Integrity*)

The person will

1. Express willingness to participate in prevention of pressure ulcers
2. Describe etiology and prevention measures
3. Demonstrate skin integrity free of pressure ulcers

INTERVENTIONS (For *High Risk for Impaired Skin Integrity*)

1. Maintain sufficient fluid intake for adequate hydration (approximately 2500 ml daily, unless contraindicated); check mucous membranes in mouth for moisture and check urine specific gravity.
2. Establish a schedule for emptying bladder (begin with q2 hour).
   If person is confused, determine what incontinence pattern is and intervene before incontinence occurs.
   Explain problem to individual and secure cooperation for plan.
3. When incontinent, wash perineum with a liquid soap that will not alter skin *p*H and apply a protective barrier to the perineal region (incontinence film barrier spray or wipes).
4. Encourage range of motion exercise and weight-bearing mobility, when possible.
5. Turn or instruct person to turn or shift weight every 30 minutes to 2 hours, depending on other causative factors present and the ability of the skin to recover from pressure.
6. Frequency of turning schedule should be increased if any reddened areas that appear do not disappear within 1 hour after turning.
7. Keep bed as flat as possible to reduce shearing forces; limit Fowler's position to only 30 minutes at a time.
8. Use enough personnel to lift person up in bed or chair rather than pull or slide skin surfaces.
9. Instruct person to lift self using chair arms every 10 minutes if possible or assist person in rising up off the chair every 10 to 20 minutes, depending on risk factors present.

10. Observe for erythema and blanching and palpate for warmth and tissue sponginess with each position change.
11. Use gentle massage over vulnerable areas with each position change. To avoid damaging the capillaries avoid deep massage.
12. Increase protein and carbohydrate intake to maintain a positive nitrogen balance; weigh the person daily and determine serum albumin level weekly to monitor status.
13. Instruct person and family in specific techniques to use at home to prevent pressure ulcers.

Oral Mucous Membrane, Altered

DEFINITION

Altered Oral Mucous Membrane: The state in which an individual experiences or is at risk of experiencing disruptions in the oral cavity.

DEFINING CHARACTERISTICS

Major (Must Be Present)

Disrupted oral mucous membranes

Minor (May Be Present)

Coated tongue
Xerostomia (dry mouth)
Stomatitis
Oral tumors
Oral lesions

Leukoplakia
Edema
Hemorrhagic gingivitis
Purulent drainage

RELATED FACTORS

Pathophysiological

Diabetes mellitus
Oral cancer
Periodontal disease

Infection
  Herpes simplex   Gingivitis

Treatment-related

NPO 24 hours
Radiation to head or neck
Prolonged use of corticosteroids or other
  immunosuppressives
Use of antineoplastic drugs
Endotrachial intubation
Nasogastric intubation

Situational (Personal, Environmental)

Chemical trauma
  Acidic foods   Alcohol
  Drugs   Tobacco
  Noxious agents
Mechanical trauma
  Broken or jagged teeth   Braces
  Ill-fitting dentures
Malnutrition
Dehydration
Mouth breathing
Inadequate oral hygiene
Lack of knowledge
Fractured mandible

OUTCOME CRITERIA

The person will

1. Demonstrate integrity of the oral cavity
2. Be free of harmful plaque to prevent secondary infection
3. Be free of oral discomfort during food and fluid intake
4. Demonstrate knowledge of optional oral hygiene

INTERVENTIONS

1. Discuss the importance of daily oral hygiene and periodic dental examinations.
2. Evaluate the person's ability to perform oral hygiene.
3. Teach correct oral care.
    a. Remove and clean dentures and bridges daily.
    b. Floss teeth (q24 hours).

    c. Brush teeth (after meals and before sleep).

    d. Inspect mouth for lesions, sores, or excessive bleeding.

4. Perform oral hygiene on person who is unconscious or at risk for aspiration as often as needed.

5. Teach preventive oral hygiene to individuals at risk to develop stomatitis.

    a. Perform the regimen after meals and before sleep (if there is excessive exudate, also perform regimen before breakfast).

    b. Floss teeth only once in 24 hours.

    c. Omit flossing if excessive bleeding occurs and use extreme caution with persons with platelet counts of less than 50,000.

    d. Avoid mouthwashes with high alcohol content, lemon/glycerine swabs, or prolonged use of hydrogen peroxide.

    e. Use an oxidizing agent to loosen thick, tenacious mucous (gargle and expectorate); for example, hydrogen peroxide and water quarter strength (avoid prolonged use) or sodium bicarbonate 1 teaspoon in 8 oz warm water (can flavor these with mouthwash or one drop of oil of wintergreen).

    f. Rinse mouth with saline solution after gargling.

    g. Apply lubricant to lips q2 hours and PRN (*e.g.,* lanolin, A&D ointment, petroleum jelly).

    h. Inspect mouth daily for lesions and inflammation and report alterations.

6. For person who is unable to tolerate brushing or swabbing, teach to irrigate mouth (q2 hours and PRN).

    a. With baking soda solution (4 teaspoons in 1 liter warm water) using an enema bag (labeled for oral use only) with a soft irrigation catheter tip.

    b. By placing catheter tip in mouth and slowly increasing flow while standing over a basin or having a basin held under chin.

    c. Remove dentures prior to irrigation and do not replace in person with severe stomatitis.

7. Inspect oral cavity three times daily with tongue blade and light; if stomatitis is severe, inspect mouth q4 hours.

8. Ensure that oral hygiene regimen is done q2 hours while awake and q6 hours (q4 if severe) during the night.

9. Instruct individual to
   a. Avoid commercial mouthwashes, citrus fruit juices, spicy foods, extremes in food temperature (hot, cold), crusty or rough foods, alcohol, mouthwashes with alcohol.
   b. Eat bland, cool foods (sherbets).
   c. Drink cool liquids q2 hours and PRN.
10. Consult with physician for an oral pain relief solution.
    a. Xylocaine Viscous 2% oral swish and expectorant q2 hours and before meals (if throat is sore, the solution can be swallowed; if swallowed, Xylocaine produces local anesthesia and may affect the gag reflex).
    b. Mix equal parts of Xylocaine Viscous, 0.5 aqueous Benadryl solution, and Maalox, swish and swallow 1 oz of mixture q2–4 hours PRN.
    c. Mix equal parts of 0.5 aqueous Benadryl solution and Kaopectate; swish and swallow q2–4 hours PRN.
11. Teach person and family the factors that contribute to the development of stomatitis and its progression.
12. Have individual describe or demonstrate home care regimen.

Respiratory Function, High Risk for Altered*

Ineffective Airway Clearance

Ineffective Breathing Patterns

Impaired Gas Exchange

* This diagnostic category is not currently on the NANDA list but has been included for clarity or usefulness.

DEFINITION

High Risk for Altered Respiratory Function (ARF): The state in which an individual is at risk of experiencing a threat to the passage of air through the respiratory tract and to the exchange of gases (O_2–CO_2) between the lungs and the vascular system.

Author's Note:

This diagnostic category has been added by the author to describe a state in which the entire respiratory system may be affected, not just isolated areas such as airway clearance or gas exchange. Smoking, allergy, and immobility are examples of factors that affect the entire system and thus make it incorrect to use Impaired Gas Exchange related to immobility, since immobility also affects airway clearance and breathing patterns. It is advised that High Risk for Altered Respiratory Function not be used to describe an actual problem, which is a collaborative problem—not a nursing diagnosis. The diagnoses Ineffective Airway Clearance and Ineffective Breathing Patterns can be used when the nurse can definitively alter the contributing factors that are influencing respiratory function; for example, ineffective cough, immobility, or stress. The nurse is cautioned not to use this diagnostic category to describe acute respiratory disorders, which are the primary responsibility of physicians and nurses together (*i.e.,* a collaborative problem). This can be labeled Potential Complication: Hypoxemia or Potential Complication: Pulmonary edema. When an individual's immobility threatens multiple systems—integumentary, musculoskeletal, vascular, and respiratory—the nurse should use High Risk for Disuse Syndrome to describe the entire situation.

RISK FACTORS

Presence of risk factors that can change respiratory function (see Related Factors)

RELATED FACTORS

The codes IAC (Ineffective Airway Clearance), and IBP (Ineffective Breathing Patterns) are used to indicate factors specific to that diagnosis. Factors without a code relate to all diagnostic categories.

Pathophysiological

Excessive or thick secretions (IAC)
    Infection (IAC)
Neuromuscular impairment (ineffective cough)
    Diseases of the nervous system (*e.g.,* Guillain-Barré syndrome, multiple sclerosis, myasthenia gravis)
    Central nervous system depression
    Cerebrovascular accident (stroke)
Allergic response
Hypertrophy or edema of the upper airway structures—tonsils, adenoids, sinuses (IAC)

Treatment-related

Medications (narcotics, sedatives, analgesics)
Anesthesia, general or spinal (IAC, IBP)
Suppressed cough reflex (IAC)
Decreased oxygen in the inspired air
Bed rest or immobility

Situational (Personal, Environmental)

Surgery or trauma
Pain, fear, anxiety
Fatigue
Mechanical obstruction (IAC)
Improper positioning (IAC)
Altered anatomic structure (IAC)
    Tracheostomy
Aspiration
Extreme high or low humidity (IAC)
Smoking
Mouth breathing (IAC, IBP)
Perception/cognitive impairment (IAC)
Severe nonrelieved cough (IAC, IBP)
Exercise intolerance

Maturational

Neonate
    Complicated delivery
    Prematurity
    Cesarean birth
    Low birthweight

Infant/child
  Asthma or allergies
  Increased emesis (potential for aspiration)
  Croup
  Cystic fibrosis
  Small airway
Elderly
  Decreased surfactant in the lungs
  Decreased elasticity of the lungs
  Immobility
  Slowing of reflexes

OUTCOME CRITERIA

The person will

1. Perform hourly deep breathing exercises (sigh) and cough sessions as needed
2. Achieve maximum pulmonary function
3. Relate importance of daily pulmonary exercises

INTERVENTIONS

1. Assess for optimal pain relief with minimal period of fatigue or respiratory depression.
2. Encourage ambulation as soon as consistent with medical plan of care.
3. If unable to walk, establish a regimen for being out of bed in a chair several times a day (*i.e.,* 1 hour after meals and 1 hour before bedtime).
4. Increase activity gradually, explaining that respiratory function will improve and dyspnea will decrease with practice.
5. Assist to reposition, turning frequently from side to side (hourly if possible).
6. Encourage deep breathing and controlled coughing exercises five times every hour.
7. Teach individual to use blow bottle or incentive spirometer every hour while awake (with severe neuromuscular impairment, the person may have to be awakened during the night as well).
8. Auscultate lung field every 8 hours; increase frequency if altered breath sounds are present.

Ineffective Airway Clearance

DEFINITION

Ineffective Airway Clearance: The state in which an individual experiences a real or potential threat to respiratory status related to inability to cough effectively.

DEFINING CHARACTERISTICS

Major (Must Be Present)

Ineffective cough
or
Inability to remove airway secretions

Minor (May Be Present)

Abnormal breath sounds
Abnormal respiratory rate, rhythm, depth

RELATED FACTORS

See *High Risk for Altered Respiratory Function.*

OUTCOME CRITERIA

The person will

1. Not experience aspiration
2. Demonstrate effective coughing and increased air exchange in the lungs

INTERVENTIONS

1. Instruct person on the proper method of controlled coughing.
   a. Breathe deeply and slowly while sitting up as high as possible.
   b. Use diaphragmatic breathing.
   c. Hold the breath for 3–5 seconds and then slowly exhale as much of this breath as possible through the mouth (lower rib cage and abdomen should sink down).

     d. Take a second breath, hold, and cough forcefully from the chest (not from the back of the mouth or throat), using two short forceful coughs.

2. Assess present analgesic regime.
   a. Assess its effectiveness: Is the individual too lethargic? Is the individual still in pain?

3. Initiate coughing when person appears to have best pain relief with optimal level of alertness and physical performance.

4. Splint abdominal or chest incisions with hand, pillow, or both.

5. Maintain adequate hydration (increase fluid intake to 2–3 quarts a day if not contraindicated by decreased cardiac output or renal disease).

6. Maintain adequate humidity of inspired air.

7. Plan and bargain for rest periods (after coughing, before meals).

8. Vigorously coach and encourage coughing, using positive reinforcement.

9. Proceed with health teaching with constant reinforcement in principles of care. Acknowledge and encourage good individual effort and progress.

Ineffective Breathing Patterns

DEFINITION

Ineffective Breathing Patterns: The state in which an individual experiences an actual or potential loss of adequate ventilation related to an altered breathing pattern.

Author's Note:

This diagnostic category has little clinical utility except to describe situations that nurses definitively treat, such as hyperventilation. Individuals with periodic apnea and hypoventilation have a collaborative problem that can be labeled Potential

(Continued)

DEFINING CHARACTERISTICS

See also *High Risk for Altered Respiratory Function.*

Major (Must Be Present)

Changes in respiratory rate or pattern (from baseline)
Changes in pulse (rate, rhythm, quality)

Minor (May Be Present)

Orthopnea
Tachypnea, hyperpnea, hyperventilation
Dysrhythmic respirations
Splinted/guarded respirations

RELATED FACTORS

See *High Risk for Altered Respiratory Function.*

OUTCOME CRITERIA

The person will

1. Demonstrate an effective respiratory rate and experience
   improved gas exchange in the lungs
2. Relate the causative factors, if known, and relate adaptive ways of coping with them

INTERVENTIONS

1. Reassure person that measures are being taken to ensure
   safety.

2. Distract person from thinking about anxious state by having person maintain eye contact with you. Say, "Now look at me and breathe slowly with me like this."
3. Consider use of paper bag as means of rebreathing expired air.
4. Stay with person and coach in taking slower, more effective breaths.
5. Explain that one can learn to overcome hyperventilation through conscious control of breathing even when the cause is unknown.
6. Discuss possible causes, physical and emotional, and methods of coping effectively (see *Anxiety*).

Impaired Gas Exchange

DEFINITION

Impaired Gas Exchange: The state in which an individual experiences an actual (or may experience a potential) decreased passage of gases (oxygen and carbon dioxide) between the alveoli of the lungs and the vascular system.

Author's Note:

This diagnostic category does not represent a situation for which nurses prescribe definitive treatment. Nurses do not treat impaired gas exchange, but nurses can treat the functional health patterns that decreased oxygenation can affect, such as activity, sleep, nutrition, and sexual function. Thus, Activity Intolerance related to insufficient oxygenation for activities of daily living better describes the nursing focus. If an individual is at risk or has experienced respiratory dysfunction, the nurse can describe the situation as Potential Complication: Respiratory, or be even more specific with Potential Complication: Emboli.

DEFINING CHARACTERISTICS

See also *High Risk for Altered Respiratory Function.*

Major (Must Be Present)

Dyspnea on exertion

Minor (May Be Present)

Tendency to assume a three-point position (sitting, one
hand on each knee, bending forward)
Pursed-lip breathing with prolonged expiratory phase
Increased anteroposterior chest diameter, if chronic
Lethargy and fatigue
Increased pulmonary vascular resistance (increased
pulmonary artery/right ventricular pressure)
Decreased gastric motility, prolonged gastric emptying
Decreased oxygen content, decreased oxygen saturation,
increased PCO_2, as measured by blood gas studies
Cyanosis

RELATED FACTORS

See *High Risk for Altered Respiratory Function.*

Role Performance, Altered

DEFINITION

Altered Role Performance: The state in which an individual
experiences or is at risk of experiencing a disruption in the
way he or she perceives his or her role performance.

Author's Note:
This nursing diagnosis had previously been a subcategory under
Self-Concept Disturbance. The use of this category in its present
state may prove problematic. If a woman were unable to continue her household responsibilities because of illness and these
responsibilities were assumed by other family members, the situations that might arise would better be described as High Risk
for Self-Concept Disturbance related to recent loss of role re-
(*Continued*)

Author's Note *(Continued)*
sponsibility secondary to illness and High Risk for Impaired
Home Maintenance Management related to lack of knowledge
of family members. Until clinical research defines this category
more definitively, use Altered Role Performance as a cause of
Self-Concept Disturbance or High Risk for Impaired Home
Maintenance Management. Should the role disturbance relate
to parenting, Parental Role Conflict should be considered.

DEFINING CHARACTERISTICS

Major (Must Be Present)

Conflict related to role perception or performance

Minor (May Be Present)

Change in self-perception of role
Denial of role
Change in others' perception of role
Change in physical capacity to resume role
Lack of knowledge of role
Change in usual patterns of responsibility

Self-Care Deficit Syndrome

DEFINITION

Self-care deficit syndrome: The state in which the individual
experiences an impaired motor function or cognitive function,
causing a decreased ability in performing each of the four self-
care activities.

DEFINING CHARACTERISTICS*

Major (One deficit must be present in each activity)

1. Self-feeding deficits
   a. Unable to cut food or open packages
   b. Unable to bring food to mouth
2. Self-bathing deficits (includes washing entire body, combing hair, brushing teeth, attending to skin and nail care, and applying makeup)
   a. Unable or unwilling to wash body or body parts
   b. Unable to obtain a water source
   c. Unable to regulate temperature or water flow
3. Self-dressing deficits (including donning regular or special clothing, not nightclothes)
   a. Impaired ability to put on or take off clothing
   b. Unable to fasten clothing
   c. Unable to groom self satisfactorily
   d. Unable to obtain or replace articles of clothing
4. Self-toileting deficits
   a. Unable or unwilling to get to toilet or commode
   b. Unable or unwilling to carry out proper hygiene
   c. Unable to transfer to and from toilet or commode
   d. Unable to handle clothing to accommodate toileting
   e. Unable to flush toilet or empty commode

RELATED FACTORS

Pathophysiological

Neuromuscular impairment
   Autoimmune alterations (arthritis, multiple sclerosis)
   Metabolic and endocrine alterations (diabetes mellitus, hypothyroidism)

---

* Evaluate each of the activities of daily living using the following coding scale:
0 = Completely independent
1 = Requires use of assistive device
2 = Needs minimal help
3 = Needs assistance and/or some supervision
4 = Needs total supervision
5 = Needs total assistance or unable to assist

Nervous system disorders (Parkinsonism, myasthenia gravis, muscular dystrophy, Guillain–Barré)
Lack of coordination
Spasticity or flaccidity
Muscular weakness
Partial or total paralysis (spinal cord injury, stroke)
Central nervous system (CNS) tumors
Increased intracranial pressure
Musculoskeletal disorders
Atrophy
Muscle contractures
Connective tissue diseases (systemic lupus erythematosus)
Edema (increased synovial fluid)
Visual disorders
Glaucoma
Cataracts
Diabetic/hypertensive retinopathy
Ocular histoplasmosis
Cranial nerve neuropathy
Visual field deficits
Depression

Treatment-related

External devices (casts, splints, braces, intravenous equipment)
Surgical procedures
Fractures
Tracheostomy
Gastrostomy
Jejunostomy
Ileostomy
Colostomy

Situational (Personal, Environmental)

Immobility
Trauma
Nonfunctioning or missing limbs
Coma

Maturational

Elderly
> Decreased visual and motor ability, muscle weakness,
> dementia

Author's Note:

Self-care encompasses the activities needed to meet daily needs,
usually called *activities of daily living* (ADL). Activities of daily
living are learned over time and become life-long habits. Enmeshed in the broad category of self-care activities are those
tasks not only that *are* to be done (hygiene, bathing, dressing,
toileting, feeding) but *how* these tasks are done, and *when*, and
where, and *with whom.** Self-Care Deficit Syndrome, not currently on the NANDA list, has been added to describe an individual with compromised ability in all four self-care activities.
The nurse will assess functioning in each of the four areas and
identify the level of participation of which the individual is capable. The goal will be to maintain that functioning or to increase
participation and independence. The syndrome distinction will
serve to cluster all four self-care deficits together to provide
clustering of interventions when indicated, *i.e.*, to assure that
the individual is wearing the corrective lenses required. It will
also permit specialized interventions for one of the four activities,
i.e., to lay out clothes in the order in which they will be put on
by the person.

The danger of Self-Care Deficit diagnoses is that the nurse
could prematurely label an individual as unable to participate
at any level. This would eliminate a rehabilitation focus. It is
important that the nurse classify the functional level of the client
to promote independence.

Self-Care Deficit Syndrome

ASSESSMENT

Subjective/Objective Data

Observed or reported inability or difficulty in performing some
activity in each of the four areas of self-care

---

* Hoskins LM: Self-Care Deficit. In McFarland G, McFarlane E (eds):
Nursing Diagnosis and Interventions. St. Louis, CV Mosby, 1989

OUTCOME CRITERIA

The person will

1. Identify preferences in self-care activities (*e.g.,* time, products, location)
2. Demonstrate optimal hygiene after assistance with care
3. Participate physically and/or verbally in feeding, dressing, toileting, bathing activities

INTERVENTIONS

1. Assess causative or contributing factors:
   a. Visual deficits
   b. Impaired cognition
   c. Decreased motivation
   d. Impaired mobility
   e. Lack of knowledge
   f. Inadequate social support
2. Promote optimal participation.
3. Promote self-esteem and self-determination:
   a. During self-care activities provide choices and request preferences
4. Evaluate ability to participate in each self-care activity.
5. Refer to interventions under each diagnosis, *Feeding, Bathing, Dressing,* and *Toileting Self-Care Deficit* as indicated.

Feeding Self-Care Deficit

DEFINITION

Feeding Self-Care Deficit: A state in which the individual experiences an impaired ability to perform or complete feeding activities for oneself.

DEFINING CHARACTERISTICS

Unable to cut food or open packages
Unable to bring food to mouth

RELATED FACTORS

See *Self-Care Deficit Syndrome.*

OUTCOME CRITERIA

The person will:
1. Demonstrate increased ability to feed self *or*
2. Report that he or she is unable to feed self
3. Demonstrate ability to make use of adaptive devices, if indicated
4. Demonstrate increased interest and desire to eat
5. Describe rationale and procedure for treatment
6. Describe causative factors for feeding deficit

INTERVENTIONS

1. Ascertain from person or family members what foods the person likes or dislikes.
2. Have meals taken in the same setting: pleasant surroundings that are not too distracting.
3. Maintain correct food temperatures (hot foods hot, cold foods cold).
4. Provide pain relief, since pain can affect appetite and ability to feed self.
5. Provide good oral hygiene before and after meals.
6. Encourage person to wear dentures and eyeglasses.
7. Place person in the most normal eating position suited to his or her physical disability (best is sitting in a chair at a table).
8. Provide social contact during eating.
9. For perceptual deficits:
   a. Choose different-colored dishes to help distinguish items (*e.g.,* red tray, white plates).
   b. Ascertain person's usual eating patterns and provide food items according to preference (or arrange food items in clocklike pattern); record on care plan the arrangement used (*e.g.,* meat, 6 o'clock; potatoes, 9 o'clock; vegetables, 12 o'clock).
   c. Encourage eating of "finger foods" (*e.g.,* bread, bacon, fruit, hot dogs) to promote independence.
10. To enhance maximum amount of independence, provide necessary adaptive devices
    a. Plate guard to avoid pushing food off plate
    b. Suction device under plate or bowl for stabilization
    c. Padded handles on utensils for a more secure grip

219

     d. Wrist or hand splints with clamp to hold eating utensils
     e. Special drinking cup
     f. Rocker knife for cutting
11. Assist with set-up if needed, opening containers, napkins, condiment packages; cutting meat; buttering bread
12. For people with cognitive deficits:
     a. Provide isolated, quiet atmosphere until person is able to attend to eating and is not easily distracted from the task.
     b. Orient person to location and purpose of feeding equipment.
     c. Place person in the most normal eating position he is physically able to assume.
     d. Encourage person to attend to the task, but be alert for fatigue, frustration, or agitation.
13. Assess to assure that both person and family understand the reason and purpose of all interventions

Bathing/Hygiene Self-Care Deficit

DEFINITION

Bathing/Hygiene Self-Care Deficit: A state in which the individual experiences an impaired ability to perform or complete bathing/hygiene activities for oneself.

DEFINING CHARACTERISTICS

Self-bathing deficits (including washing entire body, combing hair, brushing teeth, attending to skin and nail care and applying makeup)

    Unable or unwilling to wash body or body parts
    Unable to obtain a water source
    Unable to regulate temperature or water flow

RELATED FACTORS

See *Self-Care Deficit Syndrome.*

OUTCOME CRITERIA

The person will:
1. Perform bathing activity at expected optimal level *or*
2. Report satisfaction with accomplishments despite limitations
3. Relate feeling of comfort and satisfaction with body cleanliness
4. Demonstrate ability to use adaptive devices
5. Describe causative factors of bathing deficit
6. Relate rationale and procedures for treatment

INTERVENTIONS

1. Encourage person to wear prescribed corrective lenses or hearing aid.
2. Keep bathroom temperature warm; ascertain individual's preferred water temperature.
3. Provide for privacy during bathing routine.
4. Provide all bathing equipment within easy reach.
5. Provide for safety in the bathroom (nonslip mats, grab bars).
6. When person is physically able, encourage use of either tub or shower stall, depending upon which facility is at home (the person should practice in the hospital in preparation for going home).
7. Provide for adaptive equipment as needed:
   a. Chair or stool in bathtub or shower
   b. Long-handled sponge to reach back or lower extremities
   c. Grab bars on bathroom walls where needed to assist in mobility
   d. Bath board for transferring to tub chair or stool
   e. Safety treads or nonslip mat on floor of bathroom, tub, and shower
   f. Washing mitts with pocket for soap
   g. Adapted toothbrushes
   h. Shaver holders
   i. Hand-held shower spray
8. For persons with visual deficits:
   a. Place bathing equipment in location most suitable to individual.
   b. Keep call bell within reach if person is to bathe alone.

    c. Give the visually impaired individual the same degree of privacy and dignity as any other person.

    d. Verbally announce yourself before entering or leaving the bathing area.

    e. Observe the person's ability to locate all bathing utensils.

    f. Observe the person's ability to perform mouth care, hair combing, and shaving tasks.

    g. Provide place for clean clothing within easy reach.

9. For persons with affected or missing limbs:

    a. Bathe early in morning or before bed at night to avoid unnecessary dressing and undressing.

    b. Encourage person to use a mirror during bathing to inspect the skin of paralyzed areas.

    c. Encourage the person with amputation to inspect remaining foot or stump for good skin integrity.

    d. Provide only the amount of supervision or assistance necessary for relearning the use of extremity or adaptation to the handicap.

10. For persons with cognitive deficits:

    a. Provide a consistent time for the bathing routine as part of a structured program to help decrease confusion.

    b. Keep instructions simple and avoid distractions; orient to purpose of bathing equipment.

    c. If person is unable to bathe the entire body, have the individual bathe one part until it is done correctly; give positive reinforcement for success.

    d. Supervise activity until person can safely perform the task unassisted.

    e. Encourage attention to the task, but be alert for fatigue that may increase confusion.

11. Ascertain bathing facilities at home and assist in determining if there is any need to make adaptations; refer to occupational therapy or social service for help in obtaining needed home equipment.

Dressing/Grooming Self-Care Deficit

DEFINITION

Dressing/Grooming Self-Care Deficit: A state in which the individual experiences an impaired ability to perform complete dressing and grooming activities for oneself.

DEFINING CHARACTERISTICS

Self-dressing deficits (including donning regular or special clothing, not nightclothes)

Impaired ability to put on or take off clothing
Unable to fasten clothing
Unable to groom self satisfactorily
Unable to obtain or replace articles of clothing

RELATED FACTORS

See *Self-Care Deficit Syndrome.*

OUTCOME CRITERIA

The person will:
1. Demonstrate increased ability to dress self *or*
2. Report the need of having someone else assist him or her in performing the task
3. Demonstrate ability to learn how to use adaptive devices to facilitate optimal independence in the task of dressing
4. Demonstrate increased interest in wearing street clothes
5. Describe causative factors for dressing deficit
6. Relate rationale and procedures for treatments

INTERVENTIONS

1. Encourage person to wear prescribed corrective lenses or hearing aid.
2. Promote independence in dressing through continual and unaided practice.
3. Choose clothing that is loose fitting, with wide sleeves and pant legs and front fasteners.
4. Allow sufficient time for dressing and undressing, since the task may be tiring, painful, or difficult.
5. Plan for person to learn and demonstrate one part of an activity before progressing further.
6. Lay clothes out in the order in which they will be needed to dress.
7. Provide dressing aids as necessary (some commonly used aids include dressing stick, Swedish reacher, zipper

pull, buttonhook, long-handled shoehorn, and shoe fasteners adapted with elastic laces, Velcro closures, or flip-back tongues; all garments with fasteners may be adapted with Velcro closures).

8. Encourage person to wear ordinary or special clothing rather than nightclothes.
9. Provide for privacy during dressing routine.
10. For persons with visual deficits:
    a. Allow person to ascertain the most convenient location for clothing, and adapt the environment to best accomplish the task (*e.g.,* remove unnecessary barriers).
    b. Verbally announce yourself before entering or leaving the dressing area.
11. For persons with cognitive deficits:
    a. Establish a consistent dressing routine to provide a structured program to decrease confusion.
    b. Keep instructions simple and repeat them frequently; avoid distractions.
    c. Introduce one article of clothing at a time.
    d. Encourage attention to the task; be alert for fatigue, which may increase confusion.
12. Assess understanding and knowledge of individual and family for above instructions and rationale.

Toileting Self-Care Deficit

DEFINITION

Toileting Self-Care Deficit: A state in which the individual experiences an impaired ability to perform or complete toileting activities for oneself.

DEFINING CHARACTERISTICS

Unable or unwilling to get to toilet or commode
Unable or unwilling to carry out proper hygiene
Unable to transfer to and from toilet or commode
Unable to handle clothing to accommodate toileting
Unable to flush toilet or empty commode

RELATED FACTORS

See *Self-Care Deficit Syndrome.*

OUTCOME CRITERIA

The person will:

1. Demonstrate increased ability to toilet self *or*
2. Report that he is unable to toilet self.
3. Demonstrate ability to make use of adaptive devices to facilitate toileting.
4. Describe causative factors for toileting deficit.
5. Relate rationale and procedures for treatment.

INTERVENTIONS

1. Encourage person to wear prescribed corrective lenses or hearing aid.
2. Obtain bladder and bowel history from individual or significant other (see *Altered Bowel Elimination* or *Altered Patterns of Urinary Elimination*).
3. Ascertain communication system person uses to express the need to toilet.
4. Maintain bladder and bowel record to determine toileting patterns.
5. Avoid development of "bowel fixation" by less frequent discussion and inquiries about bowel movements.
6. Be alert to possibility of falls when toileting person (be prepared to ease him or her to floor without causing injury to either of you).
7. Achieve independence in toileting by continual and unaided practice.
8. Allow sufficient time for the task of toileting to avoid fatigue (lack of sufficient time to toilet may cause incontinence or constipation).
9. Avoid use of indwelling catheters and condom catheters to expedite bladder continence (if possible).
10. For persons with visual deficits:
    a. Keep call bell easily accessible so person can quickly obtain help to toilet; answer call bell promptly to decrease anxiety.
    b. If bedpan or urinal is necessary for toileting, be sure it is within person's reach.
    c. Verbally announce yourself before entering or leaving toileting area.
    d. Observe person's ability to obtain equipment or get to the toilet unassisted.
    e. Provide for a safe and clear pathway to toilet area.

11. For persons with affected or missing limbs:
    a. Provide only the amount of supervision and assistance necessary for relearning or adapting to the prosthesis.
    b. Encourage person to look at affected area or limb and use it during toileting tasks.
    c. Encourage useful transfer techniques taught by Occupational or Physical Therapy (the nurse should familiarize himself or herself with planned mode of transfer).
    d. Provide the necessary adaptive devices to enhance the maximum amount of independence and safety (commode chairs, spill-proof urinals, fracture bedpans, raised toilet seats, support side rails for toilets).
    e. Provide for a safe and clear pathway to toilet area.
12. For persons with cognitive deficits:
    a. Offer toileting reminders every 2 hours, after meals, and before bedtime.
    b. When person is able to indicate the need to toilet, begin toileting at 2 hour intervals, after meals, and before bedtime.
    c. Answer call bell immediately to avoid frustration and failure to be continent.
    d. Encourage wearing ordinary clothes (many confused individuals are continent while wearing regular clothing).
    e. Avoid the use of bedpans and urinals; if physically possible, provide a normal atmosphere of elimination in bathroom (the toilet used should remain constant to promote familiarity).
    f. Give verbal cues as to what is expected of the individual, and give positive reinforcement for success.
    g. See *Altered Patterns of Urinary Elimination* for additional information on incontinence.
13. Ascertain home toileting needs and refer to Occupational Therapy or Social Services for help in obtaining necessary equipment.

Instrumental Self-Care Deficit

DEFINITION

Instrumental Self-Care Deficit: A state in which the individual experiences an impaired ability to perform certain activities or access certain services essential for managing a household.

DEFINING CHARACTERISTICS

Observed or reported difficulty in one or more of the following:

Using a telephone
Accessing transportation
Laundering, ironing
Preparing meals
Shopping (food, clothes)
Managing money
Medication administration

RELATED FACTORS

See *Self-Care Deficit*

> **Author's Note:**
> Instrumental Self-Care Deficit is not currently on the NANDA list but has been added for clarity and usefulness. Instrumental Self-Care Deficit describes problems in performing certain activities or accessing certain services needed to live in the community (*e.g.,* phone use, shopping, money management). This diagnosis is important to consider in discharge planning and during the home visit by the community nurse.

OUTCOME CRITERIA

The person/family will:

1. Demonstrate use of adaptive devices (*e.g.,* phone, cooking aids).
2. Describe a method to ensure adherence to medication schedule.

3. Report ability to call and answer telephone.
4. Report regular laundering by self or others.
5. Report daily intake of two nutritious meals.
6. Identify transportation options to stores, physician, house of worship, social activities.
7. Demonstrate management of simple money transactions.
8. Identify individual(s) who will assist with money matters.

INTERVENTIONS

1. Assess for causative and contributing factors:
   a. Visual, hearing deficits
   b. Impaired cognition
   c. Impaired mobility
   d. Lack of knowledge
   e. Inadequate social support
2. Assist to identify self-help devices.
3. Promote self-care and safety with individuals with cognitive deficits:
   a. Evaluate activities that are achievable.
   b. Evaluate ability to procure, select, and prepare nutritious food daily.
   c. Teach hints for adherence to medicine schedule (*e.g.,* 7-day pill holder, separate pill for each time to be taken).
4. Determine sources of transportation (*e.g.,* church groups, neighbors).
5. Determine sources of social support (transportation, laundry, money matters).
6. Discuss the importance of identifying need for assistance (*e.g.,* Department of Social Services, agency on aging).

Self-Concept Disturbance*

Body Image Disturbance

* This diagnostic category is not currently on the NANDA list but has been included for clarity or usefulness.

Personal Identity Disturbance

Self-Esteem Disturbance

Chronic Low Self-Esteem

Situational Low Self-Esteem

DEFINITION

Self-Concept Disturbance: The state in which an individual experiences or is at risk of experiencing a negative state of change about the way he or she feels, thinks, or views himself or herself. It may include a change in body image, self-esteem, role performance, or personal identity.

Author's Note:

Self-Concept Disturbance represents a broad category under which more specific categories fall. Initially the nurse may not have sufficient clinical data to validate a more specific category as Chronic Low Self-Esteem or Body Image Disturbance; thus, Self-Concept Disturbance can be used until more specific categories can be supported with data.

DEFINING CHARACTERISTICS

Since a self-concept disturbance may include a change in any one or a combination of its four component parts (body image, self-esteem, role performance, personal identity), and since the nature of the change causing the alteration can be so varied, there is no "typical" response. Reactions may include the following:

Refusal to touch or look at a body part
Refusal to look into a mirror
Unwillingness to discuss a limitation, deformity, or disfigurement
Refusal to accept rehabilitation efforts

Inappropriate attempts to direct own treatment
Denial of the existence of a deformity or disfigurement
Increasing dependence on others
Signs of grieving
 Weeping
 Despair
 Anger
Refusal to participate in own care or take responsibility
 for self-care (self-neglect)
Self-destructive behavior (alcohol, drug abuse)
Displaying hostility toward the healthy
Withdrawal from social contacts
Changing usual patterns of responsibility
Showing change in ability to estimate relationship of body
 to environment

RELATED FACTORS

A self-concept disturbance can occur as a response to a variety
of health problems, situations, and conflicts. Some common
sources include the following:

Pathophysiological

Loss of body part(s)
Loss of body function(s)
Severe trauma
Chronic disease

Treatment-related

Hospitalization: chronic or terminal illness
Surgery

Situational (Personal, Environmental)

Divorce, separation from or death of a significant other
Loss of job or ability to work
Pain
Obesity
Pregnancy
Immobility or loss of function
Need for placement in a nursing home

Maturational

Infant and preschool
Deprivation
Young adult
Peer pressure
Puberty
Middle-aged
Signs of aging (graying or loss of hair)
Reduced hormonal levels (menopause)
Elderly
Losses (people, function, financial, retirement)

Other

Women's movement
Sexual revolution

OUTCOME CRITERIA

The person will

1. Describe changes in feelings regarding self
2. Identify resources available for assistance

INTERVENTIONS

1. Encourage person to express feelings, especially about the way person feels, thinks, or views self.
2. Encourage person to ask questions about health problem, treatment, progress, prognosis.
3. Provide reliable information and reinforce information already given.
4. Clarify any misconceptions the person has about self, care, or caregivers.
5. Avoid negative criticism.
6. Provide privacy and a safe environment.
7. If indicated, refer to *Self-Esteem Disturbance* or *Body Image Disturbance* for interventions under the category.
8. Teach person what community resources are available, if needed (*e.g.,* mental health centers, self-help groups such as Reach for Recovery, Make Today Count).

Body Image Disturbance

DEFINITION

Body Image Disturbance: The state in which an individual experiences or is at risk of experiencing a disruption in the way one perceives one's body image.

DEFINING CHARACTERISTICS

Major (Must Be Present)

Verbal or nonverbal negative response to actual or perceived change in structure and/or function

Minor (May Be Present)

Not looking at body part
Not touching body part
Hiding or overexposing body part
Change in social involvement
Negative feelings about body, feelings of helplessness, hopelessness, powerlessness
Preoccupation with change or loss
Refusal to verify actual change
Depersonalization of part or loss

RELATED FACTORS

Pathophysiological

Chronic disease
Loss of body part
Loss of body function
Severe trauma

Treatment-related

Hospitalization
Surgery
Chemotherapy
Radiation

Situational

Pain
Obesity

Pregnancy
Infertility
Immobility
Cultural influences

Maturational

Adolescent
  Puberty
Middle age
  Signs of aging (graying, menopause)
Elderly
  Loss of function

OUTCOME CRITERIA

The person will

1. Share feelings about view of self
2. Achieve or maintain control of body
3. Begin to assume role-related responsibilities
4. Develop confidence in ability to accomplish what is desired

INTERVENTIONS

1. Encourage person to express feelings, especially about the way he or she feels, thinks, or views self.
2. Encourage person to ask questions about health problem, treatment, progress, prognosis.
3. Provide reliable information and reinforce information already given.
4. Clarify any misconceptions the person has about self, care, or caregivers.
5. Support family as they adapt.
6. Encourage visits from peers and significant others.
7. Encourage contact (letters, telephone) with peers and family.
8. Provide opportunity to share with persons going through similar experiences.
9. For loss of body part or function:
   a. Assess the meaning of the loss for the individual and significant others, as related to visibility of loss, function of loss, and emotional investment.
   b. Expect the individual to respond to the loss with denial, shock, anger, and depression.

    c. Be aware of the effect of the responses of others to the loss; encourage sharing of feelings between significant others.

    d. Allow individual to ventilate feelings and to grieve.

    e. Use role-playing to assist with sharing.

    f. Explore realistic alternatives and provide encouragement.

    g. Explore strengths and resources with person.

10. Assist with the resolution of a surgically created alteration of body image.

    a. Replace the lost body part with prosthesis as soon as possible.

    b. Encourage viewing of site.

    c. Encourage touching of site.

11. For changes associated with chemotherapy (Cooley).*

    a. Discuss the possibility of hair loss, absence of menses, temporary or permanent sterility, decreased estrogen levels, vaginal dryness, mucosititis.

    b. Encourage person to share concerns, fears and perception of the impact of these changes on the person's life.

    c. Explain where hair loss may occur (head, eyelashes, eyebrows, auxiliary hair, pubic and leg hair).

    d. Explain that hair will grow back after treatment but may change in color and texture.

    e. Select a wig prior to hair loss, wear it before hair loss. Consult a beautician for tips on how to vary the look (*e.g.,* combs, clips, etc.).

    f. Encourage the wearing of scarves, turbans when wig is not on.

    g. Teach to minimize the amount of hair loss by:
- Avoiding excessive shampooing, using a conditioner twice weekly
- Patting hair dry gently
- Avoiding electric curlers, dryers and curling irons

---

* Cooley ME, Yeomans AC, Cobb SC: Sexual and reproductive issues for women with Hodgkin's disease. II. Application of PLISSIT model. Cancer Nurs 9:248–255, 1986

- Avoiding pulling hair with bands, clips, or bobby pins
- Avoiding hair spray and hair dye
- Using wide-tooth comb, avoiding vigorous brushing

h. Refer to American Cancer Society for information regarding new or used wigs. Inform that the wig is a tax-deductible item.

12. Discuss the difficulty that others (spouse, friends, co-workers) may have with visible changes.
13. Allow significant others opportunities to share feelings and fears.
14. Assist significant others to identify positive aspects of the client and ways this can be shared.
15. Teach person what community resources are available, if needed (*e.g.,* mental health centers, such self-help groups as Reach for Recovery, Make Today Count).

Personal Identity Disturbance

DEFINITION

Personal Identity Disturbance: The state in which an individual experiences or is at risk of experiencing an inability to distinguish between self and nonself.

Author's Note:

This diagnostic category is a subcategory under Self-Concept Disturbance. Until clinical research defines and differentiates this category from others, refer to Self-Concept Disturbance or Altered Growth and Development for assessment criteria and interventions.

DEFINING CHARACTERISTICS

See Defining Characteristics for *Self-Concept Disturbance* or *Altered Growth and Development.*

Self-Esteem Disturbance

DEFINITION

Self-Esteem Disturbance: The state in which an individual experiences or is at risk of experiencing negative self-evaluation about self or capabilities.

Author's Note:

Self-Esteem is one of the four components of Self-Concept. Self-Esteem Disturbance is the general diagnostic category. Chronic Low Self-Esteem and Situational Low Self-Esteem represent specific types of Self-Esteem Disturbances, thus involving more specific interventions. Initially the nurse may not have sufficient clinical data to validate a more specific diagnosis such as Chronic Low Self-Esteem or Situational Low Self-Esteem. Refer to the major defining characteristics under these categories for validation.

DEFINING CHARACTERISTICS*

Overt or covert:
   Self-negating verbalization
   Expressions of shame or guilt
   Evaluates self as unable to deal with events
   Rationalizes away/rejects positive feedback and
      exaggerates negative feedback about self
   Hesitant to try new things/situations
   Denial of problems obvious to others
   Projection of blame/responsibility for problems
   Rationalizes personal failures
   Hypersensitivity to slight criticism
   Grandiosity

* Norris J, Kunes–Connell M: Self-Esteem disturbance: A clinical validation study. In McLane A (ed): Classification of Nursing Diagnoses: Proceedings of the Seventh Conference. St. Louis, CV Mosby, 1987

RELATED FACTORS

Self-Esteem Disturbance can be either an episodic event or a
chronic problem. Failure to resolve a problem or multiple se-
quential stresses can result in chronic low self-esteem. Those
factors that occur over time and are associated with chronic
low self-esteem are indicated by CLSE.

Pathophysiological

Loss of body part(s)
Loss of body function(s)
Disfigurement (trauma, surgery, birth defects)

Situational (Personal, Environmental)

Hospitalization
Loss of job or ability to work
Death of significant other
Separation from significant other
Increase/decrease in weight
Pregnancy
Unemployment
Financial problems
Relationship problems
   Marital discord
   Separation
   Step-parents
   In-laws
Failure in school
History of ineffective relationship with own parents
  (CLSE)
History of abusive relationships (CLSE)
Unrealistic expectations of child by parent (CLSE)
Unrealistic expectations of self (CLSE)
Unrealistic expectations of parent by child (CLSE)
Parental rejection (CLSE)
Overpassivity (CLSE)
Inconsistent punishment (CLSE)
Legal difficulties
Institutionalization
   Mental health facility
   Jail
   Orphanage
   Halfway house

Cultural Influences
 Ethnic group
 Minority
Drug/alcohol abuse by self or family member

Maturational

Infant/toddler/preschool
 Lack of stimulation (CLSE)
 Separation from parents/significant others (CLSE)
 Restriction of activity (CLSE)
 Inadequate parental support (CLSE)
 Inability to trust significant other (CLSE)
School age
 Loss of significant others
 Failure to achieve grade level objectives
 Loss of peer group
Adolescent
 Loss of independence and autonomy
 Disruption of peer relationships
 Disruption in body image
 Interruption of intellectual achievement
 Loss of significant others
 Career choices
Middle age
 Signs of graying
 Menopause
 Career pressures
Elderly
 Losses (people, function, financial, retirement)

OUTCOME CRITERIA

The person will

1. Verbalize feelings and thinking about self
2. Identify two positive attributes about self

INTERVENTIONS

1. Establish a trusting nurse/client relationship.
 a. Encourage person to express feelings, especially about the way he or she thinks, or views self.
 b. Encourage person to ask questions: about health problem, treatment, progress, prognosis.

    c. Provide reliable information and reinforce information already given.

    d. Clarify any misconceptions the person has about self, care, or caregivers.

    e. Avoid negative criticism.

    f. Provide privacy and a safe environment.

2. Promote social interaction.

    a. Assist person to accept help from others.

    b. Avoid overprotection while still limiting the demands made on the individual.

    c. Encourage movement.

    d. Support family as they adapt.

3. Explore strengths and resources with person.

4. Discuss expectations.

    a. Discuss if realistic.

    b. Explore realistic alternatives.

5. Refer to community resources as indicated (*e.g.,* counseling, assertiveness courses).

Chronic Low Self-Esteem

DEFINITION

Chronic Low Self-Esteem: The state in which an individual experiences a long-standing negative self-evaluation about self or capabilities.

DEFINING CHARACTERISTICS*

Major (80%–100%)

    Long-standing or chronic:

        Self-negating verbalization

        Expressions of shame/guilt

        Evaluates self as unable to deal with events

        Rationalizes away/rejects positive feedback and exaggerates negative feedback about self

        Hesitant to try new things/situations

---

* Norris J, Kunes–Connell M: Self-Esteem disturbance: A clinical validation study. In McLane A (ed): Classification of Nursing Diagnoses: Proceedings of the Seventh Conference. St. Louis, CV Mosby, 1987

Minor (50%–79%)

Frequent lack of success in work or other life events
Overly conforming, dependent on opinions of others
Lack of eye contact
Nonassertive/passive
Indecisive
Excessively seeks reassurance

RELATED FACTORS

See *Self-Esteem Disturbance.*

OUTCOME CRITERIA

The individual will

1. Verbalize realistic perceptions of self
2. Identify positive aspects about self
3. Interact appropriately with others
4. Participate in activities

INTERVENTIONS

1. Assist the person to reduce present anxiety level.
2. Enhance the person's sense of self.
    a. Be attentive.
    b. Respect individual's personal space.
    c. Validate your interpretation of what person is saying or experiencing ("Is this what you mean?").
3. Provide encouragement as a task or skill is attempted.
4. Assist person in expressing thoughts and feelings.
5. Encourage visits/contact with peers and significant others (letters, telephone).
6. Be a role model in one-to-one interactions.
7. Involve in activities, especially when strengths can be used.
8. Do not allow person to isolate self (refer to *Social Isolation* for further interventions)
9. Set limits on problematic behavior such as aggression, poor hygiene, ruminations and suicidal preoccupation. Refer to *High Risk for Self Harm* and/or *High Risk for Violence* if these are assessed as problems.
10. Provide for development of social and vocational skills.
11. Refer for vocational counseling, if indicated.

Situational Low Self-Esteem

DEFINITION

Situational Low Self-Esteem: The state in which an individual who previously had positive self-esteem experiences negative feelings about self in response to an event (loss, change).

> **Author's Note:**
> Although situational low self-esteem is an episodic event, repeated occurrences and/or the continuation of these negative self-appraisals over time can lead to chronic low self-esteem (Willard).

DEFINING CHARACTERISTICS*

Major (80%–100%)

Episodic occurrence of negative self-appraisal in response to life events in a person with a previous positive self-evaluation

Verbalization of negative feelings about self (helplessness, uselessness)

Minor (50%–79%)

Self-negating verbalizations

Expressions of shame/guilt

Evaluates self as unable to handle situations/events

Difficulty making decisions

RELATED FACTORS

See *Self-Esteem Disturbance.*

---

* Norris J, Kunes–Connell M: Self-Esteem disturbance: A clinical validation study. In McLane A (ed): Classification of Nursing Diagnoses: Proceedings of the Seventh Conference. St. Louis, CV Mosby, 1987

OUTCOME CRITERIA

The person will

1. Identify positive aspects of self
2. Express a positive outlook for the future
3. Analyze own behavior and its consequences
4. Identify ways of exerting control and influencing outcomes

INTERVENTIONS

1. Assist the individual in identifying and expressing feelings.
2. Assist in identifying positive self-evaluations.
3. Examine and reinforce positive abilities and traits (*e.g.*, hobbies, skills, school, relationships, appearance, loyalty, industriousness, etc.).
4. Help individual accept both positive and negative feelings.
5. Encourage examination of current behavior and its consequences (*e.g.*, dependency, procrastination, isolation).
6. Help to identify negative automatic thoughts and overgeneralizing.
7. Assist in identifying own responsibility and control in a situation (*e.g.*, when continually blaming others for problems).
8. Assess and mobilize current support system.
9. Refer to community resources as indicated (*e.g.*, Reach for Recovery).

Self-Harm, High Risk for*

DEFINITION

High Risk for Self-Harm: The state in which an individual is at risk for inflicting direct harm on himself or herself.

* This diagnostic category is not currently on the NANDA list but has been included for clarity or usefulness.

Author's Note:
High Risk for Self-Harm is not currently on the NANDA list but has been added for clarity. High Risk for Violence to Self is included under High Risk for Violence. The term violence is described as a swift and intense force or a rough or injurious physical force. Suicide can be violent but it can also be non-violent (overdose of barbiturates). Using the term violence can unfortunately cause the risk for suicide to be undetected because of the belief that an individual is not capable of violence.

High Risk for Self-Harm clearly denotes an individual at high risk for suicide and of the need for protection. The treatment of the diagnosis comprises validation, contracting, and protection. The treatment of the underlying depression and hopelessness should be addressed with other nursing diagnoses, e.g., Ineffective Individual Coping, Hopelessness.

RISK FACTORS

Major (Must Be Present)

Suicidal ideation
Previous suicidal attempts

Minor (See also Related Factors)

RELATED FACTORS

High Risk for Self-Harm can occur as a response to a variety of health problems, situations, and conflicts. Some sources are the following:

Pathophysiological

Terminal illness
Chronic illness (*e.g.,* diabetes, hypertension)
Alcoholism
Organic mental disorder
Ingestion of prescribed or nonprescribed drugs

Treatment-related

Dialysis
Insulin injections or any ongoing treatments
Cancer chemotherapy/radiation

Situational (Personal, Environmental)

Parental/marital conflict
Job loss
Divorce/separation
Threatened or actual financial loss
Alcoholism/drug abuse in family
Wish to reunite with loved one who has died
Depression
Death of significant other
Loss of status, prestige
Inadequate coping skills
Someone leaving home
Child abuse
Threat of abandonment by significant other

Maturational

Adolescent
  Separation from family
  Peer pressure
  Role changes
  Identity crisis
  Loss of significant support person
Adult
  Marital conflict
  Parenting
  Loss of family member
  Role changes
Elderly
  Retirement
  Social isolation
  Loss of spouse

OUTCOME CRITERIA

The person will

1. Not harm self
2. Accept help from significant others and community
3. Use effective coping mechanisms in handling stress

INTERVENTIONS

1. Assess level of present risk:
     a. High   Moderate   Low

2. Assess level of long-term risk:
   a. Life-style Lethality of plan Usual coping mechanisms
3. Provide immediate management for high-risk person: Closely supervised environment.
   a. Restrict glass, nail files, scissors, nail polish remover, mirrors, needles, razors, soda cans, plastic bags, lighters, electric equipment, belts, hangers, knives, tweezers, alcohol, guns.
   b. Meals should be provided in a closely supervised area.
   c. When administering oral medications, check to ensure that all medications are swallowed.
   d. Provide checks on the person as designated by institution's policy.
   e. Restrict the individual to the unit unless specifically ordered by physician. When off unit, provide a staff member to accompany the person.
   f. Instruct visitors on restricted items.
   g. The acutely suicidal person may be required to wear a hospital gown to prevent elopement.
   h. Room searches should be done periodically according to institution policy.
   i. Utilize seclusion and restraint if necessary (refer to *High Risk for Violence* for discussion).
   j. Notify police if the person elopes and is at risk for suicide.
4. Notify all staff that this person is at risk for self-harm.
5. Make a no-suicide contract with the individual (include family if person is at home).
   a. Use a written contract
   b. Mutual agreement
6. Encourage appropriate expression of anger and hostility.
7. Set limits on ruminations about suicide or previous attempts.
8. Assist in recognizing predisposing factors: "What was happening before you started having these thoughts?"
9. Facilitate examination of life stresses and past coping mechanisms.
10. Explore alternative behaviors.
11. Anticipate future stresses and assist in planning alternatives.

12. Involve person in planning the treatment goals and evaluating progress.
13. Instruct significant others in how to recognize an increase in risk: change in behavior, verbal, nonverbal communication, withdrawal, signs of depression.
14. Supply phone numbers of 24-hour emergency hotlines.
15. Refer to community agency and/or ongoing therapy.

Sensory–Perceptual Alteration

DEFINITION

Sensory–Perceptual Alteration: The state in which an individual/group experiences or is at risk of experiencing a change in the amount, pattern, or interpretation of incoming stimuli.

Author's Note:
Sensory–Perceptual Alterations describe an individual with altered perception and cognition influenced by physiological factors, *e.g.*, pain, sleep deprivation, immobility, and excessive or decreased meaningful stimuli from the environment. Altered Thought Processes can also manifest with altered perception and cognition. Sensory–Perceptual Alterations result when barriers or factors interfere with a person's ability to accurately interpret stimuli. When personality or mental disorders interfere with one's ability to accurately interpret stimuli, Altered Thought Processes is more accurate than Sensory–Perceptual Alterations.

The diagnosis Sensory–Perceptual Alterations has six subcategories: visual, auditory, kinesthetic, gustatory, tactile, and olfactory. When an individual has a visual or hearing deficit, how does the nurse intervene with the diagnosis Sensory–Perceptual Alterations: visual related to effects of glaucoma? What would the outcome criteria be? The nurse should assess for the individual's response to the visual loss and specifically label the response, not the deficit.

(Continued)

Author's Note (Continued)
Sensory-Perceptual Alterations is more clinically useful without the addition of the sensory deficit. Examples of responses to sensory deficits may be:

Visual
   High risk for injury
   Self-care deficit
Auditory
   Impaired communicaton
   Social isolation
Kinesthetic
   High Risk for injury
Olfactory
   Altered nutrition
Tactile
   High Risk for injury
Gustatory
   Altered nutrition

DEFINING CHARACTERISTICS

Major (Must Be Present)

Inaccurate interpretation of environmental stimuli
or
Negative change in amount or pattern of incoming stimuli

Minor (May Be Present)

Disoriented about time or place
Disoriented about people
Altered problem-solving ability
Altered behavior or communication pattern
Sleep pattern disturbances
Restlessness
Reports auditory or visual hallucinations
Fear
Anxiety
Apathy

RELATED FACTORS

Many factors in an individual's life can contribute to sensory–perceptual alterations. Some common factors are listed below.

Pathophysiological

Sensory organ alterations (visual, gustatory, auditory, olfactory, and tactile deficits)
Neurological alterations
    Cerebrovascular accident   Neuropathies
    Encephalitis/meningitis
Metabolic alterations
    Fluid and electrolyte   Acidosis
      imbalance   Alkalosis
    Elevated blood urea
      nitrogen
Impaired oxygen transport
    Cerebral   Respiratory
    Cardiac   Anemia
Musculoskeletal changes
    Paraplegia   Quadriplegia

Treatment-related

Amputation
Medications (sedatives, tranquilizers)
Surgery (glaucoma, cataract, detached retina)
Physical isolation (reverse isolation, communicable disease, prison)
Radiation therapy
Immobility
Mobility restrictions (bed rest, traction, casts, Stryker frame, Circoelectric bed)

Situational (Personal, Environmental)

Social isolation (patient with terminal or infectious disease)
Pain
Stress
Environment ("noise pollution")

OUTCOME CRITERIA

The person will

1. Demonstrate decreased symptoms of sensory overload as evident by (specify)

2. Identify and eliminate the potential risk factors if possible
3. Describe the rationale for the treatment modality

INTERVENTIONS

1. Reduce excess noise or light.
2. Share with person the source of the noise.
3. Discuss the use of a radio with earplugs to provide soft, relaxing music.
4. Share with personnel the need to reduce noise and provide individuals with uninterrupted sleep for at least 2–4 hours' duration.
5. Attempt to reduce fears and concerns by explaining equipment, its purpose and noises.
6. Encourage person to share perceptions of noises.
7. Orient to all three spheres (person, place, time).
8. Offer simple explanations of each task.
9. Allow person to participate in task, such as washing own face.
10. Promote movement in and out of bed.

Sexuality Patterns, Altered

Sexual Dysfunction

DEFINITION

Altered Sexuality Patterns: The state in which an individual experiences or is at risk of experiencing a change in sexual health.

Author's Note:

The diagnoses Altered Sexuality Patterns and Sexual Dysfunction are difficult to differentiate. Altered Sexuality Patterns is a

(*Continued*)

Author's Note (Continued)
broad diagnosis of which sexual dysfunction can be one part. Sexual health is the integration of somatic, emotional, intellectual, and social aspects of sexual being in ways that are enriching and that enhance personality communication and love (World Health Organization).

Sexual Dysfunction may be more appropriately used by a nurse with advanced preparation in sex therapy. Until Sexual Dysfucntion is differentiated from Altered Sexuality Patterns, it is unnecessary for most nurses to use this diagnosis.

DEFINING CHARACTERISTICS

Major (Must Be Present)

Identification of sexual difficulties, limitations, or changes

RELATED FACTORS

Altered sexuality patterns can occur as a response to a variety of health problems, situations, and conflicts. Some common sources are indicated below.

Pathophysiological

Endocrine
  Diabetes mellitus
  Decreased hormone
    production
  Myxedema

Hyperthyroidism
Addison's disease
Acromegaly

Genitourinary
  Chronic renal failure
  Premature or retarded
    ejaculation
  Priapism
  Chronic vaginal infection

Decreased vaginal
  lubrication
Vaginismus
Altered structures
Venereal disease

Neuromuscular and skeletal
  Arthritis
  Multiple sclerosis
  Amyotrophic lateral
    sclerosis

Disturbances of the
  nerve supply to the
  brain, spinal cord,
  sensory nerves, and
  autonomic nerves

Cardiorespiratory
  Myocardial infarction
  Congestive heart failure

Peripheral vascular
  disorders
Chronic respiratory
  disorders

Cancer
Liver disease

Treatment-related

Medications
Radiation treatment
Altered self-concept from change in appearance (trauma,
  radical surgery)

Situational (Personal, Environmental)

Partner
  Unwilling
  Uninformed
  Abusive
Environment
  Unfamiliar
  No privacy
Stressors
  Job problems
  Financial worries
Lack of knowledge
Fatigue
Obesity
Pain
Alcohol ingestion
Drug abuse
Fear of sexual failure
Fear of pregnancy
Depression
Anxiety
Guilt
Fear of sexually transmitted disease

Not available
Separated
Divorced

Hospital

Conflicting values
Religious conflict

Maturational

Ineffective role models
Negative sexual teaching
Absence of sexual teaching
Aging (separation, isolation)

OUTCOME CRITERIA

The person will

1. Share concerns regarding sexual functioning
2. Express increased satisfaction with sexual patterns
3. Identify stressors in life
4. Resume previous sexual activity
5. Report a desire to resume sexual activity

INTERVENTIONS

1. Acquire a sexual history.
   a. Usual sexual pattern
   b. Satisfaction (individual, partner)
   c. Sexual knowledge
   d. Problems
   e. Expectations
2. If stressors or a stressful life-style have negatively impacted functioning:
   a. Assist person in modifying life-style to reduce stress.
   b. Encourage identification of present stressors in life; group as those person can control and those person cannot
      • *Can Control*
         Personal lateness
         Involvement in community activities
      • *Cannot Control*
         Report due
         Daughter's illness
   c. Initiate a regular exercise program for stress reduction. See *Health Seeking Behaviors* for interventions.
3. Identify alternative methods for dispersing sexual energy when partner is unavailable or unwilling.
   a. Use masturbation, if acceptable to individual.
   b. Teach the physical and psychological benefits of regular physical activity (at least three times a week for 30 minutes).
   c. If partner is deceased, explore opportunities to meet and socialize with others (night school, singles club, community work).
4. If a change or loss of body part has negatively impacted functioning:

    a. Assess the stage of adaptation of the individual and partner to the loss (denial, depression, anger, resolution; see *Grieving*).

    b. Explain the normalcy of the foregoing responses to loss.

    c. Explain the need to share concerns with partner.
- The imagined response of partner
- The fear of rejection
- Fear of future losses
- Fear of physically hurting partner

    d. Encourage the partner to discuss the strengths of their relationship and to assess the influence of the loss on their strengths.

    e. Encourage person to resume sexual activity as close to previous pattern as possible.

5. Identify barriers to satisfying sexual functioning (*e.g.,* hypoxia, pain, impaired mobility, pregnancy).

6. Teach techniques to:

    a. Reduce oxygen consumption
- Use oxygen during sexual activity if indicated.
- Engage in sexual activity after intermittent positive-pressure breathing treatment or postural drainage.
- Plan sexual activities for time of day person is most rested.
- Use positions for intercourse that are comfortable and permit unrestricted breathing (side to side; compromised individual on top).

    b. Reduce cardiac workload
- Cardiac patients should avoid sexual activity:
  In extremes of temperature
  Directly after eating or drinking
  When intoxicated
  When tired
  With unfamiliar partner (when other stressors are present, *e.g.,* alcohol, fatigue)
- Rest before engaging in sexual activity (mornings are best).
- Cardiac patients should terminate sexual activity if chest discomfort or dyspnea occurs.

    c. Reduce or eliminate pain
- If vaginal lubrication is decreased, use a water-soluble lubricant.

- Take medication for pain before beginning sexual activity.
- Use whatever relaxes individual before beginning sexual activity (hot packs, hot showers).

7. For pregnant woman:
   a. Discuss the effects of stress, fatigue, and the other changes that pregnancy and motherhood bring on libido and sexual function.
   b. Allow her to verbalize her concerns and beliefs about pregnancy and coitus.
   c. Advise that coital positions may need to be varied according to the woman's contour (side-lying during 8th and 9th months).
   d. Orgasms from intercourse or masturbation should be discouraged if spotting or bleeding occurs, fetal membranes rupture prematurely, or there is a repeated history of miscarriage.
   e. Vaginal discomfort during coitus can be reduced with the use of a water-soluble lubricant.

8. Initiate health teaching and referrals as indicated; discuss with individuals or couples the availability of self-help groups (*e.g.,* Reach for Recovery, United Ostomy Association).

Sexual Dysfunction

DEFINITION

Sexual Dysfunction: The state in which an individual experiences or is at risk of experiencing a change in sexual function that is viewed as unrewarding or inadequate.

DEFINING CHARACTERISTICS

Major (Must Be Present)

Verbalization of problem with sexual function
or
Reports limitations on sexual performance imposed by disease or therapy

Minor (May Be Present)

Fears future limitations on sexual performance
Misinformed about sexuality

Lacks knowledge about sexuality and sexual function
Value conflicts involving sexual expression (cultural, religious)
Altered relationship with significant other
Dissatisfaction with sex role (perceived or actual)

Author's Note:
Refer to *Altered Sexuality Patterns.*

Sleep Pattern Disturbance

DEFINITION

Sleep Pattern Disturbance: The state in which an individual experiences or is at risk of experiencing a change in the quantity or quality of his or her rest pattern as related to the person's biological and emotional needs.

DEFINING CHARACTERISTICS
Adults
Major (Must Be Present)

Difficulty falling or remaining asleep

Minor (May Be Present)

Fatigue on awakening or during the day
Dozing during the day
Agitation
Mood alterations

Children

Sleep disturbances in children are frequently related to fear, enuresis, or inconsistent responses of parents to the child's requests for changes in sleep rules, such as requests to stay up late.

Reluctance to retire
Frequent awakening during the night
Desire to sleep with parents

RELATED FACTORS

Many factors in life can contribute to sleep pattern disturbances. Some common factors are listed below.

Pathophysiological

Impaired oxygen transport
    Angina
    Peripheral
     arteriosclerosis
    Respiratory disorders
    Circulatory disorders

Impaired elimination (bowel or bladder)
    Diarrhea
    Constipation
    Incontinence
    Retention
    Dysuria
    Frequency

Impaired metabolism
    Hyperthyroidism
    Gastric ulcers
    Hepatic disorders

Treatment-related

Immobility (imposed by casts, traction)
Medications
    Tranquilizers
    Sedatives
    Hypnotics
    Antidepressants
    Antihypertensives
    Amphetamines
    Corticosteroids
    Soporifics
    Monoamine oxidase
     inhibitors
    Anesthetics
    Barbiturates

Situational (Personal, Environmental)

Lack of exercise
Pain
Anxiety response

Pregnancy
Life-style disruptions
    Occupational   Sexual
    Emotional   Financial
    Social
Environmental changes
    Hospitalization (noise,   Travel
      disturbing roommate,
      fear)

OUTCOME CRITERIA

The person will

1. Describe factors that prevent or inhibit sleep
2. Identify techniques to induce sleep
3. Report an optimal balance of rest and activity

INTERVENTIONS

1. Reduce noise.
2. Organize procedures to provide the fewest number of disturbances during sleep period (*e.g.,* when individual awakens for medication also administer treatments and obtain vital signs).
3. If voiding during the night is disruptive, have person limit nighttime fluids and void before retiring.
4. Establish with person a schedule for a daytime program of activity (walking, physical therapy).
5. Limit amount and length of daytime sleeping if excessive (*i.e.,* more than 1 hour).
6. Assess with person, family, or parents the usual bedtime routine—time, hygiene practices, rituals (reading, toy)—and adhere to it as closely as possible.
7. For children:
   a. Explain night to the child (stars and moon).
   b. Discuss how some people (nurses, factory workers) work at night.
   c. Compare the contrast that when night comes for them, day is coming for other people somewhere else.
   d. If a nightmare occurs, encourage the child to talk about it if possible. Reassure child that it is a dream, even if it seems so real. Share with child that you have dreams too.

> e. Provide child with a nightlight and/or a flashlight to use to give child control over the dark.
> f. Reassure child that you will be nearby all night.

8. Explain to person and significant others the causes of sleep/rest disturbance and possible ways to avoid them.

Social Interaction, Impaired

DEFINITION

Impaired Social Interaction: The state in which an individual experiences or is at risk of experiencing negative, insufficient, or unsatisfactory responses from interactions.

DEFINING CHARACTERISTICS

Major (Must Be Present)

Reports inability to establish and/or maintain stable supportive relationships

Minor (May Be Present)

Lack of motivation
Severe anxiety
Dependent behavior
Hopelessness
Delusions/hallucinations
Disorganized thinking
Lack of self-care skills
Distractibility/inability to concentrate
Social isolation
Superficial relationships
Poor impulse control
Difficulty holding a job
Lack of self-esteem

RELATED FACTORS

Impaired social interactions can result from a variety of situations and health problems that are related to the inability to establish and maintain rewarding relationships. Some common sources are as follows:

Pathophysiological

Loss of body function
Hearing deficits
Mental retardation
Terminal illness
Loss of body part
Visual deficits
Speech impediments
Chronic illness (Crohn's disease, renal failure, epilepsy)

Treatment-related

Surgical disfigurement
Dialysis
Medication reaction

Situational (Personal, Environmental)

Depression
Language/cultural barriers
Social isolation
Lack of vocational skills
Substance abuse
Anxiety (phobias)
Divorce/death of spouse
Institutionalization
Thought disturbances

Maturational

Child/adolescent
  Altered appearance
  Speech impediments
  Separation from family
Adult
  Loss of ability to practice vocation
Elderly
  Death of spouse
  Retirement

OUTCOME CRITERIA

The person will

1. Acknowledge problems with socialization
2. Identify new behaviors to promote effective socialization
3. Report or role play the use of a constructive substitute behavior

INTERVENTIONS

1. Provide an individual, supportive relationship.
2. Help to identify how stress precipitates problems.
3. Support healthy defenses.
4. Help to identify alternative courses of action.
5. Assist in analyzing approaches that work best.
6. Role-play situations that are problematic. Discuss feelings.
7. If in group therapy:
   a. Focus on here and now.
   b. Establish group norms that discourage inappropriate behavior.
   c. Encourage testing of new social behavior.
   d. Use snacks or coffee to decrease anxiety during sessions.
   e. Role-model certain accepted social behaviors (*e.g.,* responding to a friendly greeting versus ignoring it).
   f. Foster development of relationships among members through self-disclosure and genuineness.
   g. Use questions and observations to encourage persons with limited interaction skills.
   h. Encourage members to validate their perception with others.
   i. Identify strengths among members and ignore selected weaknesses.
8. For chronic mental illness.
   a. Assist family members in understanding and providing support.
   b. Provide factual information concerning illness, treatment, and progress to family members.
   c. Validate family members' feelings of frustration in dealing with daily problems.

d. Provide guidance on overstimulating or under-stimulating environments.
e. Allow families to discuss their feelings of guilt and how their behavior affects the person.
f. Develop an alliance with family.
g. Arrange for periodic respite care.
9. For individuals with chronic mental illness, teach (McFarland):*
   a. Responsibilities of his or her role as a client (making requests clearly known, participating in therapies)
   b. To outline activities of the day and to focus on accomplishing them
   c. How to approach others in order to communicate
   d. To identify which interactions encourage others to give him or her consideration and respect
   e. To identify how he or she can participate in for-mulating family roles and responsibility to com-ply
   f. To recognize signs of anxiety and methods to re-lieve them
   g. To identify his or her positive behavior and to experience satisfaction with self in selecting con-structive choices
10. As indicated, refer to community agencies (*e.g.,* social service, occupational counseling, family therapy, crisis intervention).

Social Isolation

DEFINITION

Social Isolation: The state in which an individual or group experiences a need or desire for contact with others but is unable to make that contact.

---

* McFarland G, Wasli E: Manipulation in nursing diagnoses and process. In Johnson BS: Psychiatric–Mental Health Nursing, p. 92. Philadelphia, JB Lippincott, 1986

Author's Note:

Isolation can be viewed as one extreme of a continuum of loneliness with intimacy at the other extreme. The term *social isolation* as a nursing diagnosis is problematic. Loneliness can occur without isolation. The nurse should view Social Isolation as a nursing diagnosis that represents loneliness. Social Isolation is the cause of loneliness but there are other causes, *e.g.,* emotional isolation. Social Isolation is not a response but it produces responses such as loneliness and unhappiness. Loneliness is a subjective state that exists whenever a person says it does and is perceived as imposed by others. Social isolation is *not* the voluntary solitude that is necessary for personal renewal, nor is it the creative aloneness of the artist or the aloneness—and possible suffering—one may experience as a result of seeking individualism and independence (*e.g.,* moving to a new city, going away to college).

DEFINING CHARACTERISTICS

Since social isolation is a subjective state, all inferences made regarding a person's feelings of aloneness must be validated. Because the causes vary and people show their aloneness in different ways, there are no absolute cues to this diagnosis.

Major (Must Be Present)

Expressed feelings of aloneness and/or desire for more social contact

Minor (May Be Present)

Time passing slowly ("Mondays are so long for me.")
Inability to concentrate and make decisions
Feelings of uselessness
Doubts about ability to survive
Feelings of rejection
Behavior changes
Increased irritability or restlessness
Underactivity (physical or verbal)
Inability to make decisions
Increased signs and symptoms of illness (a change from previous state of good health)
Appearing depressed, anxious, or angry

Postponing important decision-making
Failure to interact with others nearby
Sleep disturbance (too much or insomnia)
Change in eating habits (overeating or anorexia)

RELATED FACTORS

A state of social isolation can result from a variety of situations and health problems that are related to a loss of established relationships or to a failure to generate these relationships. Some common sources follow.

Pathophysiological

Obesity
Cancer (disfiguring surgery of head or neck, superstitions of others)
Physical handicaps (paraplegia, amputation, arthritis, hemiplegia)
Emotional handicaps (extreme anxiety, depression, paranoia, phobias)
Incontinence (embarrassment, odor)
Communicable diseases (acquired immunodeficiency syndrome [AIDS], hepatitis)

Situational (Personal, Environmental)

Death of a significant other
Divorce
Extreme poverty
Hospitalization or terminal illness (dying process)
Moving to another culture (*e.g.,* unfamiliar language)
Drug or alcohol addiction
Homosexuality
Loss of usual means of transportation

Maturational

Child
    In protective isolation or with a communicable disease
Elderly
    Sensory losses
    Motor losses
    Loss of significant others

OUTCOME CRITERIA

The person will

1. Identify the reasons for feelings of isolation
2. Discuss ways of increasing meaningful relationships
3. Identify appropriate diversional activities

INTERVENTIONS

1. Support the individual who has experienced a loss as person works through grief (see *Grieving*).
2. Encourage person to talk about feelings of loneliness and the reasons they exist.
3. Mobilize person's support system of neighbors and friends.
4. Determine available transportation in the community (public, church-related, volunteer).
5. Identify activities that help keep people busy, especially during times of high risk of loneliness (see *Diversional Activity Deficit*).
6. Assist with the management of esthetic problems (*e.g.,* consult enterostomal therapist if ostomy odor is a problem; teach those with cancer to control odor of tumors by packing area with yogurt or pouring in buttermilk, then rinsing well with saline solution).
7. Identify strategies for socialization:
   a. Senior centers and church groups
   b. Day care centers for the elderly
   c. Retirement communities
   d. House sharing
   e. College classes opened to older persons
   f. Pets
   g. Telephone contact

Spiritual Distress

DEFINITION

Spiritual Distress: The state in which an individual or group experiences or is at risk of experiencing a disturbance in the belief or value system that provides strength, hope, and meaning to one's life.

DEFINING CHARACTERISTICS

Major (Must Be Present)

Experiences a disturbance in belief system

Minor (May Be Present)

Questions credibility of belief system
Demonstrates discouragement or despair
Is unable to practice usual religious rituals
Has ambivalent feelings (doubts) about beliefs
Expresses that he or she has no reason for living
Feels a sense of spiritual emptiness
Shows emotional detachment from self and others
Expresses concern—anger, resentment, fear—over the
  meaning of life, suffering, death
Requests spiritual assistance for a disturbance in belief
  system

RELATED FACTORS

Pathophysiological

Loss of body part or function
Terminal illness
Debilitating disease
Pain
Trauma
Miscarriage, stillbirth

Treatment-related

Abortion   Isolation
Surgery   Amputation
Blood transfusion   Medications
Dietary restrictions   Medical procedures

Situational (Personal, Environmental)

Death or illness of significant other
Embarrassment at practicing spiritual rituals

Hospital barriers to practicing spiritual rituals

Intensive care restrictions	Lack of privacy
Confinement to bed or room	Lack of availability of special foods/diet

Beliefs opposed by family, peers, health care providers
Childbirth
Divorce, separation from loved ones

OUTCOME CRITERIA

The person will

1. Continue spiritual practices not detrimental to health
2. Express decreasing feelings of guilt and anxiety
3. Express satisfaction with spiritual condition

INTERVENTIONS

1. Communicate acceptance of various spiritual beliefs and practices.
2. Convey nonjudgmental attitude.
3. Acknowledge importance of spiritual needs.
4. Express willingness of health care team to help in meeting spiritual needs.
5. Provide privacy and quiet as needed for daily prayer, for visit of spiritual leader, and for spiritual reading and contemplation.
6. Contact spiritual leader to clarify practices and perform religious rites or services if desired.
7. Maintain diet with spiritual restrictions when not detrimental to health.
8. Encourage spiritual rituals not detrimental to health.
9. Provide opportunity for individual to pray with others or be read to by members of own religious group or member of the health care team who feels comfortable with these activities.
10. For parent conflict regarding treatment of child:
    a. If parents refuse treatment of child, encourage consideration of alternate methods of therapy* (*e.g.,* utilization of Christian Science nurses and practitioners; special surgeons and techniques for

* May require a physician's order.

surgery without blood transfusions); support individual making informed decision—even if decision conflicts with own values.

   b. If treatment is still refused, physician or hospital administrator may obtain court order appointing temporary guardian to consent to treatment.*

   c. Call spiritual leader to support parents (and possibly child).

   d. Encourage expression of negative feelings.

11. Give "permission" to discuss spiritual matters with nurse by bringing up subject of spiritual welfare if necessary.

12. Use questions about past beliefs and spiritual experiences to assist person in putting this life event into wider perspective.

13. Offer to pray/meditate/read with client if you are comfortable with this or arrange for another member of health care team if more appropriate.

14. Be available and willing to listen when client expresses self-doubt, guilt, or other negative feelings.

15. Offer to contact other spiritual support person (such as pastoral care, hospital chaplain, etc.) if person cannot share feelings with usual spiritual leader.

Thought Processes, Altered

DEFINITION

Altered Thought Processes: The state in which an individual experiences a disruption in such mental activities as conscious thought, reality orientation, problem-solving, judgment, and comprehension related to coping.

---

* May require a physician's order.

Author's Note:
Altered Thought Processes describes an individual with altered perception and cognition that interferes with daily living. Causes are physiological dysfunctions, *e.g.*, dementia, or psychological disturbances, *e.g.*, depression, personality disorders, bipolar disorders. The focus of nursing is to reduce disturbed thinking and/or promote reality orientation.

The nurse should be cautioned in using this diagnosis as a "waste-basket" diagnosis for all clients with disturbed thinking or confusion. Frequently confusion in older adults is erroneously attributed to aging. Confusion in the elderly can be caused by a single factor or multiple factors, *e.g.*, dementia, medication side-effects, depression, or metabolic disorder. Depression causes impaired thinking in older adults more frequently than dementia (Miller).*

DEFINING CHARACTERISTICS

Major (Must Be Present)

Inaccurate interpretation of stimuli, internal and/or external

Minor (May Be Present)

Cognitive deficits, including abstraction, memory deficits
Suspiciousness
Delusions
Hallucinations
Phobias
Obsessions
Distractibility
Lack of consensual validation
Language
Confusion/disorientation
Suicidal/homicidal thoughts

RELATED FACTORS

Pathophysiological

Personality and mental disorders related to alteration in biochemical compounds

* Miller CA: Nursing Care of Older Adults. Glenview, IL, Scott Foresman, 1990

Genetic disorder
Progressive dementia
Hormonal changes

Situational (Personal, Environmental)

Depression or anxiety
Substance abuse (alcohol, drugs)
Fear of the unknown
Actual loss (of control, routine, income, significant others, familiar object or surroundings)
Emotional trauma
Rejection or negative appraisal by others
Negative response from others
Isolation
Unclear communication
Abuse (physical, sexual, mental)
Torture

Maturational

Adolescent
   Peer pressure
   Conflict
   Separation
Adult
   Marital conflict
   Family additions or deaths
Elderly
   Isolation, late-life depression, dementia

OUTCOME CRITERIA

The person will

1. Identify situations that evoke anxiety
2. Express delusional material less frequently
3. Describe problems in relating with others
4. Differentiate between reality and fantasy
5. Demonstrate an increase in self-care activities

INTERVENTIONS

1. Approach in a calm, nurturing manner.
2. Recognize when person is testing the trustworthiness of others.
3. Avoid making promises that cannot be fulfilled.

4. Initial staff contact minimal and brief with suspicious person; increase time as suspicion decreases.
5. Verify your interpretation of what person is experiencing ("I understand you are fearful of others.").
6. Use communication that helps person maintain own individuality (*e.g.,* "I" instead of "we").
7. For hallucinations:
    a. Observe for verbal and nonverbal hallucinations—inappropriate laughter, delayed verbal response, eye movements, moving lips without sound, increased motor movements, grinning.
    b. Direct the focus from delusional expression to discussion of reality-centered situations.
    c. Encourage differentiation of stimuli arising from inner sources from those from outside (*e.g.,* in response to "I hear voices," say: "Those are the voices of people on TV" or "I hear no one speaking now; they are your own thoughts.").
    d. Avoid the impression that you confirm or approve reality distortions; tactfully express doubt.
    e. Set limits for discussing repetitive delusional material ("You've already told me about that; let's talk about something realistic.").
    f. Identify the underlying needs being met by the delusions/hallucinations.
8. Assist in communicating more effectively.
    a. Ask for the meaning of what is said; do not assume that you understand.
    b. Validate your interpretation of what is being said ("Is this what you mean?").
    c. Clarify all global pronouns—we, they ("Who is *they?*").
    d. Refocus when person changes the subject in the middle of an explanation or thought.
    e. Tell the person when you are not following his or her train of thought.
    f. Do not mimic or restate words, phrases that you do not understand.
    g. Teach the person to consensually validate with others.
9. Assist person to set limits on own behavior.
    a. Discuss alternative methods of coping (*e.g.,* taking a walk instead of crying).

    b. Confront person with the attitude that regression is not acceptable behavior.

    c. Help delay gratification (*e.g.,* "I want you to wait 5 minutes before you repeat your request for help in making your bed.").

    d. Encourage person to achieve realistic expectations.

    e. Pace expectations to avoid frustration.

10. Encourage and support person in the decision-making process.

    a. Compliment the person who assumes more responsibility.

    b. Provide opportunity for person to contribute to own treatment plan.

    c. Help establish future goals that are realistic; examine problems in achieving a goal and suggest various alternatives.

11. Assist person to differentiate between needs and demands.

    a. Explain the difference between needs and demands (*e.g.,* food and clothing are needs; expectations that others dress and feed person, if he or she can do it, are demands).

    b. Assist person to examine the effects of behavior on others; encourage a change in behavior if it evokes negative responses.

12. Help person recognize behaviors that stimulate rejection.

    a. Identify activities that reduce interpersonal anxiety (*e.g.,* exercise, controlled breathing exercises).

    b. Set limits firmly and kindly on destructive behavior.

    c. Allow expression of negative emotions, verbally or in constructive activity.

    d. Help person accept responsibility for responses he or she elicits from others.

    e. Encourage discussion of problems in relating after visits with family members.

    f. Help person test new skills in relating to others in role-playing situations.

13. Anticipate difficulties in adjusting to community living; discuss concerns about returning to community and elicit family reaction to individual's discharge.

14. Provide health teaching that will prepare person to deal with life stresses (methods of relaxation, problem-solving skills, how to negotiate with others, how to express feelings constructively).

15. Inform individual of social agencies that offer help in adjusting to community living.

16. Provide sensory input that is sufficient and meaningful.
    a. Keep person oriented to time and place.
       - Refer to time of day and place each morning.
       - Provide person with a clock and calendar large enough to see.
       - Provide person with opportunity to see daylight and dark through a window or take person outdoors.
       - Single out holidays with cards or pins (*e.g.,* wear a red heart for Valentine's Day).
    b. Encourage family to bring in familiar objects from home (photographs, afghan).
    c. Discuss current events, seasonal events (snow, water activities); share your interests (travel, crafts).
    d. Assess if person can perform an activity with own hands (*e.g.,* latch rugs, wood crafts).
       - Provide reading materials, audio tapes, puzzles (manual, computer, crossword).
       - Encourage person to keep own records if possible (*e.g.,* intake and output).
       - Provide tasks to perform (addressing envelopes, occupational therapy).

17. In teaching a task or activity—for example, eating—break it into small, brief steps by giving only one instruction at a time.

18. Discourage the use of nightclothes during the day; have person wear shoes, not slippers and encourage self-care and grooming activities.

19. Use various modalities to promote stimulation for the individual.
    a. Music therapy
       - Provide soft, familiar music during meals.
       - Arrange group song fests.
       - Play music during other therapies (physical, occupational).
       - Have person exercise to music.

    b. Recreation therapy
- Encourage arts and crafts (knitting and crocheting).
- Suggest creative writing.
- Provide puzzles.
- Organize group games.

    c. Remotivation therapy
- Topics for remotivation sessions are chosen based on suggestions from group leaders and the interest of the group. Examples are pets, bodies of water, canning fruits and vegetables, transportation, holidays (Janssen).*
- Use associations and analogies
  "If ice is cold, then fire is . . . ?"
  "If day is light, then night is . . . ?"

    d. Sensory training
- Stimulate vision (with mirrors, brightly colored items of different shapes, pictures, colored decorations, kaleidoscopes).
- Stimulate smell (with flowers, coffee, cologne).

20. Discourage the use of restraints; explore other alternatives.
    a. Put person in a room with others who can help watch him or her.
    b. Enlist aid of family or friends to watch person during confused periods.
    c. If person is pulling out tubes, use mitts instead of wrist restraints.

21. Refer to *High Risk for Injury* for strategies for assessing and manipulating the environment for hazards.

---

* Janssen J, Giberson D: Remotivation therapy. J. Gerontol Nurs 14(6):31–34, 1988

Tissue Perfusion, Altered: (Specify)

DEFINITION

Altered Tissue Perfusion: The state in which an individual experiences or is at risk of experiencing a decrease in nutrition and respiration at the cellular level because of a decrease in capillary blood supply.

Altered Peripheral Tissue Perfusion: The state in which an individual experiences or is at risk of experiencing a decrease in nutrition and respiration at the peripheral cellular level because of a decrease in capillary blood supply.

Author's Note:

This nursing diagnosis is restricted in use to represent only diminished peripheral tissue perfusion situations in which nurses prescribe definitive treatment to reduce, eliminate, or prevent the problem. In the other situations of diminished cardiopulmonary, cerebral, renal, or gastrointestinal tissue perfusion, the nurse should focus on the functional abilities of the individual that are or may be compromised because of the decreased tissue perfusion. The nurse should also monitor to detect for physiological complications of decreased tissue perfusion and label these situations as collaborative problems. The following illustrates examples of a compromised functional health problem (nursing diagnosis) and a potential complication (collaborative problem) for an individual with compromised cerebral tissue perfusion:

> *High Risk for Injury* related to vertigo secondary to recent head injury (nursing diagnosis)
> *Potential Complication: Increased Intracranial Pressure* (collaborative problem)

Refer to Chapter 2 of Carpenito LJ: Nursing Diagnosis: Application to Clinical Practice, 3rd ed. Philadelphia, JB Lippincott, 1989 for additional information on collaborative problems. For additional examples of nursing diagnoses and collaborative problems grouped under medical conditions, refer to Section II of this handbook.

DEFINING CHARACTERISTICS*

Major (Must Be Present)

Presence of one of the following types:
Claudication   Aching pain
Rest pain
Diminished or absent arterial pulses
Skin color changes
Pallor (arterial)   Reactive hyperemia
Cyanosis (venous)   (arterial)
Skin temperature changes
Cooler (arterial)   Warmer (venous)
Decreased blood pressure changes (arterial)
Capillary refill less than three seconds (arterial)

Minor (May Be Present)

Edema (venous)
Loss of sensory function (arterial)
Loss of motor function (arterial)
Trophic tissue changes (arterial)
Hard, thick nails
Loss of hair
Lack of lanugo (newborn)

RELATED FACTORS

Pathophysiological

Vascular disorders
Arteriosclerosis   Leriche syndrome
Hypertension   Raynaud's disease/
Aneurysm   syndrome
Arterial thrombosis   Varicosities
Deep vein thrombosis   Buerger's disease

---

* Tissue perfusion depends on many physical and physiological factors within the systems of the body and in the structures and functions of the cells. When an alteration in peripheral tissue perfusion exists, the nurse must take into account the nature of the alteration in perfusion. The two major components of the peripheral vascular system are the arterial and the venous systems. Signs, symptoms, etiologies, and nursing interventions are different for problems occurring in each of these two systems and are therefore addressed separately when appropriate.

Collagen vascular disease   Sickle cell crisis
Rheumatoid arthritis   Cirrhosis
                                      Alcoholism
Diabetes Mellitus
Hypotension
   Sympathetic stress response (vasospasm/
     vasoconstriction)
Blood dyscrasias (platelet disorders)
Renal failure
Cancer/tumor

Treatment-related

Immobilization
Presence of invasive lines
Pressure sites/constriction (Ace bandages, stockings)
Medications (diuretics, tranquilizers, anticoagulants)
Anesthesia
Blood vessel trauma or compression

Situational (Personal, Environmental)

Pregnancy
Heredity
Obesity
Diet (hyperlipidemia)
Anorexia/malnutrition
Dehydration
Dependent venous pooling
Hypothermia
Frequent exposure to vibrating tools/equipment
Tobacco use
Exercise

Maturational

Neonate
   Immature peripheral circulation
   Rh incompatibility (erythroblastosis fetalis)
   Hypothermia
Elderly
   Sensory–perceptual changes
   Atherosclerotic plaques
   Capillary fragility

OUTCOME CRITERIA

The individual will

1. Identify factors that improve peripheral circulation
2. Identify necessary life-style changes
3. Identify medical regimen, diet, medications, activities that promote vasodilation
4. Report decrease in pain
5. Describe when to contact physician/health care professional

INTERVENTIONS

1. Teach person to:
   a. Keep extremity in a dependent position
   b. Keep extremity warm (Do not use heating pad or hot water bottle, since the individual with a peripheral vascular disease may have a disturbance in sensation and will not be able to determine if the temperature is hot enough to damage tissue; the use of external heat may also increase the metabolic demands of the tissue beyond its capacity.)
   c. Reduce risk for trauma
      • Change positions at least every hour
      • Avoid leg crossing
      • Reduce external pressure points (inspect shoes daily for rough lining)
      • Avoid sheepskin heel protectors (they increase heel pressure and pressure across dorsum of foot)
      • Encourage range of motion exercises
2. Plan a daily walking program.
   a. Instruct individual in reasons for program.
   b. Teach individual to avoid fatigue.
   c. Instruct to avoid increase in exercise until assessed by physician for cardiac problems.
   d. Reassure individual that walking does not harm the blood vessels or the muscles; "walking into the pain," resting and resuming walking, assists in developing collateral circulation.
3. Teach factors that improve venous blood flow.

    a. Elevate extremity above the level of the heart (may be contraindicated if severe cardiac or respiratory disease is present).
    b. Avoid standing or sitting with legs dependent for long periods of time.
    c. Consider the use of Ace bandages or below-knee elastic stockings to prevent venous stasis.
    d. Reduce or remove external venous compression that impedes venous flow.
       • Avoid pillows behind the knees or Gatch bed that is elevated at the knees.
       • Avoid leg crossing.
       • Change positions, move extremities or wiggle fingers and toes every hour.
       • Avoid garters and tight elastic stockings above the knees.
4. Measure baseline circumference of calves and thighs if individual is at risk for deep venous thrombosis, or if it is suspected.
5. Teach person to:
    a. Avoid long car or plane rides (get up and walk around at least every hour)
    b. Keep dry skin lubricated (cracked skin eliminates the physical barrier to infection)
    c. Wear warm clothing during cold weather
    d. Wear cotton or wool socks
    e. Avoid dehydration in warm weather
    f. Give special attention to feet and toes
       • Wash feet and dry well daily
       • Do not soak feet
       • Avoid harsh soaps or chemicals (including iodine) on feet
       • Keep nails trimmed and filed smooth
    g. Inspect feet and legs daily for injuries and pressure points
    h. Wear clean socks
    i. Wear shoes that offer support and fit comfortably
    j. Inspect the inside of shoes daily for rough lining
6. Teach risk factor modification.
    a. Diet:
       • Avoid foods high in cholesterol
       • Modify sodium intake to control hypertension
       • Refer to dietitian
    b. Relaxation techniques to reduce effects of stress

   c. Smoking cessation
   d. Exercise program

Unilateral Neglect

DEFINITION

Unilateral Neglect: The state in which an individual is unable to attend to or "ignores" the hemiplegic side of his or her body and/or objects, persons, or sounds on the affected side of the individual's environment.

DEFINING CHARACTERISTICS

Major (Must Be Present)

   Neglect of involved body parts and/or extrapersonal space and/or denial of the existence of the affected limb or side of the body

Minor (May Be Present)

   Left homonymous hemianopsia
   Difficulty with spatial–perceptual tasks
   Hemiplegia (usually left side)

RELATED FACTORS

Pathophysiological

   Neurological disease/damage
      Cerebrovascular accident (CVA)
      Cerebral tumors
      Brain injury/trauma
      Cerebral aneurysms

OUTCOME CRITERIA

The person will

   1. Demonstrate an ability to scan the visual field to compensate for loss of function/sensation in affected limb(s)

2. Identify safety hazards in the environment
3. Describe the deficit and rationale for treatment

INTERVENTIONS

1. Initially adapt the environment to the deficit.
   a. Position person, call light, bedside stand, television, telephone, and personal items on the unaffected side.
   b. Position person's bed so unaffected side is toward the door.
   c. Approach and speak to person from unaffected side.
   d. If you must approach person from affected side, announce your presence as soon as you enter the room to avoid startling the person.
2. Gradually change the person's environment as you teach person to compensate and learn to recognize the forgotten field; move furniture and personal items out of visual field.
3. For a person in a wheelchair, obtain a lapboard (preferably Plexiglas) and position affected arm on lapboard with fingertips at midline; encourage person to look for arm on board.
4. For an ambulatory person, obtain an arm sling to prevent the arm from dangling and causing shoulder subluxation.
5. Constantly cue person to the environment.
6. Encourage person to wear prescribed corrective lens or hearing aids.
7. For bathing, dressing, and toileting:
   a. Instruct person to attend to affected extremity/side first when performing activities of daily living (ADLs).
   b. Instruct person always to look for affected extremity when performing ADLs, to know where it is at all times.
   c. Encourage person to integrate affected extremity during bathing, encourage person to feel extremity by rubbing and massage.
8. For eating:
   a. Instruct person to eat in small amounts; place food on unaffected side of mouth.
   b. Instruct person to use tongue to sweep out

> "pockets" of food from affected side after every bite.

c. After meals/medications check oral cavity for pocketed food/medication.

d. Provide oral care tid and PRN.

e. Initially place food in visual field, gradually move food out of field and teach person to scan entire visual field.

9. Retrain person to scan entire environment.

10. Have person stroke involved side with uninvolved hand; the person should watch arm or leg as he or she strokes it.

11. Assess to ensure that both person and family understand the purpose and rationale of all interventions.

Urinary Elimination, Altered Patterns of

Maturational Enuresis*

Functional Incontinence

Reflex Incontinence

Stress Incontinence

Total Incontinence

Urge Incontinence

Urinary Retention

* This diagnostic category is not currently on the NANDA list but has been included for clarity or usefulness.

DEFINITION

Altered Patterns of Urinary Elimination: The state in which
an individual experiences or is at risk of experiencing urinary
elimination dysfunction.

DEFINING CHARACTERISTICS

Major (Must Be Present)

Reports or experiences a urinary elimination problem,
such as

Urgency	Dribbling
Frequency	Bladder distention
Hesitancy	Incontinence
Nocturia	Large residual urine
Enuresis	volumes

RELATED FACTORS

Pathophysiological

Congenital urinary tract anomolies

Strictures	Bladder neck
Hypospadias	contractures
Epispadias	Megalocystis (large-
Ureterocele	capacity bladder
	without tone)

Disorders of the urinary tract

Infection	Calculi

Trauma   Carcinoma
Urethritis
Neurogenic disorders or injuries
    Cord injury/tumor/   Multiple sclerosis
      infection   Diabetic neuropathy
    Brain injury/tumor/   Alcoholic neuropathy
      infection   Tabes dorsalis
    Cerebrovascular accident   Parkinsonism
    Demyelinating diseases
Prostatic enlargement
Estrogen deficiency
    Atrophic vaginitis   Atrophic urethritis
Herpes zoster

Treatment-related

Surgical
    Postprostatectomy   Extensive pelvic
                                dissection

Diagnostic instrumentation
General or spinal anesthesia
Drug therapy (iatrogenic)
    Antihistamines   Immunosuppressant
    Epinephrine   therapy
    Anticholinergics   Diuretics
    Sedatives   Tranquilizers
                                Muscle relaxants

Post–indwelling catheters

Situational (Personal, Environmental)

Loss of perineal tissue
    Obesity   Childbirth
    Aging
    Recent substantial
      weight loss
Irritation to perineal area
    Sexual activity   Poor personal hygiene
Pregnancy
Inability to communicate needs
Fecal impaction
Dehydration
Stress or fear
Decreased attention to bladder cues
    Depression   Confusion

Intentional suppression (self-induced deconditioning)
Environmental barriers to bathroom

Distant toilets	Bed too high
Poor lighting	Siderails
Unfamiliar surroundings	

Impaired mobility

Maturational

Child
Small bladder capacity
Lack of motivation
Elderly
Motor and sensory losses
Loss of muscle tone
Inability to communicate needs
Depression

OUTCOME CRITERIA

The person will

1. Be continent (specify during day, night, 24 hours)
2. Be able to identify the cause of incontinence and rationale for treatment

INTERVENTIONS

1. Maintain optimal hydration.
   a. Increase fluid intake to 2000–3000 ml/day, un-
      less contraindicated.
   b. Space fluids every 2 hours.
   c. Decrease fluid intake after 7 p.m. and provide
      only minimal fluids during the night.
   d. Reduce intake of coffee, tea, dark colas, alcohol,
      and grapefruit juice because of their diuretic ef-
      fect.
   e. Avoid large amounts of tomato and orange juice
      because they tend to make the urine more al-
      kaline.
2. Maintain adequate nutrition to ensure bowel elimination at least once every 3 days.
3. Promote micturition.
   a. Ensure privacy and comfort.

      b. Use toilet facilities, if possible, instead of bed-pans.

      c. Provide male with opportunity to stand, if possible.

      d. Assist person on bedpan to flex knees and support back.

      e. Teach postural evacuation (bend forward while sitting on toilet).

4. Promote personal integrity and provide motivation to increase bladder control.

5. Convey to person that incontinence can be cured or at least controlled to maintain dignity.

6. Expect person to be continent, not incontinent (*e.g.,* encourage street clothes, discourage use of bedpans, protective pads).

7. Promote skin integrity.

      a. Identify individuals at risk of developing pressure ulcers.

      b. Wash area, rinse, and dry well after incontinent episode.

      c. Use a protective ointment if needed (for area burns, use hydrocortisone cream; for fungal irritations, use antifungal ointment).

8. Assess the person's potential for participation in a bladder retraining program (cognition, willingness to participate, desire to change behavior).

9. Provide individual with rationale for plan and acquire informed consent.

10. Encourage individual to continue program by providing accurate information concerning reasons for success or failure.

11. Assess voiding pattern.

      a. Time and amount of fluid intake

      b. Type of fluid

      c. Amount of incontinence

      d. Amount of void, whether it was voluntary or involuntary

      e. Presence of sensation of need to void

      f. Amount of retention

      g. Amount of residual

      h. Amount of triggered urine

      i. Identify certain activities that precede voiding (*e.g.,* restlessness, yelling, exercise)

12. Schedule fluid intake and voiding times.

13. Schedule intermittent catheterization program, if indicated.
14. Teach intermittent catheterization to person and family for long-term management of bladder.
    a. Explain the reasons for the catheterization program.
    b. Explain the relationship of fluid intake and the frequency of catheterization.
    c. Explain the importance of emptying the bladder at the prescribed time regardless of circumstances because of the hazards of an overdistended bladder (*e.g.,* circulation contributes to infection, and stasis of urine contributes to bacterial growth).
15. Teach prevention of urinary tract infections (UTI).
    a. Encourage regular complete emptying of the bladder.
    b. Ensure adequate fluid intake.
    c. Keep urine acidic; avoid citrus juices, dark colas, and coffee.
    d. Monitor urine *p*H.
16. Teach individual to monitor for signs and symptoms of UTI.
    a. Increase in mucus and sediment
    b. Blood in urine (hematuria)
    c. Change in color (from normal straw-colored) or odor
    d. Elevated temperature, chills, and shaking
    e. Changes in urine properties
    f. Suprapubic pain
    g. Painful urination
    h. Urgency
    i. Frequent small voids or frequent small incontinences
    j. Increased spasticity in spinal cord injured individuals
    k. Increase in urine *p*H
    l. Nausea/vomiting
    m. Lower back and/or flank pain
17. Refer to community nurses for assistance in bladder reconditioning, if indicated.

Maturational Enuresis*

DEFINITION

Maturational Enuresis: The state in which a child experiences involuntary voiding during sleep, which is not pathophysiological in origin.

Author's Note:
This diagnostic category would represent enuresis that is not caused by pathophysiological or structural deficits such as strictures.

DEFINING CHARACTERISTICS
Major (Must Be Present)

Reports or demonstrates episodes of involuntary voiding during sleep

RELATED FACTORS
Situational (Personal, Environmental)

Stressors (school, siblings)
Inattention to bladder cues
Unfamiliar surroundings

Maturational

Child
Small bladder capacity
Lack of motivation
Attention-seeking behavior

OUTCOME CRITERIA

1. The child will remain dry during the sleep cycle

---

* This diagnostic category is not currently on the NANDA list but has been included for clarity or usefulness.

2. The child or family will be able to state the nature and causes of enuresis

INTERVENTIONS

1. Explain the nature of enuresis to parents and child.
2. Explain to parents that disapproval (shaming, punishing) is useless in stopping enuresis but can make child shy, ashamed, and afraid.
3. Offer reassurance to child that other children wet the bed at night and child is not bad or sinful.
4. Teach:
   a. After child drinks fluids, encourage him or her to postpone voiding to help stretch the bladder
   b. To have child void prior to retiring
   c. To restrict fluids at bedtime
   d. If child is awakened later (about 11 P.M.) to void, attempt to awaken child fully for positive reinforcement.
   e. Child awareness of sensations that occur when it is time to void
   f. Child ability to control urination (have child start and stop the stream; have child "hold" the urine during the day, even if for only a short time)
5. Have child keep a record of progress; emphasize dry days or nights (*e.g.,* stars on a calendar).
6. If child wets, have him or her explain or write down, if possible, why child thinks it happened.
7. Teach child and family techniques to control the adverse effects of enuresis (*e.g.,* use of plastic mattress covers, use of child's own sleeping bag (machine washable) when staying overnight away from home).
8. Seek out opportunities to teach the public about enuresis and incontinence (*e.g.,* school and parent organizations, self-help groups).

Functional Incontinence

DEFINITION

Functional Incontinence: The state in which an individual experiences difficulty in reaching or inability to reach the toilet prior to urination because of environmental barriers, disorientation, and physical limitations.

DEFINING CHARACTERISTICS

Major (Must Be Present)

Incontinence before or during an attempt to reach the toilet

RELATED FACTORS
Pathophysiological

Neurogenic disorders
  Brain injury/tumor/infection
  Cerebrovascular accident
  Demyelinating diseases
  Multiple sclerosis
  Alcoholic neuropathy
  Parkinsonism
Progressive dementia

Treatment-related

Drug therapy (iatrogenic)
  Antihistamines
  Epinephrine
  Anticholinergics
  Sedatives
  Immunosuppressant therapy
  Diuretics
  Tranquilizers
  Muscle relaxants

Situational (Personal, Environmental)

Impaired mobility
Stress or fear
Decreased attention to bladder cues
  Depression
  Confusion
  Intentional suppression (self-induced deconditioning)
Environmental barriers to bathroom
  Distant toilets
  Poor lighting

Unfamiliar surroundings
Bed too high
Siderails

Maturational

Elderly
Motor and sensory losses
Loss of muscle tone
Inability to communicate needs
Depression

OUTCOME CRITERIA

The person will

1. Eliminate or reduce incontinent episodes (specify number of hours)
2. Remove or minimize environmental barriers from home
3. Use proper adaptive equipment to assist with voiding, transfers, and dressing
4. Describe causative factors for incontinence

INTERVENTIONS

1. Determine if there is another cause contributing to incontinence (*e.g.*, stress, urge or reflex incontinence, urinary retention, or infection).
2. Assess for sensory/cognitive deficits.
3. Assess for motor/mobility deficits.
4. Reduce environmental barriers.
   a. Obstacles, lighting, and distance
   b. Adequacy of toilet height and need for grab bars
5. Provide a commode between bathroom and bed, if needed.
6. For an individual with cognitive deficits offer toileting reminders every 2 hours, after meals, and before bedtime.
7. For persons with limited hand function:
   a. Assess person's ability to remove and replace clothing
   b. Clothing that is loose is easier to manipulate
   c. Provide dressing aids as necessary: Velcro closures in seams for wheelchair patients, zipper pulls; all

garments with fasteners may be adapted with Velcro closures
8. Initiate referral to visiting nurse (occupational therapy
department) for assessment of bathroom facilities at
home.

Reflex Incontinence

DEFINITION

Reflex Incontinence: The state in which an individual experiences an involuntary loss of urine caused by damage to the
spinal cord between the cortical and sacral (S1–S3) bladder
centers.

DEFINING CHARACTERISTICS

Major (Must Be Present)

Uninhibited bladder contractions
Involuntary reflexes produce spontaneous voiding
Partial or complete loss of sensation of bladder fullness or
urge to void

RELATED FACTORS
Pathophysiological

Cord injury/tumor/infection

OUTCOME CRITERIA

The person will

1. Report a state of dryness that is personally satisfactory
2. Have a residual urine volume of less than 50 ml
3. Use triggering mechanisms to initiate reflex voiding

INTERVENTIONS

1. Explain to person rationale for treatment.
2. Teach cutaneous triggering mechanisms:
   a. Repeated deep, sharp suprapubic tapping (most
      effective)

    b. Instruct individual to:
- Position self in a half-sitting position
- Tapping is aimed directly at bladder wall
- Rate is 7–8 times/5 seconds (50 single blows)
- Use only one hand
- Shift site of stimulation over bladder to find most successful site
- Continue stimulation until a good stream starts
- Wait approximately 1 minute, repeat stimulation until bladder is empty
- One or two series of stimulations without response signifies that nothing more will be expelled

    c. If the above is ineffective perform each of the following for 2–3 minutes each.

    d. Wait 1 minute between facilitation attempts.
- Stroking glans penis
- Punching abdomen above inguinal ligaments (lightly)
- Stroking inner thigh

3. Encourage person to void or trigger at least every 3 hours.
4. Persons with abdominal muscle control should use the Valsalva maneuver during triggered voiding.
5. Indicate on intake and output sheet which mechanism was used to induce voiding.
6. Teach person that if fluid intake is increased, he or she also needs to increase the frequency of triggering to prevent overdistention.
7. If needed, schedule intermittent catheterization program.
8. Instruct person in signs and symptoms of dysreflexia:
   a. Elevated blood pressure, decreasing pulse
   b. Flushing and sweating above the level of the lesion
   c. Cool and clammy below the level of the lesion
   d. Pounding headache
   e. Nasal stuffiness
   f. Anxiety, "feeling of impending doom"
   g. Goose pimples
   h. Blurred vision
   i. Instruct person in measures to reduce or eliminate symptoms

j. Elevate head
k. Check blood pressure
l. Rule out bladder distention; empty bladder by catheter (do not trigger); use lidocaine lubricant for catheter

9. If condition persists after emptying bladder, check for bowel distention. If stool is present in the rectum, use a Nupercainal suppository to desensitize the area before removing stool.

10. If condition persists or person has not been able to identify cause, notify physician immediately or seek help in an emergency room.

11. Instruct person to carry an identification card that states signs, symptoms, and management in the event that the person would not be able to direct others.

Stress Incontinence

DEFINITION

Stress Incontinence: The state in which an individual experiences an immediate involuntary loss of urine upon an increase in intra-abdominal pressure.

DEFINING CHARACTERISTICS

Major (Must Be Present)

The individual reports
Loss of urine (usually less than 50 ml) occurring with increased abdominal pressure from standing, sneezing, or coughing

RELATED FACTORS

Pathophysiological

Congenital urinary tract anomalies
Strictures
Hypospadias
Epispadias
Ureterocele
Bladder neck contractures
Megalocystis (large-capacity bladder without tone)

Disorders of the urinary tract
　Infection
　Trauma
　Urethritis
Estrogen deficiency
　Atrophic vaginitis
　Atrophic urethritis

Situational (Personal, Environmental)

Loss of perineal tissue
　Obesity
　Aging
　Recent substantial weight loss
　Childbirth
Irritation to perineal area
　Sexual activity
　Poor personal hygiene
Pregnancy
Stress or fear

Maturational

Elderly
　Loss of muscle tone

OUTCOME CRITERIA

The person will

1. Report a reduction or elimination of stress incontinence
2. Be able to explain the cause of incontinence and rationale for treatment

INTERVENTIONS

1. Assess pattern of voiding/incontinence and fluid intake.
2. Explain to the person the effect of incompetent floor muscles on continence.
3. Teach person to identify her pelvic floor muscles and strengthen them with exercise (Kegel exercises).
   a. "For posterior pelvic floor muscles, imagine you are trying to stop the passage of stool and tighten your anal muscles without tightening your legs or your abdominal muscles."

  b. "For anterior pelvic floor muscles, imagine you are trying to stop the passage of urine, tighten the muscles (back and front) for 4 seconds and then release them; repeat ten times, four times a day." (Can be increased to four times an hour if indicated)

  c. Instruct person to stop and start the urine stream several times during voiding.

 4. Teach to decrease abdominal pressure with pregnancy

  a. Teach to avoid prolonged periods of standing.

  b. Teach the benefit of frequent voidings at least every 2 hours.

  c. Teach Kegel exercises.

 5. Explain the relationship of obesity and stress incontinence and teach:

  a. Kegel exercises

  b. If person desires to lose weight, refer to community programs.

  c. Void every 2 hours

  d. Avoid prolonged periods of standing

Total Incontinence

DEFINITION

Total Incontinence: The state in which an individual experiences continuous, unpredictable loss of urine.

Author's Note:

This category is used only after the other types of incontinence have been ruled out.

DEFINING CHARACTERISTICS

Major (Must Be Present)

Constant flow of urine without distention
Nocturia more than two times during sleep
Incontinence refractory to other treatments

Minor (May Be Present)

Unaware of bladder cues to void
Unaware of incontinence

RELATED FACTORS
Pathophysiological

Congenital urinary tract anomalies
    Strictures
    Hypospadias
    Epispadias
    Ureterocele
    Megalocystis (large-capacity bladder without tone)
Disorders of the urinary tract
    Infection
    Trauma
    Urethritis
Neurogenic disorders or injury
    Cord injury/tumor/infection
    Brain injury/tumor/infection
    Cerebrovascular accident
    Demyelinating diseases
    Multiple sclerosis
    Diabetic neuropathy
    Alcoholic neuropathy
    Tabes dorsalis

Treatment-related

Surgical
    Postprostatectomy
    Extensive pelvic dissection
General or spinal anesthesia
Post-indwelling catheters

Situational (Personal, Environmental)

Inability to communicate needs
Dehydration
Stress or fear
Decreased attention to bladder cues
    Depression
    Confusion

Maturational

Elderly
    Motor and sensory losses
    Loss of muscle tone
    Inability to communicate needs
    Depression

OUTCOME CRITERIA

The person will

1. Be continent (specify during day, night, 24 hours)
2. Be able to identify the cause of incontinence and rationale for treatment

INTERVENTIONS

1. Maintain optimal hydration
   a. Increase fluid intake to 2000–3000 ml/day, unless contraindicated.
   b. Space fluids every 2 hours.
   c. Decrease fluid intake after 7 P.M. and provide only minimal fluids during the night.
   d. Reduce intake of coffee, tea, dark colas, alcohol, and grapefruit juice because of their diuretic effect.
   e. Avoid large amounts of tomato and orange juice because they tend to make the urine more alkaline.
2. Maintain adequate nutrition to ensure bowel elimination at least once every 3 days
3. Promote micturition.
   a. Ensure privacy and comfort.
   b. Use toilet facilities, if possible, instead of bedpans.
   c. Provide male with opportunity to stand, if possible.
   d. Assist person on bedpan to flex knees and support back.
   e. Teach postural evacuation (bend forward while sitting on toilet).
4. Promote personal integrity and provide motivation to increase bladder control.
5. Convey to person that incontinence can be cured or at least controlled to maintain dignity.

6. Expect person to be continent, not incontinent (*e.g.,* encourage street clothes, discourage use of bedpans, protective pads).
7. Promote skin integrity.
    a. Identify individuals at risk of developing pressure ulcers.
    b. Wash area, rinse, and dry well after incontinent episode.
    c. Use a protective ointment if needed (for area burns, use hydrocortisone cream; for fungal irritations, use antifungal ointment).
8. Assess the person's potential for participation in a bladder retraining program (cognition, willingness to participate, desire to change behavior).
9. Provide individual with rationale for plan and acquire informed consent.
10. Encourage individual to continue program by providing accurate information concerning reasons for success or failure.
11. Assess voiding pattern.
    a. Time and amount of fluid intake
    b. Type of fluid
    c. Amount of incontinence
    d. Amount of void, whether it was voluntary or involuntary
    e. Presence of sensation of need to void
    f. Amount of retention
    g. Amount of residual
    h. Amount of triggered urine
    i. Identify certain activities that precede voiding (*e.g.,* restlessness, yelling, exercise)
12. Schedule fluid intake and voiding times.
13. Schedule intermittent catheterization program, if indicated.
14. Teach intermittent catheterization to person and family for long-term management of bladder.
    a. Explain the reasons for the catheterization program.
    b. Explain the relationship of fluid intake and the frequency of catheterization.
    c. Explain the importance of emptying the bladder at the prescribed time regardless of circumstances because of the hazards of an overdistended blad-

der (*e.g.,* circulation contributes to infection, and stasis of urine contributes to bacterial growth).

15. Teach prevention of urinary tract infections (UTI).
    a. Encourage regular complete emptying of the bladder.
    b. Ensure adequate fluid intake.
    c. Keep urine acidic; avoid citrus juices, dark colas, and coffee.
    d. Monitor urine pH.
16. Teach individual to monitor for signs and symptoms of UTI.
    a. Increase in mucus and sediment
    b. Blood in urine (hematuria)
    c. Change in color (from normal straw-colored) or odor
    d. Elevated temperature, chills, and shaking
    e. Changes in urine properties
    f. Suprapubic pain
    g. Painful urination
    h. Urgency
    i. Frequent small voids or frequent small incontinences
    j. Increased spasticity in spinal cord injured individuals
    k. Increase in urine pH
    l. Nausea/vomiting
    m. Lower back and/or flank pain
17. Refer to community nurses for assistance in bladder reconditioning, if indicated.

Urge Incontinence

DEFINITION

Urge Incontinence: The state in which an individual experiences an involuntary loss of urine associated with a strong sudden desire to void.

DEFINING CHARACTERISTICS

Major (Must Be Present)

Urgency followed by incontinence

RELATED FACTORS

Pathophysiological

Disorders of the urinary tract
    Infection
    Trauma
    Urethritis
Neurogenic disorders or injury
    Brain injury/tumor/infection
    Cerebrovascular accident
    Demyelinating diseases
    Diabetic neuropathy
    Alcoholic neuropathy
    Parkinsonism

Treatment-related

Diagnostic instrumentation
General or spinal anesthesia
Post-indwelling catheters

Situational (Personal, Environmental)

Loss of perineal tissue
    Obesity
    Aging
    Recent substantial weight loss
    Childbirth
Irritation to perineal area
    Sexual activity
    Poor personal hygiene
Intentional suppression (self-induced deconditioning)

Maturational

Child
    Small bladder capacity

OUTCOME CRITERIA

The person will

1. Report an absence or decreased episodes of incontinence (specify)
2. Explain causes of incontinence

INTERVENTIONS

1. Explain the causative or contributing factors.
    a. Bladder irritants
        • Infection
        • Inflammation
        • Alcohol, caffeine, or dark cola ingestion
        • Concentrated urine
    b. Diminished bladder capacity
        • Self-induced deconditioning (frequent small voids)
        • Post-indwelling catheter
    c. Overdistended bladder
        • Increased urine production (diabetes mellitus, diuretics)
        • Intake of alcohol and/or large quantities of fluids
    d. Uninhibited bladder contractions
        • Neurologic disorders
            Cerebrovascular accident
            Brain tumor/trauma/infection
            Parkinson's disease
2. Explain the risk of insufficient fluid intake and its relation to infection and concentrated urine.
3. Explain the relationship between incontinence and intake of alcohol, caffeine and dark colas (irritants).
4. Determine amount of time between urge to void and need to void (record how long person can hold off urination).
5. For a person with difficulty prolonging waiting time, communicate to personnel the need to respond rapidly to request for assistance for toileting (note on care plan).
6. Teach person to increase waiting time by increasing bladder capacity.
    a. Determine volume of each void.
    b. Ask person to "hold off" urinating as long as possible.
    c. Give positive reinforcement.
    d. Discourage frequent voiding that is result of habit, not need.
    e. Develop bladder reconditioning program.
7. For uninhibited bladder contractions provide an opportunity to void on awakening, after meals, physical exercise, bathing, and drinking coffee or tea, and before going to sleep.

Urinary Retention

DEFINITION

Urinary Retention: The state in which an individual experiences a chronic inability to void followed by involuntary voiding (overflow incontinence).

> **Author's Note:**
> This category is not recommended for use with individuals with acute episodes of urinary retention (*e.g.,* focal impaction, postanesthesia, postdelivery), in which cases catheterization, treatment of the cause, or surgery (prostatic hypertrophy) cure urinary retention. These situations are collaborative problems: PC: Urinary retention.

DEFINING CHARACTERISTICS

Major (Must Be Present)

Bladder distention (not related to acute, reversible etiology)
or
Bladder distention with small frequent voids or dribbling (overflow incontinence)
100 ml or more residual urine

Minor (May Be Present)

The individual states that it feels as though the bladder is not empty after voiding.

RELATED FACTORS

Pathophysiological

Congenital urinary tract anomalies
    Strictures
    Ureterocele
    Bladder neck contractures
    Megalocystis (large-capacity bladder without tone)

Neurogenic disorders or injury
    Cord injury/tumor/infection
    Brain injury/tumor/infection
    Cerebrovascular accident
    Demyelinating diseases
    Multiple sclerosis
    Diabetic neuropathy
    Alcoholic neuropathy
    Tabes dorsalis
Prostatic enlargement

Treatment-related

Surgical
    Postprostatectomy
    Extensive pelvic dissection
Diagnostic instrumentation
General or spinal anesthesia
Drug therapy (iatrogenic)
    Antihistamines
    Epinephrine
    Anticholinergics
    Theophylline
    Isoproterenol
Post-indwelling catheters

Situational (Personal, Environmental)

Loss of perineal tissue
    Obesity
    Aging
    Recent substantial weight loss
    Childbirth
Irritation to perineal area
    Sexual activity
    Poor personal hygiene
Pregnancy
Inability to communicate needs
Fecal impaction
Dehydration
Stress or fear
Decreased attention to bladder cues
    Depression
    Confusion
    Intentional suppression (self-induced deconditioning)

303

Environmental barriers to bathroom
    Distant toilets
    Poor lighting
    Unfamiliar surroundings
    Bed too high
    Siderails

Maturational

Child
    Small bladder capacity
    Lack of motivation
Elderly
    Motor and sensory losses
    Loss of muscle tone
    Inability to communicate needs
    Depression

OUTCOME CRITERIA

The person will

1. Empty the bladder using the Credé's and/or Valsalva maneuvers with residual urine of less than 50 ml, if indicated
2. Void voluntarily
3. Achieve a state of dryness that is personally satisfactory

INTERVENTIONS

1. Develop a bladder retraining or reconditioning program (see Total Incontinence for general interventions).
2. Teach person abdominal strain and Valsalva maneuver, if indicated.
   a. Lean forward on thighs.
   b. Contract abdominal muscles if possible and strain or "bear down"; hold breath while straining (Valsalva maneuver).
   c. Hold strain or breath until urine flow stops; wait 1 minute and strain again as long as possible.
   d. Continue until no more urine is expelled.
3. Teach person Credé's maneuver, if indicated.
   a. Place hands flat (or place fist) just below umbilical area.
   b. Place one hand on top of the other.
   c. Press firmly down and in toward the pelvic arch.

    d. Repeat six or seven times until no more urine can be expelled.

    e. Wait a few minutes and repeat to ensure complete emptying.

4. Teach person anal stretch maneuver, if indicated.

    a. Sit on commode or toilet.

    b. Lean forward on thighs.

    c. Place one gloved hand behind buttocks.

    d. Insert one to two lubricated fingers into the anus to the anal sphincter.

    e. Spread fingers apart, or pull to posterior direction.

    f. Gently stretch the anal sphincter and hold it distended.

    g. Bear down and void.

    h. Take a deep breath and hold it while straining (Valsalva).

    i. Relax and repeat the procedure until the bladder is empty

5. Instruct individual to try all three techniques or a combination of techniques to determine which is most effective in emptying the bladder.

6. Indicate on the intake and output record which technique was used to induce voiding.

7. Obtain postvoid residuals after attempts at emptying bladder; if residual urine volumes are greater than 100 ml, schedule intermittent catheterization program.

Violence, High Risk for

DEFINITION

High Risk for Violence: The state in which an individual is or may be assaultive toward others or the environment.

Author's Note:

This diagnostic category can be made more specific by adding High Risk for Violence directed at others or self-directed. High
(Continued)

> **Author's Note** (*Continued*)
> Risk for Self-Harm has been added by the author to describe individuals at risk for self-inflicted injuries; thus, the descriptor *self-directed* is not needed. Therefore, the content for High Risk for Violence will focus exclusively on violence directed at others.

RISK FACTORS

Presence of risk factors (See also Related Factors.)

RELATED FACTORS

Pathophysiological

Temporal lobe epilepsy
Progressive central nervous system deterioration (brain tumor)
Head injury
Hormonal imbalance
Viral encephalopathy
Mental retardation
Minimal brain dysfunction
Toxic response to alcohol or drugs
Mania

Treatment-related

Toxic reaction to medication

Situational (Personal, Environmental)

History of overt aggressive acts
Increase in stressors within a short period
Physical immobility
Suicidal behavior
Environmental controls
Perceived threat to self-esteem
Hallucination
Argumentative
Acute agitation
Suspiciousness
Persecutory delusions

Verbal threats of physical assault
Low frustration tolerance
Poor impulse control
Feelings of helplessness
Excessively controlled, inflexible
Fear of the unknown
Response to catastrophic event
Rage reaction
Misperceived messages from others
Antisocial character
Response to dysfunctional family throughout
  developmental stages
Dysfunctional communication patterns
Drug or alcohol abuse

Maturational

Adolescent
    Role identity
    Peer pressure
    Separation from family

OUTCOME CRITERIA

The person will

1. Experience control of behavior with assistance from others
2. Have a decreased number of violent responses
3. Describe causation and possible preventive measures

INTERVENTIONS

1. Acknowledge the individual's feelings, be genuine and empathetic.
2. Tell individual that you will help control behavior and not let him or her do anything destructive.
3. Set limits when individual presents a risk to others. Refer to *Anxiety* for further interventions on limit-setting.
4. Offer the individual choices and options. At times, it is necessary to give in on some demands to avoid a power struggle.
5. Encourage individual to express anger and hostility verbally instead of "acting out."

6. Remain calm; if you are becoming upset, leave the situation in the hands of others, if possible.

7. Allow the acutely agitated individual space that is five times greater than that for an individual who is in control. Do not touch the person unless you have a trusting relationship. Avoid physical entrapment of individual or staff.

8. Do not approach a violent individual alone. Often the presence of three to four staff members will be enough to reassure the individual that you will not let him or her lose control.

9. When assault is imminent, quick, coordinated action is essential.

10. Approach individual in a calm, self-assured manner so as not to communicate your anxiety or fear.

11. Establish an environment that reduces agitation.
    a. Decrease noise level.
    b. Give short, concise explanations.
    c. Control the number of persons present at one time.
    d. Provide single or semiprivate room.

12. Establish the expectation that person can control behavior, and continue to reinforce the expectation.

13. Provide positive feedback when person is able to exercise restraint.

14. Allow appropriate verbal expressions of anger. Give positive feedback.

15. Set limits on verbal abuse. Do not take insults personally. Support others (clients, staff) who may be targets of abuse.

16. Plan for unpredictable violence.
    a. Assess person's potential for violence and past history.
    b. Ensure availability of staff prior to potential violent behavior (never try to assist person alone when physical restraint is necessary).
    c. Determine who will be in charge of directing personnel to intervene in violent behavior if it occurs.
    d. Ensure protection for oneself (door nearby for withdrawal, pillow to protect face).

17. Use seclusion and/or restraint, according to policy.
    a. Remove individual from situation if environment is contributing to aggressive behavior, using the

least amount of control needed (*e.g.*, ask others to leave, and take individual to quiet room).

b. Reinforce that you are going to help person control self.

c. Repeatedly tell the person what is going to happen before external control is begun. When using seclusion, institutional policy will provide specific guidelines; the following are general.

- Observe individual at least every 15 minutes.
- Search the individual before secluding to remove harmful objects.
- Check seclusion room to see that safety is maintained.
- Offer fluids and food periodically (in non-breakable containers).
- When approaching an individual to be secluded, have sufficient staff present.
- Explain concisely what is going to happen ("You will be placed in a room by yourself until you can better control your behavior") and give person a chance to cooperate.
- Assist person in toileting and personal hygiene (assess ability to be out of seclusion; a urinal or commode may need to be used).
- If person is taken out of seclusion, someone must be present continually.
- Maintain verbal interaction during seclusion (provides information necessary to assess person's degree of control).
- When person is allowed out of seclusion, a staff member needs to be in constant attendance to determine whether person can handle additional stimulation.

18. Assist individual in developing alternative coping strategies when crisis has passed and learning can occur.

19. Practice negotiation skills with significant others and people in authority.

20. Encourage an increase in recreational activities.

21. Use group therapy to decrease sense of aloneness and increase communication skills.

Section II

Diagnostic Clusters
(Medical Conditions
With Associated Nursing
Diagnoses and Collaborative
Problems)

Medical Conditions

Cardiovascular/ Hematological/Peripheral Vascular Disorders

Cardiac Conditions

ANGINA PECTORIS

Nursing Diagnoses*

Anxiety related to chest pain secondary to effects of cardiac ischemia

Fear related to present status and unknown future

Sleep Pattern Disturbances related to treatments and environment

High Risk for Constipation related to bed rest, change in life-style, and medications

Activity Intolerance related to fear of recurrent angina

High Risk for Self-Concept Disturbance related to perceived or actual role changes

Possible Impaired Home Maintenance Management related to angina or fear of angina

High Risk for Altered Family Processes related to impaired ability of person to assume role responsibilities

High Risk for Altered Sexuality Patterns related to fear of angina and altered self-concept

Grieving related to actual or perceived losses secondary to cardiac condition

High Risk for Altered Health Maintenance related to insufficient knowledge of condition, home activities, diet, and medications

* List includes nursing diagnoses that may be associated with the medical diagnosis.

CONGESTIVE HEART FAILURE WITH PULMONARY EDEMA

Collaborative Problems

Potential Complications (PC):* Deep vein thrombosis
PC: Severe hypoxia
PC: Cardiogenic shock
PC: Hepatic failure

Nursing Diagnoses

Activity Intolerance related to insufficient oxygen for activities of daily living

Altered Nutrition: Less Than Body Requirements related to nausea; anorexia secondary to venous congestion of gastrointestinal tract and fatigue

Altered Peripheral Tissue Perfusion related to venous congestion

Anxiety related to breathlessness

Fear related to progressive nature of condition

High Risk for Impaired Home Maintenance related to inability to perform activities of daily living secondary to breathlessness and fatigue

(Specify) Self-Care Deficit related to dyspnea and fatigue

Sleep Pattern Disturbance related to nocturnal dyspnea and inability to assume usual sleep position

High Risk for Fluid Volume Excess: Edema related to compensatory kidney mechanisms

High Risk for Altered Health Maintenance related to insufficient knowledge of low-salt diet, drug therapy (diuretic, digitalis), activity program, and signs and symptoms of complications

Powerlessness related to progressive nature of condition

ENDOCARDITIS, PERICARDITIS
(Rheumatic, Infectious)

See also *Corticosteroid Therapy.*
If child, see *Rheumatic Fever.*

---

* PC: (Potential complications) are collaborative problems, not nursing diagnoses.

Collaborative Problems

PC: Congestive heart failure
PC: Valve stenosis
PC: Cerebrovascular accident
PC: Emboli (pulmonary, cerebral, renal, splenic, heart)
PC: Cardiac tamponade

Nursing Diagnoses

Activity Intolerance related to insufficient oxygenation
    secondary to decreased cardiac output
High Risk for Altered Respiratory Function related to
    decreased respiratory depth secondary to pain
Pain related to friction rub and inflammation process
High Risk for Altered Health Maintenance related to
    insufficient knowledge of etiology, prevention, antibiotic
    prophylaxis, and signs and symptoms of complications

MYOCARDIAL INFARCTION (Uncomplicated)

Collaborative Problems

PC: Dysrhythmias
PC: Cardiac arrest
PC: Cardiogenic shock
PC: Thromboembolism
PC: Angina

Nursing Diagnoses

Anxiety related to acute pain secondary to cardiac tissue
    ischemia
Fear related to pain, present status and unknown future
Sleep Pattern Disturbances related to treatments and
    environment
High Risk for Colonic Constipation related to decreased
    peristalsis secondary to medication effects, decreased
    activity, and change in diet
Activity Intolerance related to impaired oxygen transport
    secondary to decreased cardiac output and fear of
    recurrent angina
High Risk for Self-Concept Disturbances related to
    perceived or actual role changes
Possible Impaired Home Maintenance Management related
    to angina or fear of angina

High Risk for Altered Family Processes related to impaired
ability of ill person to assume role responsibilities

High Risk for Altered Sexuality Patterns related to fear of
angina and altered self-concept

Grieving related to actual or perceived losses secondary to
cardiac condition

High Risk for Altered Health Maintenance related to
insufficient knowledge of condition, home activities, diet,
and medications

Hematological Conditions

ANEMIA

Collaborative Problems

PC: Transfusion reaction
PC: Cardiac failure
PC: Iron overload (repeated transfusion)

Nursing Diagnoses

Activity Intolerance related to impaired oxygen transport
secondary to diminished red blood cell count

High Risk for Infection related to decreased resistance
secondary to tissue hypoxia and/or abnormal white blood
cells (neutropenia, leukopenia)

High Risk for Injury: Bleeding Tendencies related to
thrombocytopenia and splenomegaly

High Risk for Altered Oral Mucous Membrane related to
gastrointestinal mucosal atrophy

High Risk for Altered Health Maintenance related to
insufficient knowledge of condition, nutritional
requirements, and drug therapy

APLASTIC ANEMIA

Collaborative Problems

PC: Fatal aplasia
PC: Pancytopenia
PC: Hemorrhage
PC: Hypoxia
PC: Sepsis

Nursing Diagnoses

Activity Intolerance related to insufficient oxygen secondary to diminished red blood cell count

High Risk for Infection related to increased susceptibility secondary to leukopenia

High Risk for Altered Oral Mucous Membrane related to tissue hypoxia and vulnerability

High Risk for Altered Health Maintenance related to insufficient knowledge of causes, prevention, and signs and symptoms of complications

PERNICIOUS ANEMIA

See also *Anemia.*

Nursing Diagnoses

Altered Oral Mucous Membrane related to sore red tongue secondary to papillary atrophy and inflammatory changes

Diarrhea/Constipation related to gastrointestinal mucosal atrophy

High Risk for Altered Nutrition: Less Than Body Requirements related to anorexia secondary to sore mouth

High Risk for Altered Health Maintenance related to insufficient knowledge of chronicity of disease, vitamin B treatment, and familial propensity

DISSEMINATED INTRAVASCULAR COAGULATION (DIC)

See also *Underlying Disorders (e.g., Obstetric, Infections, Burns).*
See also *Anticoagulant Therapy.*

Collaborative Problems

PC: Hemorrhage
PC: Renal failure
PC: Microthrombi (renal, cardiac, pulmonary, cerebral, gastrointestinal)

Nursing Diagnoses

Fear related to treatments, environment, and risk of death

Altered Family Processes related to critical nature of the situation and uncertain prognosis

High Risk for Altered Health Maintenance related to insufficient knowledge of causes and treatment

POLYCYTHEMIA VERA

Collaborative Problems

PC: Thrombus formation
PC: Hemorrhage
PC: Hypertension
PC: Congestive heart failure
PC: Peptic ulcer
PC: Gout

Nursing Diagnoses

Altered Nutrition: Less Than Body Requirements related to anorexia, nausea, and vasocongestion

Activity Intolerance related to insufficient oxygenation secondary to pulmonary congestion and tissue hypoxia

High Risk for Infection related to hypoxia secondary to vasocongestion

High Risk for Altered Health Maintenance related to insufficient knowledge of fluid requirements, exercise program, and signs and symptoms of complications

Peripheral Vascular Conditions

DEEP VEIN THROMBOSIS

See also *Anticoagulant Therapy,* if indicated.

Collaborative Problems

PC: Embolism
PC: Chronic leg edema
PC: Chronic stasis ulcers

Nursing Diagnoses

High Risk for Colonic Constipation related to decreased peristalsis secondary to immobility

High Risk for Altered Respiratory Function related to
   immobility
High Risk for Impaired Skin Integrity related to chronic ankle
   edema
Pain related to impaired circulation
High Risk for Altered Health Maintenance related to
   insufficient knowledge of prevention of recurrence,
   implications of anticoagulant therapy, exercise program,
   and prevention of sequelae

HYPERTENSION

Collaborative Problems

PC: Retinal hemorrhage
PC: Cerebrovascular accident
PC: Cerebral hemorrhage
PC: Renal failure

Nursing Diagnoses

High Risk for Noncompliance related to negative side
   effects of prescribed therapy versus the belief that no
   treatment is needed without the presence of symptoms
High Risk for Altered Sexuality Patterns related to
   decreased libido or erectile dysfunction secondary to
   medication side effects
High Risk for Altered Health Maintenance related to
   insufficient knowledge of diet restriction, medications,
   signs of complications, risk factors (obesity, smoking),
   follow-up care, and stress reduction activities

VARICOSE VEINS

Collaborative Problems

PC: Vascular rupture
PC: Hemorrhage

Nursing Diagnoses

Chronic Pain related to engorgement of veins
High Risk for Altered Health Maintenance related to
   insufficient knowledge of condition, treatment options,
   and risk factors

PERIPHERAL VASCULAR DISEASE
(Atherosclerosis, Arteriosclerosis)

Collaborative Problems

PC: Stroke (cerebrovascular accident)
PC: Ischemic ulcers
PC: Claudication
PC: Acute arterial thrombosis, embolus
PC: Hypertension

Nursing Diagnoses

High Risk for Impaired Tissue Integrity related to compromised circulation

Chronic Pain related to muscle ischemia during prolonged activity

High Risk for Injury related to decreased sensation secondary to chronic atherosclerosis

High Risk for Infection related to compromised circulation

High Risk for Injury related to effects of orthostatic hypotension

Activity Intolerance related to claudication

High Risk for Altered Health Maintenance related to insufficient knowledge of condition, risk factors (obesity, smoking, cold), signs and symptoms of complications, prevention of complications, exercise program, foot care, and diet

RAYNAUD'S DISEASE/RAYNAUD'S SYNDROME

Collaborative Problems

PC: Acute arterial occlusion
PC: Ischemic ulcers
PC: Gangrene

Nursing Diagnoses

Pain related to ischemia secondary to acute vasospasm

Altered Peripheral Tissue Perfusion related to cold environment

High Risk for Impaired Tissue Integrity: Ischemic Ulcers related to vasospasm

Fear related to potential loss of work secondary to work-related aggravating factors

High Risk for Altered Health Maintenance related to insufficient knowledge of condition, stress, cold, stress reduction techniques, and risk factors (smoking, vibrations)

STASIS ULCERS (Postphlebitis Syndrome)

Collaborative Problem

PC: Cellulitis

Nursing Diagnoses

Altered Peripheral Tissue Perfusion related to dependent position of legs

High Risk for Infection related to compromised circulation

Self-Concept Disturbance related to chronic open wounds

Chronic Pain related to ulcers and treatments

High Risk for Altered Health Maintenance related to insufficient knowledge of etiology of ulcers, risk factors, prevention of injury, infection, exercise program, dressings, and need for compression

Respiratory Disorders

ADULT RESPIRATORY DISTRESS SYNDROME (ARDS)

See also *Mechanical Ventilation* (under *Diagnostic and Therapeutic Procedures*).

Collaborative Problems

PC: Electrolyte imbalance
PC: Hypoxemia

Nursing Diagnoses

Anxiety related to implications of condition and critical care setting

Powerlessness related to condition and treatments (ventilator, monitoring)

CHRONIC OBSTRUCTIVE PULMONARY DISEASE—COPD (Emphysema, Bronchitis)

Collaborative Problems

PC: Hypoxemia
PC: Electrolyte imbalance
PC: Acid–base imbalance
PC: Inadequate cardiac output
PC: Right-sided heart failure

Nursing Diagnoses

Ineffective Airway Clearance related to excessive and tenacious mucus secretions

High Risk for Altered Nutrition: Less Than Body Requirements related to anorexia secondary to dyspnea, halitosis, and fatigue

Activity Intolerance related to insufficient oxygenation for activities of daily living

Impaired Verbal Communication related to dyspnea

Anxiety related to breathlessness and fear of suffocation

Powerlessness related to loss of control and the restrictions that this condition places on life-style

Sleep Pattern Disturbance related to cough, inability to assume recumbent position, and environmental stimuli

High Risk for Altered Health Maintenance related to insufficient knowledge of condition, pharmacologic therapy, nutritional therapy, prevention of infection, rest versus activity, breathing exercises, and home care (*e.g.,* equipment)

PLEURAL EFFUSION

See also underlying disorders *(Congestive Heart Disease, Cirrhosis, Malignancy).*

Collaborative Problems

PC: Respiratory failure
PC: Pneumothorax (post-thoracentesis)
PC: Hypoxemia
PC: Hemothorax

Nursing Diagnoses

Activity Intolerance related to insufficient oxygenation for activities of daily living

High Risk for Altered Nutrition: Less Than Body
Requirements related to anorexia secondary to pressure
on abdominal structures

Altered Comfort related to accumulation of fluid in pleural
space

(Specify) Self-Care Deficits related to fatigue and dyspnea

PNEUMONIA

Collaborative Problems

PC: Hyperthermia
PC: Respiratory insufficiency
PC: Septic shock
PC: Paralytic ileus

Nursing Diagnoses

High Risk for Hyperthermia related to infectious process

Activity Intolerance related to insufficient oxygenation for
activities of daily living

High Risk for Altered Oral Mucous Membrane related to
mouth breathing and frequent expectoration and
decreased fluid intake secondary to malaise

High Risk for Fluid Volume Deficit related to increased
insensible fluid loss secondary to fever and
hyperventilation

High Risk for Altered Nutrition: Less Than Body
Requirements related to anorexia, dyspnea, and
abdominal distention secondary to air swallowing

Ineffective Airway Clearance related to pain, increased
tracheobronchial secretions, and fatigue

High Risk for Infection Transmission related to
communicable nature of the disease

Altered Comfort related to hyperthermia, malaise,
secondary to pulmonary pathology

High Risk for Impaired Skin Integrity related to prescribed
bed rest

High Risk for Altered Health Maintenance related to
insufficient knowledge of fluid requirements, caloric
requirements, spread of infection, signs and symptoms
of recurrence, prevention of recurrence, and medication
regimen

PULMONARY EMBOLISM

See also *Anticoagulant Therapy*.

Collaborative Problem

PC: *Hypoxemia*

Nursing Diagnoses

High Risk for Impaired Skin Integrity related to immobility
and prescribed bed rest

High Risk for Altered Health Maintenance related to
insufficient knowledge of anticoagulant therapy and signs
and symptoms of complications

Metabolic/Endocrine Disorders

ADDISON'S DISEASE

Collaborative Problems

PC: *Addisonian crisis (shock)*
PC: *Electrolyte imbalances (sodium, potassium)*
PC: *Hypoglycemia*

Nursing Diagnoses

High Risk for Altered Nutrition: Less Than Body
Requirements related to anorexia and nausea

High Risk for Fluid Volume Deficit related to excessive loss
of sodium and water secondary to polyuria

Diarrhea related to increased excretion of sodium and water

High Risk for Self-Concept Disturbance related to
appearance changes secondary to increased skin
pigmentation and decreased axillary and pubic hair
(female)

High Risk for Injury related to postural hypotension
secondary to fluid/electrolyte imbalances

High Risk for Altered Health Maintenance related to
insufficient knowledge of disease, signs and symptoms
of complications, risks for crisis (infection, diarrhea,
decreased sodium intake, diaphoresis), overexertion,

dietary management, identification (card, medallion), emergency kit, and pharmacologic management and titration dose, as needed

ALDOSTERONISM, PRIMARY

Collaborative Problems

PC: Hypokalemia
PC: Alkalosis
PC: Hypertension
PC: Hypernatremia

Nursing Diagnoses

Altered Comfort related to excessive urine excretion and polydipsia
High Risk for Fluid Volume Deficit related to excessive urinary excretion
High Risk for Altered Health Maintenance related to insufficient knowledge of condition, surgical treatment, and effects of corticosteroid therapy

CIRRHOSIS (Laënnec's Disease)

See also *Substance Abuse,* if indicated.

Collaborative Problems

PC: Hemorrhage
PC: Hypokalemia
PC: Portal systemic encephalopathy
PC: Negative nitrogen balance
PC: Drug toxicity (opiates, short-acting barbiturates, major tranquilizers)
PC: Renal failure
PC: Anemia
PC: Esophageal varices

Nursing Diagnoses

Chronic Pain related to liver enlargement and ascites
Diarrhea related to excessive secretion of fats in stool secondary to liver dysfunction
High Risk for Injury related to decreased prothrombin

production and synthesis of substances used in blood
coagulation

Altered Nutrition: Less Than Body Requirements related to
anorexia, impaired utilization, and storage of vitamins (A,
C, K, D, E)

High Risk for Altered Respiratory Function related to
pressure on diaphragm secondary to ascites

High Risk for Self-Concept Disturbance related to
appearance changes (jaundice, ascites)

High Risk for Infection related to leukopenia secondary to
enlarged, overactive spleen and hypoproteinemia

Altered Comfort related to pruritus secondary to
accumulation of bilirubin pigment and bile salts

Fluid Volume Excess: Peripheral Edema related to portal
hypertension, lowered plasma colloidal osmotic pressure,
and sodium retention

High Risk for Altered Health Maintenance related to
insufficient knowledge of pharmacological
contraindication, nutritional requirements, signs and
symptoms of complications, and risks of alcohol
ingestion

CUSHING'S SYNDROME

Collaborative Problems

PC: Hypertension
PC: Congestive heart failure
PC: Psychosis
PC: Electrolyte imbalance (sodium, potassium)

Nursing Diagnoses

Self-Concept Disturbance related to physical changes
secondary to disease process (moon face, thinning of
hair, truncal obesity, virilism)

High Risk for Infection related to excessive protein
catabolism and depressed leukocytic phagocytosis
secondary to hyperglycemia

High Risk for Injury: Fractures related to osteoporosis

High Risk for Impaired Skin Integrity related to loss of tissue,
edema, and dryness

Altered Sexuality Patterns related to loss of libido and
cessation of menses (female) secondary to excessive
adrenocorticotropic hormone production

High Risk for Altered Health Maintenance related to
   insufficient knowledge of disease and diet therapy (high
   protein, low cholesterol, low sodium)

DIABETES MELLITUS

Collaborative Problems

Acute complications:
   PC: Ketoacidosis (DKA)
   PC: Hyperosmolar hyperglycemic nonketotic coma (HHNK)
   PC: Hypoglycemia
   PC: Infections
Chronic complications:
   Macrovascular
   PC: Cardiac artery disease
   PC: Peripheral vascular disease
   Microvascular
   PC: Retinopathy
   PC: Neuropathy
   PC: Nephropathy

Nursing Diagnoses

High Risk for Injury related to decreased tactile sensation,
   diminished visual acuity, and hypoglycemia
Altered Comfort related to insulin injections, capillary blood
   glucose (CBG) testing, and diabetic peripheral
   neuropathy
Anxiety/Fear (individual, family) related to diagnosis of
   diabetes, potential complications of diabetes, and self-
   care regimens
High Risk for Ineffective Coping (individual, family) related to
   chronic disease, complex self-care regimen, and
   decreased support systems
Altered Nutrition: Greater Than Body Requirements related
   to intake in excess of need, lack of knowledge, and
   ineffective coping
High Risk for Altered Sexuality Patterns (male) related to
   peripheral neuropathy and/or psychological problems
High Risk for Altered Sexuality Patterns (female) related to
   physical and psychological stressors of diabetes
Powerlessness related to complications of diabetes
   (blindness, amputations, kidney failure, neuropathy)
Social Isolation related to visual impairment/blindness

High Risk for Noncompliance related to the complexity and chronicity of the prescribed regimen

High Risk for Altered Health Maintenance related to insufficient knowledge of ADA exchange diet, weight control, weight maintenance, benefits/risks of exercise, self-monitoring of blood glucose (SMBG), medications, sick day care, foot care, hypoglycemia, and available resources

HEPATITIS (Acute, Viral)

Collaborative Problems

PC: Hepatic failure
PC: Coma
PC: Subacute hepatic necrosis
PC: Fulminant hepatitis
PC: Portal systemic encephalopathy
PC: Hypokalemia
PC: Hemorrhage
PC: Drug toxicity
PC: Renal failure

Nursing Diagnoses

Fatigue related to weakness secondary to reduced energy metabolism by liver

High Risk for Infection Transmission related to contagious agents

Altered Nutrition: Less Than Body Requirements related to anorexia, epigastric distress, and nausea

High Risk for Fluid Volume Deficit related to lack of desire to drink

Altered Comfort related to pruritus secondary to bile salt accumulation

High Risk for Injury related to reduced prothrombin synthesis and reduced vitamin K absorption

Pain related to swelling of inflamed liver

Diversional Activity Deficit related to the monotony of confinement and isolation precautions

High Risk for Altered Health Maintenance related to insufficient knowledge of condition, rest requirements, precautions to prevent transmission, nutritional requirements, and contraindications (certain medications, alcohol)

327

HYPERTHYROIDISM
(Thyrotoxicosis, Graves' Disease)

Collaborative Problems

PC: Thyroid storm
PC: Cardiac dysrhythmias

Nursing Diagnoses

Altered Nutrition: Less Than Body Requirements related to intake less than metabolic needs secondary to excessive metabolic rate

Activity Intolerance related to fatigue and exhaustion secondary to excessive metabolic rate

Diarrhea related to increased peristalsis secondary to excessive metabolic rate

Altered Comfort related to heat intolerance and profuse diaphoresis

High Risk for Impaired Tissue Integrity: Corneal related to inability to close eyelids secondary to exophthalmos

High Risk for Injury related to tremors

High Risk for Hyperthermia related to lack of metabolic compensatory mechanism secondary to hyperthyroidism

High Risk for Altered Health Maintenance related to insufficient knowledge of condition, treatment regimen, pharmacologic therapy, eye care, dietary management, and signs and symptoms of complications

HYPOTHYROIDISM (Myxedema)

Collaborative Problems

PC: Atherosclerotic heart disease
PC: Normochromic, normocytic anemia
PC: Acute organic psychosis
PC: Myxedemic coma
PC: Metabolic
PC: Hematological

Nursing Diagnoses

Altered Nutrition: More Than Body Requirements related to intake greater than metabolic needs secondary to slowed metabolic rate

Activity Intolerance related to insufficient oxygenation secondary to slowed metabolic rate

Colonic Constipation related to decreased peristaltic action secondary to decreased metabolic rate and decreased physical activity

Impaired Skin Integrity related to edema and dryness secondary to decreased metabolic rate and infiltration of fluid into interstitial tissues

Altered Comfort related to cold intolerance secondary to decreased metabolic rate

High Risk for Impaired Social Interactions related to listlessness and depression

Impaired Verbal Communication related to slowed speech secondary to enlarged tongue

High Risk for Altered Health Maintenance related to insufficient knowledge of condition, treatment regimen, dietary management, signs and symptoms of complications, pharmacological therapy, and sensitivity to narcotics, barbiturates, and anesthetic agents

OBESITY

Nursing Diagnoses

Altered Health Maintenance related to imbalance between caloric intake and energy expenditure

Ineffective Individual Coping related to increase in food consumption as a response to stressors

Chronic Low Self-Esteem related to feelings of self-degradation and the response of others to the condition

PANCREATITIS

Collaborative Problems

PC: Shock
PC: Hemorrhagic pancreatitis
PC: Respiratory failure
PC: Pleural effusion
PC: Hypocalcemia
PC: Hyperglycemia
PC: Delirium tremens

Nursing Diagnoses

Pain related to nasogastric suction, distention of pancreatic capsule, and local peritonitis

High Risk for Fluid Volume Deficit related to decreased intake secondary to nausea and vomiting

Altered Nutrition: Less Than Body Requirements related to vomiting and diet restrictions

Diarrhea related to excessive excretion of fats in stools secondary to insufficient pancreatic enzymes

High Risk for Altered Health Maintenance related to insufficient knowledge of disease, contraindications (alcohol, coffee, large meals), dietary management, and follow-up care

Ineffective Denial related to acknowledgement of alcohol abuse or dependency

Gastrointestinal Disorders

ESOPHAGEAL DISORDERS (Esophagitis, Hiatal Hernia)

Collaborative Problems

PC: Hemorrhage
PC: Gastric ulcers

Nursing Diagnoses

High Risk for Altered Nutrition: Less Than Body Requirements related to anorexia, heartburn, and dysphagia

Altered Comfort: Heartburn related to regurgitation and eructation

High Risk for Altered Health Maintenance related to insufficient knowledge of condition, dietary management, hazards of alcohol and tobacco, positioning after meals, pharmacological therapy, and weight reduction (if indicated)

GASTROENTERITIS

Collaborative Problem

PC: Fluid/electrolyte imbalance

Nursing Diagnoses

> High Risk for Fluid Volume Deficit related to vomiting and
> diarrhea
> Altered Comfort related to abdominal cramps, diarrhea, and
> vomiting
> High Risk for Altered Health Maintenance related to
> insufficient knowledge of condition, dietary restrictions,
> and signs and symptoms of complications

HEMORRHOIDS/ANAL FISSURE (Nonsurgical)

Collaborative Problems

> *PC: Bleeding*
> *PC: Strangulation*
> *PC: Thrombosis*

Nursing Diagnoses

> Altered Comfort related to pain on defecation
> High Risk for Constipation related to fear of pain on
> defecation
> High Risk for Altered Health Maintenance related to
> insufficient knowledge of condition, bowel routine, diet
> instructions, exercise program, and perianal care

INFLAMMATORY INTESTINAL DISORDERS
(Diverticulosis, Diverticulitis, Regional Enteritis,
Ulcerative Colitis)

Collaborative Problems

> *PC: Gastrointestinal bleeding*
> *PC: Anal fissure*
> *PC: Perianal abscess, fissure, fistula*
> *PC: Fluid/electrolyte imbalances*
> *PC: Toxic megacolon*
> *PC: Anemia*
> *PC: Intestinal obstruction*
> *PC: Urolithiasis*
> *PC: Growth retardation*

Nursing Diagnoses

> Altered Comfort related to intestinal inflammatory process

Diarrhea related to intestinal inflammatory process

Colonic Constipation related to inadequate dietary intake of fiber

High Risk for Impaired Skin Integrity (Perianal) related to diarrhea and chemical irritants

High Risk for Ineffective Individual Coping related to the chronicity of the condition and the lack of definitive treatment

Altered Nutrition: Less Than Body Requirements related to diarrhea, dietary restrictions, and pain with or after eating and/or painful ulcers in the mouth

High Risk for Altered Health Maintenance related to insufficient knowledge of condition, dietary restrictions, treatment, and signs and symptoms of complications

PEPTIC ULCER

Collaborative Problems

PC: Hemorrhage
PC: Perforation
PC: Pyloric obstruction

Nursing Diagnoses

Altered Comfort related to lesions secondary to increased gastric secretions

High Risk for Colonic Constipation related to diet restrictions and side effects of medications

High Risk for Altered Health Maintenance related to insufficient knowledge of condition, dietary restrictions, contraindications (certain medications, tobacco, caffeine, alcohol), and signs and symptoms of complications

Renal/Urinary Tract Disorders

NEUROGENIC BLADDER

Collaborative Problems

PC: Renal calculi
PC: Autonomic dysreflexia

Nursing Diagnoses

High Risk for Impaired Skin Integrity related to constant irritation from urine

High Risk for Infection related to retention of urine and/or introduction of urinary catheter

High Risk for Social Isolation related to embarrassment and fear of offending others with odor from urine

Urinary Retention related to chronically overfilled bladder with loss of sensation of bladder distention

Reflex Incontinence related to absence of sensation to void and loss of ability to inhibit bladder contraction

High Risk for Dysreflexia related to reflex stimulation of sympathetic nervous system secondary to loss of autonomic control

Urge Incontinence related to disruption of the inhibitory efferent impulses secondary to brain or spinal cord dysfunction.

High Risk for Altered Health Maintenance related to insufficient knowledge of etiology, treatment/bladder retraining programs, signs and symptoms of complications, and prevention of complications

RENAL FAILURE (Acute)

Collaborative Problems

PC: Fluid overload
PC: Hyperphosphatemia
PC: Hyperkalemia
PC: Metabolic acidosis
PC: Electrolyte imbalances

Nursing Diagnoses

Altered Nutrition: Less Than Body Requirements related to anorexia, nausea, vomiting, loss of taste, loss of smell, stomatitis, and unpalatable diet

High Risk for Infection related to invasive procedures

Anxiety related to present status and unknown prognosis

RENAL FAILURE (Chronic, Uremia)

See also *Peritoneal Dialysis and Hemodialysis,* if indicated.

Collaborative Problems

PC: *Fluid/electrolyte imbalance*
PC: *Gastrointestinal bleeding*
PC: *Hyperparathyroidism*
PC: *Pathological fractures*
PC: *Malnutrition*
PC: *Anemia, thrombocytopenia*
PC: *Fluid overload*
PC: *Hypoalbuminemia*
PC: *Polyneuropathy (peripheral)*
PC: *Congestive heart failure*
PC: *Pulmonary edema*
PC: *Metabolic acidosis*
PC: *Pleural effusion*
PC: *Pericarditis*

Nursing Diagnoses

Altered Nutrition: Less Than Body Requirements related to anorexia, nausea/vomiting, loss of taste/smell, stomatitis, and/or unpalatable diet

Altered Sexuality Patterns related to (examples) decreased libido, impotence, amenorrhea, sterility

Self-Concept Disturbance related to effects of limitation on achievement of developmental tasks

High Risk for Social Isolation (Individual, Family) related to disability and treatment requirements

Altered Comfort related to (examples) fatigue, headaches, fluid retention, anemia

Fatigue related to insufficient oxygenation secondary to anemia

Altered Comfort related to pruritus secondary to abnormal deposition of calcium

High Risk for Infection related to invasive procedures

Powerlessness related to progessively disabling nature of disorder

High Risk for Altered Health Maintenance related to insufficient knowledge of condition, fluid and sodium restrictions, dietary restrictions (protein, potassium, sodium), daily recording of intake, output and weights, pharmacological therapy, signs and symptoms of complications, follow-up visits, and community resources (support groups)

URINARY TRACT INFECTIONS
(Cystitis, Pyelonephritis, Glomerulonephritis)

See also *Acute Renal Failure.*

Nursing Diagnoses

Chronic Pain related to inflammation and tissue trauma
Altered Comfort related to inflammation and infection
High Risk for Altered Nutrition: Less Than Body
  Requirements related to anorexia secondary to malaise
High Risk for Ineffective Individual Coping related to the
  chronicity of the condition
High Risk for Altered Health Maintenance related to
  insufficient knowledge of prevention of recurrence
  (adequate fluid intake, frequent voiding, hygiene
  measures [personal post-toileting], and voiding after
  sexual activity), signs and symptoms of recurrence, and
  pharmacological therapy

UROLITHIASIS (Renal Calculi)

Collaborative Problems

PC: Pyelonephritis
PC: Acute renal failure

Nursing Diagnoses

Altered Comfort related to inflammation secondary to
  irritation of stone
Diarrhea related to renointestinal reflexes
High Risk for Altered Health Maintenance related to
  insufficient knowledge of prevention of recurrence,
  dietary restrictions, and fluid requirements

Neurological Disorders

BRAIN TUMOR

Because this disorder can cause alterations varying
from minimal to profound, the following possible
nursing diagnoses reflect individuals with varying
degrees of involvement.

See also *Surgery (General, Cranial).*
See also *Cancer.*

Collaborative Problems

PC: *Increased intracranial pressure*
PC: *Paralysis*
PC: *Hyperthermia*
PC: *Motor losses*
PC: *Sensory losses*
PC: *Cognitive losses*

Nursing Diagnoses

High Risk for Injury related to gait disorders, vertigo and/or visual disturbances, secondary to compression/displacement of brain tissue

Anxiety related to implications of condition and uncertain future

(Specify) Self-Care Deficit related to inability to perform/difficulty in performing activities of daily living secondary to sensory–motor impairments

Altered Nutrition: Less Than Body Requirements related to dysphagia and fatigue

Grieving related to actual/perceived loss of function and uncertain future

Impaired Physical Mobility related to sensory–motor impairment

Altered Comfort: Headache related to compression/displacement of brain tissue and increased intracranial pressure

Altered Family Processes related to the nature of the condition, role disturbances, and uncertain future

Self-Concept Disturbance related to interruption in achieving/failure to achieve developmental tasks (childhood, adolescence, young adulthood, middle age)

High Risk for Fluid Volume Deficit related to vomiting secondary to increased intracranial pressure

High Risk for Injury related to impaired/uncontrolled sensory–motor function

CEREBROVASCULAR ACCIDENT

Because this disorder can cause alterations varying from minimal to profound, the following possible nursing diagnoses reflect individuals with varying degrees of involvement.

Collaborative Problems

PC: Increased intracranial pressure
PC: Pneumonia
PC: Atelectasis

Nursing Diagnoses

Sensory–Perceptual Alterations: (specify) related to hypoxia and compression or displacement of brain tissue

Impaired Physical Mobility related to decreased motor function of (specify) secondary to damage to upper motor neurons

High Risk for Colonic Constipation related to prolonged periods of immobility, inadequate fluid intake, and inadequate nutritional intake

Impaired Verbal Communication related to dysarthria and/or aphasia

High Risk for Injury related to visual field deficits, motor deficits, perception deficits, and/or inability to perceive environmental hazards

Activity Intolerance related to deconditioning secondary to fatigue and weakness

High Risk for Disuse Syndrome related to effects of immobility

(Specify type) Incontinence related to (examples) loss of bladder tone, loss of sphincter control, or inability to perceive bladder cues

(Specify) Self-Care Deficit related to (specify)

Impaired Swallowing related to (specify)

Grieving (Family, Individual) related to actual or perceived loss of function and inability to meet role responsibilities

High Risk for Impaired Social Interactions related to difficulty communicating and embarrassment regarding disabilities

High Risk for Fluid Volume Deficit related to dysphagia and difficulty in obtaining fluids secondary to fatigue, weakness or sensory–motor deficits

High Risk for Impaired Home Maintenance Management related to altered ability to maintain self at home secondary to sensory–motor/cognitive deficits

Unilateral Neglect related to (specify site) secondary to effects of cerebral pathology

High Risk for Altered Health Maintenance related to insufficient knowledge of condition, pharmacological therapy, self-care activities of daily living, home care, speech therapy, exercise program, community resources, self-help groups, and signs and symptoms of complications

High Risk for Impaired Skin Integrity related to immobility, incontinence, sensory deficits, and/or motor deficits

High Risk for Self-Concept Disturbance related to effects of prolonged debilitating condition on achieving developmental tasks and life-style

NERVOUS SYSTEM DISORDERS (Degenerative, Demyelinating, Inflammatory, Myasthenia Gravis, Multiple Sclerosis, Muscular Dystrophy, Parkinson's Disease, Guillain-Barré Syndrome, Amyotrophic Lateral Sclerosis)

Because the alterations associated with these disorders can range from minimal to profound, the following possible nursing diagnoses reflect individuals with varying degrees of involvement.

Collaborative Problems

PC: Renal failure
PC: Pneumonia
PC: Atelectasis

Nursing Diagnoses

Self-Concept Disturbance related to prolonged debilitating condition and interruption in achieving developmental tasks (adolescence, young adulthood, middle age)

High Risk for Injury related to visual disturbances, unsteady gait, weakness, and/or uncontrolled movements

Impaired Verbal Communication related to dysarthrias secondary to cranial nerve impairment

High Risk for Altered Nutrition: Less Than Body Requirements related to dysphagia/chewing difficulties secondary to cranial nerve impairment

Activity Intolerance related to fatigue and difficulty in performing activities of daily living

High Risk for Disuse Syndrome related to effects of immobility

Urinary Retention related to sensory–motor deficits.

Grieving (Client, Family) related to nature of disease and uncertain prognosis

Altered Sexuality Patterns (Female) related to loss of libido, fatigue, and decreased perineal sensation

High Risk for Injury related to decreased perception of pain, touch, and temperature

Altered Family Processes related to nature of disease, role disturbances, and uncertain future

High Risk for Diversional Activity Deficits related to inability to perform usual job-related/recreational activities

High Risk for Social Isolation related to mobility difficulties and associated embarrassment

Impaired Home Maintenance Management related to inability to care for/difficulty in caring for self/home secondary to disability or unavailable or inadequate caregiver

Parental Role Conflict related to disruptions secondary to disability

Ineffective Individual Coping related to implications of disease and its prognosis

(Specify) Self-Care Deficits related to (examples) headaches, muscular spasms, joint pain, fatigue, paresis/paralysis

Powerlessness related to inability to control symptoms and the unpredictable nature of the condition (*i.e.,* remissions/exacerbations)

Incontinence: (specify type) related to (specify)

Ineffective Airway Clearance related to impaired ability to cough

High Risk for Altered Health Maintenance related to insufficient knowledge of condition, risks (severe fatigue, infection, cold, fever, pregnancy), exercise program, medications, nutritional requirements, and community services

PRESENILE DEMENTIA (Alzheimer's Disease, Huntington's Disease)

See also *Nervous System Diseases.**

* Because these disorders can cause alterations similar to those in the nervous system disorder category, the reader is referred to the latter section to review additional possible diagnoses.

Nursing Diagnoses

High Risk for Injury related to lack of awareness of
environmental hazards

Altered Thought Processes related to an inability to evaluate
reality secondary to cerebral neuron degeneration

Impaired Physical Mobility related to gait instability

High Risk for Altered Family Processes related to effects of
condition on relationships, role responsibilities, and
finances

Impaired Home Maintenance Management related to
inability to care for/difficulty in caring for self/home or
inadequate/unavailable caregiver

Unilateral Neglect related to (specify site) secondary to
neurological pathology

(Specify) Self-Care Deficit related to (specify)

Decisional Conflict related to placement of person in a care
facility

SEIZURE DISORDERS (Epilepsy)

If the client is a child, see also *Developmental
Problems/Needs.*

Nursing Diagnoses

High Risk for Injury related to uncontrolled tonic/clonic
movements during seizure episode

High Risk for Ineffective Airway Clearance related to
relaxation of tongue and gag reflexes secondary to
disruption in muscle innervation

High Risk for Social Isolation related to fear of
embarrassment secondary to having a seizure in public

High Risk for Altered Growth and Development related to
interruption in achieving/failure to achieve developmental
tasks (childhood, adolescence, young adulthood, middle
age)

High Risk for Altered Oral Mucous Membrane related to
effects of drug therapy on oral tissue

Fear related to unpredictable nature of seizures and
embarrassment

High Risk for Altered Health Maintenance related to
insufficient knowledge of condition, medication, activity
versus rest (balance), care during seizure, community

resources, possible environmental hazards (swimming, diving, operating machinery), and identification (medallion, card)

SPINAL CORD INJURY*

Collaborative Problems

PC: Accidental extension of injury (acute)
PC: Autonomic dysreflexia (postacute)
PC: Electrolyte imbalance
PC: Spinal shock
PC: Hemorrhage
PC: Respiratory complications
PC: Paralytic ileus
PC: Sepsis
PC: Hydronephrosis
PC: Gastrointestinal bleeding
PC: Thrombophlebitis (deep vein)
PC: Postural hypotension
PC: Fracture dislocation
PC: Cardiovascular
PC: Hypoxemia
PC: Urinary retention
PC: Pyelonephritis
PC: Renal insufficiency

Nursing Diagnoses

(Specify) Self-Care Deficit related to sensory-motor deficits secondary to level of spinal cord injury

Impaired Verbal Communication related to impaired ability to speak words secondary to tracheostomy

Fear related to possible abandonment by others, changes in role responsibilities, effects of injury on life-style, multiple tests, and procedures and/or separation from support systems

---

* Because disabilities associated with spinal cord injuries can be varied (hemiparesis, quadriparesis, diplegia, monoplegia, triplegia, paraplegia), the nurse will have to specify clearly the individual's limitations in the diagnostic statement.

Altered Family Processes related to adjustment requirements for the situation (time, energy, financial, physical care, prognosis)

High Risk for Aspiration related to inability to cough secondary to level of injury

High Risk for Impaired Home Maintenance Management related to inadequate resources, housing, or impaired caregiver(s)

Anxiety related to perceived effects of injury on life-style and unknown future

Grieving related to loss of body function and its effects on life-style

High Risk for Social Isolation (Individual/Family) related to disability or requirements for the caregiver(s)

High Risk for Altered Parenting related to inadequate resources and coping mechanisms

Self-Concept Disturbance related to effects of limitations on achievement of developmental tasks

High Risk for Fluid Volume Deficit related to difficulty obtaining liquids

High Risk for Altered Nutrition: More Than Body Requirements related to imbalance of intake versus activity expenditures

High Risk for Altered Nutrition: Less Than Body Requirements related to anorexia and increased metabolic requirements

High Risk for Diversional Activity Deficit related to effects of limitations on ability to participate in recreational activities

Reflex Incontinence or Urinary Retention related to bladder atony secondary to sensory-motor deficits

High Risk for Disuse Syndrome related to effects of immobility

High Risk for Injury related to impaired ability to control movements and sensory-motor deficits

High Risk for Infection related to urinary stasis, repeated catheterizations, and invasive procedures (skeletal tongs, tracheostomy, venous lines, surgical sites)

High Risk for Altered Sexuality Patterns related to (examples) inability to achieve or sustain an erection for intercourse, limitations on sexual performance, value conflicts regarding sexual expression, depression/ anxiety, decreased libido, altered self-concept, unwilling/ uninformed partner

Bowel Incontinence: Reflexic related to lack of voluntary

sphincter control secondary to spinal cord injury
above T_{11}
Bowel Incontinence: Areflexia related to lack of voluntary
sphincter control secondary to spinal cord injury involving
sacral reflex arc (S_2–S_4)
High Risk for Altered Health Maintenance related to
insufficient knowledge of condition, treatment regimen,
rehabilitation, and assistance devices

UNCONSCIOUS INDIVIDUAL

See also *Mechanical Ventilation,* if indicated.

Collaborative Problems

PC: Respiratory insufficiency
PC: Pneumonia
PC: Atelectasis
PC: Fluid/electrolyte imbalance
PC: Negative nitrogen balance
PC: Bladder distention
PC: Seizures
PC: Stress ulcers
PC: Increased intracranial pressure
PC: Sepsis
PC: Thrombophlebitis
PC: Renal calculi

Nursing Diagnoses

High Risk for Infection related to immobility and invasive
devices (tracheostomy, Foley catheter, venous lines)
High Risk for Impaired Tissue Integrity: Corneal related to
corneal drying secondary to open eyes and lower tear
production
Anxiety/Fear (Family) related to present state of individual
and uncertain prognosis
High Risk for Altered Oral Mucous Membrane related to
inability to perform mouth care on self and pooling of
secretions
Self-Care Deficit Syndrome related to unconscious state
Total Incontinence related to unconscious state
High Risk for Disuse Syndrome related to effects of
immobility

High Risk for Ineffective Airway Clearance related to stasis
of secretions secondary to inadequate cough and
decreased mobility

Sensory Disorders

OPHTHALMIC DISORDERS (Cataracts, Detached
Retina, Glaucoma, Inflammations)

See also *Cataract Extractions*
See also *Scleral Buckle/Vitrectomy*

Collaborative Problem

PC: Increased intraocular pressure

Nursing Diagnoses

High Risk for Injury related to impaired vision secondary to
condition or eye patches

Pain related to (examples) inflammation (lid, lacrimal
structures, conjunctiva, uveal tract, retina, cornea,
sclera), infection, increased intraocular pressure, ocular
tumors

High Risk for Noncompliance related to side effects of
medications, difficulty remembering, and financial impact

High Risk for Social Isolation related to fear of injury or
embarrassment outside home environment

High Risk for Impaired Home Maintenance Management
related to impaired ability to perform activities of daily
living secondary to impaired vision

(Specify) Self-Care Deficit related to impaired vision

Anxiety related to the actual or possible loss of vision and/
or surgical procedure

High Risk for Altered Health Maintenance related to
insufficient knowledge of condition, eye care,
medications, safety measures, activity restrictions, and
follow-up care

High Risk for Self-Concept Disturbance related to effects of
visual limitations

OTIC DISORDERS (Infections, Mastoiditis, Trauma)

Nursing Diagnoses

High Risk for Injury related to disturbances of balance and impaired ability to detect environmental hazards

Impaired Verbal Communication related to difficulty understanding others secondary to impaired hearing

High Risk for Impaired Social Interactions related to difficulty in participating in conversations

Social Isolation related to the lack of contact with others secondary to fear and embarrassment of hearing losses

Pain related to inflammation, infection, tinnitus, and/or vertigo

Fear related to actual or possible loss of hearing

High Risk for Altered Health Maintenance related to insufficient knowledge of condition, medications, prevention of recurrence, hazards (swimming, air travel, showers), signs and symptoms of complications, and hearing aids

Integumentary Disorders

DERMATOLOGICAL DISORDERS (Dermatitis, Psoriasis, Eczema)

Nursing Diagnoses

Impaired Skin Integrity related to lesions and inflammatory response

Pruritus related to dermal eruptions

High Risk for Impaired Social Interaction related to fear of embarrassment and negative reactions of others

High Risk for Self-Concept Disturbance related to appearance and response of others

High Risk for Altered Health Maintenance related to insufficient knowledge of condition, topical agents, and contraindications

PRESSURE ULCERS*

Collaborative Problem

PC: Septicemia

Nursing Diagnoses

High Risk for Infection related to susceptibility of open wound

Impaired Tissue Integrity: Pressure Ulcers related to (examples) skin deficits (edema, obesity, dryness), impaired oxygen transport (edema, peripheral anemia), chemical/mechanical irritants (casts, radiation, incontinence), nutritional deficits, systemic deficits (infection, cancer, renal or hepatic disorders, diabetes mellitus), sensory deficits (confusion, cord injury, neuropathy), immobility

Impaired Home Maintenance Management related to complexity of care or unavailable caregiver

The following are some situations that contribute to pressure sore development. If the situation is present in the client, the nursing diagnosis can be used.

Altered Nutrition: Less Than Body Requirements related to anorexia secondary to (specify)

Impaired Physical Mobility related to (specify)

Fluid Volume Excess: Edema related to (specify)

Total Incontinence related to (specify)

Sensory–Perceptual Alterations: Tactile related to (specify)

High Risk for Altered Health Maintenance related to insufficient knowledge of causes, preventive measures, and treatment

SKIN INFECTIONS (Impetigo, Herpes Zoster, Fungal Infections)

Collaborative Problems (Herpes Zoster)

PC: Postherpetic neuralgia
PC: Keratitis

---

* The factors that can contribute to the development of pressure sores are varied and complex; therefore, the nurse must assess for and identify the specific related factors for the individual.

PC: *Uveitis*
PC: *Corneal ulceration*
PC: *Blindness*

Nursing Diagnoses

Impaired Skin Integrity related to lesions and pruritus
Altered Comfort related to dermal eruptions and pruritus
High Risk for Infection Transmission related to contagious
nature of the organism
High Risk for Altered Health Maintenance related to
insufficient knowledge of condition (causes, course),
prevention, treatment, and skin care

THERMAL INJURIES (Burns, Severe Hypothermia)
Acute Period
Collaborative Problems

PC: *Death*
PC: *Fluid-loss shock*
PC: *Fluid overload*
PC: *Anemia*
PC: *Negative nitrogen balance*
PC: *Electrolyte imbalance*
PC: *Metabolic acidosis*
PC: *Respiratory*
PC: *Thromboembolism*
PC: *Septicemia*
PC: *Emboli*
PC: *Graft rejection*
PC: *Hypothermia*
PC: *Hypokalemia/hyperkalemia*
PC: *Curling's ulcer*
PC: *Paralytic ileus*
PC: *Convulsive disorders*
PC: *Stress diabetes*
PC: *Adrenocortical insufficiency*
PC: *Pneumonia*
PC: *Renal failure*
PC: *Compartmental syndrome*

Nursing Diagnoses

High Risk for Infection related to loss of protective layer
secondary to thermal injury

Altered Nutrition: Less Than Body Requirements related to increased caloric requirement secondary to thermal injury and inability to ingest increased requirements

Impaired Physical Mobility related to acute pain secondary to thermal injury and treatments

(Specify) Self-Care Deficit related to impaired range of motion ability secondary to pain and contractures

Fear related to painful procedures and possibility of death

High Risk for Social Isolation related to infection control measures and separation from family and support systems

High Risk for Disuse Syndrome related to effects of pain and immobility

Sleep Pattern Disturbances related to position restrictions, pain, and treatment interruptions

High Risk for Sensory–Perceptual Alterations related to (examples) excessive environmental stimuli, stress, imposed immobility, sleep deprivation, protective isolation

Grieving (Family, Individual) related to actual or perceived impact of injury on life (appearance, relationships, occupation)

Anxiety related to sudden injury, treatments, uncertainty of outcome, and pain

Anxiety related to pain secondary to thermal injury treatments and immobility

Postacute Period

If individual is a child, see also *Developmental Problems/Needs*.

Collaborative Problem

PC: Same as in acute period

Nursing Diagnoses

Diversional Activity Deficit related to monotony of confinement

High Risk for Social Isolation related to embarrassment and the response of others to injury

Powerlessness related to inability to control present situation

Self-Concept Disturbance related to effects of thermal injury on achieving developmental tasks (child, adolescent, adult)

Fear related to uncertain future and effects of injury on life-style, relationships, occupation

Impaired Home Maintenance Management related to long-term requirements of treatments

High Risk for Altered Health Maintenance related to insufficient knowledge of condition, treatments, nutritional requirements, pain management, home care, rehabilitation, and community services

Musculoskeletal/ Connective Tissue Disorders

FRACTURED JAW

Nursing Diagnoses

High Risk for Aspiration related to inadequate cough secondary to pain and fixative devices

Altered Oral Mucous Membrane related to difficulty in performing oral hygiene secondary to fixation devices

Impaired Verbal Communication related to fixation devices

Altered Comfort related to tissue trauma and fixation device

High Risk for Altered Nutrition: Less Than Body Requirements related to inability to ingest solid food secondary to fixation devices

High Risk for Altered Health Maintenance related to insufficient knowledge of mouth care, nutritional requirements, signs and symptoms of infection, and procedure for emergency wire cutting (*e.g.,* vomiting)

FRACTURES

See also *Casts.*

Collaborative Problems

PC: Neurovascular (paresis, paralysis)
PC: Fat embolism syndrome

PC: Shock (hemorrhagic, hypovolemic)
PC: Osteomyelitis
PC: Compartmental syndrome
PC: Contracture
PC: Thromboemboli

Nursing Diagnoses

Altered Comfort related to tissue trauma and immobility
High Risk for Impaired Skin Integrity related to mechanical irritants/compression secondary to casts and traction
High Risk for Disuse Syndrome related to effects of immobility secondary to casts/traction
High Risk for Infection related to invasive fixation devices
(Specify) Self-Care Deficits related to impaired ability to use upper/lower limb secondary to immobilization device
Diversional Activity Deficit related to boredom of confinement secondary to immobilization devices
High Risk for Impaired Home Maintenance Management related to (examples) fixation device, impaired physical mobility, unavailable support system
Altered Family Processes related to difficulty of ill person in assuming role responsibilities secondary to limited motion
High Risk for Altered Health Maintenance related to insufficient knowledge of condition, cast care, use of assistive devices, signs and symptoms of complications (numbness, pallor, decreased sensation) and limitations
High Risk for Altered Respiratory Function related to immobility secondary to traction or their fixation devices

LOW BACK PAIN

Collaborative Problems

PC: Pulposus
PC: Herniated nucleus pulposus

Nursing Diagnoses

Pain related to (examples) acute lumbosacral strain, weak muscles, osteoarthritis of spine, unstable lumbosacral ligaments, spinal stenosis, intervertebral disk problem
Impaired Physical Mobility related to decreased mobility and flexibility secondary to muscle spasm

350

High Risk for Ineffective Individual Coping related to effects of chronic pain on life-style

High Risk for Altered Family Processes related to impaired ability to meet role responsibilities (financial, home, social)

High Risk for Altered Health Maintenance related to insufficient knowledge of condition, exercise program, noninvasive pain relief methods (relaxation, imagery), and proper posture and body mechanics

OSTEOMYELITIS

Collaborative Problem

PC: Bone abscess

Nursing Diagnoses

Pain related to soft tissue edema secondary to infection

Impaired Physical Mobility related to limited range of motion of affected bone

High Risk for Altered Health Maintenance related to insufficient knowledge of condition, etiology, course, pharmacological therapy, nutritional requirements, pain management, and signs and symptoms of complications

OSTEOPOROSIS

Collaborative Problems

PC: Fractures
PC: Kyphosis
PC: Paralytic ileus

Nursing Diagnoses

Pain related to muscle spasm and fractures

Altered Health Maintenance related to insufficient daily physical activity

Altered Nutrition: Less Than Body Requirements related to inadequate dietary intake of calcium, protein, and vitamin D

Impaired Physical Mobility related to limited range of motion secondary to skeletal changes

Fear related to unpredictable nature of condition

High Risk for Altered Health Maintenance related to insufficient knowledge of condition, nutritional therapy, activity program, safety precautions, and prevention

INFLAMMATORY JOINT DISEASE

Collaborative Problems

PC: Septic arthritis
PC: Sjögren's syndrome
PC: Neuropathy
PC: Anemia, leukoplenea

Nursing Diagnoses

Pain related to inflammatory response and joint immobility (stiffness)

(Specify) Self-Care Deficits related to loss of motion, muscle weakness, pain, stiffness, or fatigue

Fatigue related to decreased mobility, stiffness

Powerlessness related to physical and psychological changes imposed by the disease

Ineffective Individual Coping related to the stress imposed by exacerbations (unpredictable)

Self-Concept Disturbance related to physical and psychological changes imposed by the disease

Fatigue related to effects of chronic inflammatory process

High Risk for Altered Oral Mucous Membrane related to medications and/or Sjögren's syndrome

Impaired Home Maintenance Management related to impaired ability to perform household responsibilities secondary to limited mobility

Sleep Pattern Disturbance related to pain and/or secondary to fibrositis

Impaired Physical Mobility related to pain and limited motion of limbs

Altered Sexuality Patterns related to difficulty assuming position (female), fatigue, pain, or decreased lubrication

High Risk for Social Isolation related to ambulation difficulties and fatigue

Altered Family Processes related to difficulty in assuming/ inability to assume role responsibilities secondary to fatigue and limited motion

High Risk for Altered Health Maintenance related to insufficient knowledge of condition, rest versus exercise, self-help groups, assistive devices, quackery, heat therapy, and pharmacological therapy

Infectious/ Immunodeficient Disorders

LUPUS ERYTHEMATOSUS (Systemic)

See also *Rheumatic Diseases.*
See also *Corticosteroid Therapy.*

Collaborative Problems

PC: Polymyositis
PC: Vasculitis
PC: Hematological
PC: Raynaud's disease
PC: Renal failure secondary to corticosteroid therapy
PC: Pericarditis
PC: Pleuritis

Nursing Diagnoses

Powerlessness related to unpredictable course (remissions, exacerbations)

Ineffective Individual Coping related to unpredictable course and altered appearance

High Risk for Social Isolation related to embarrassment and the response of others to appearance

High Risk for Self-Concept Disturbance related to inability to achieve developmental tasks secondary to disabling condition

High Risk for Injury related to increased dermal vulnerability

Fatigue related to decreased mobility and effects of chronic inflammation

High Risk for Altered Health Maintenance related to insufficient knowledge of condition, rest/activity balance, and pharmacological therapy

MENINGITIS/ENCEPHALITIS

Collaborative Problems

PC: Fluid/electrolyte imbalance
PC: Cerebral edema
PC: Adrenal damage

353

PC: *Circulatory collapse*
PC: *Hemorrhage*
PC: *Seizures*
PC: *Septicemia*
PC: *Alkalosis*
PC: *Increased intracranial pressure*

Nursing Diagnoses

High Risk for Infection transmission related to contagious nature of organism

Altered Comfort related to headache, fever, neck pain secondary to meningeal irritation

Activity Intolerance related to fatigue and malaise secondary to infection

High Risk for Impaired Skin Integrity related to immobility, dehydration, and diaphoresis

High Risk for Altered Oral Mucous Membrane related to dehydration and impaired ability to perform mouth care

High Risk for Altered Nutrition: Less Than Body Requirements related to anorexia, fatigue, nausea, and vomiting

High Risk for Altered Respiratory Function related to immobility and pain

High Risk for Injury related to restlessness and disorientation secondary to meningeal irritation

Altered Family Processes related to critical nature of situation and uncertain prognosis

Anxiety related to treatments, environment, and risk of death

High Risk for Altered Health Maintenance related to insufficient knowledge of condition, treatments, pharmacological therapy, rest/activity balance, signs and symptoms of complications, follow-up care, and prevention of recurrence

SEXUALLY TRANSMITTED INFECTIOUS DISEASES (Venereal Diseases, Herpes)

Nursing Diagnoses

High Risk for Infection Transmission related to lack of knowledge of the contagious nature of the disease

Fear related to nature of the condition and its implications for life-style

Grieving related to chronicity of condition (herpes)
Altered Comfort related to inflammatory process
Hopelessness related to incurable nature of condition
Social Isolation related to fear of transmitting disease to
    others
High Risk for Altered Health Maintenance related to
    insufficient knowledge of condition, modes of
    transmission, consequences of repeated infections, and
    prevention of recurrences

ACQUIRED IMMUNODEFICIENCY SYNDROME (AIDS) (Adult)

See also *End-Stage Cancer.*

Collaborative Problems

PC: Encephalopathy
PC: Septicemia
PC: Gastrointestinal bleeding
PC: Pneumocystis carinii pneumonia
PC: Meningitis
PC: Esophagitis
PC: Electrolyte imbalances
PC: Opportunistic infections
PC: Malignancies
PC: Myelosuppression

Nursing Diagnoses

Altered Comfort related to headache, fever secondary to
    inflammation of cerebral tissue
Fatigue related to pulmonary insufficiency, chronic
    infections, malnutrition secondary to chronic diarrhea and
    gastrointestinal malabsorption
High Risk for Impaired Skin Integrity related to perineal and
    anal tissue excoriation secondary to diarrhea and chronic
    genital candida or herpes lesions
Altered Nutrition: Less Than Body Requirements related to
    chronic diarrhea, gastrointestinal malabsorption, fatigue,
    anorexia, and/or oral/esophageal lesions
High Risk for Infection Transmission related to contagious
    nature of blood and body excretions
Social Isolation related to rejection of others after diagnosis

Hopelessness related to nature of the condition and poor prognosis

Powerlessness related to unpredictable nature of condition

Altered Family Processes related to the nature of the AIDS condition, role disturbance, and uncertain future

Anxiety related to perceived effects of illness on life-style and unknown future

Grieving related to loss of body function and its effects on life-style

High Risk for Altered Health Maintenance related to insufficient knowledge of condition, medication therapy, modes of transmission, infection control, and community services

Powerlessness related to change from curative to palliative status

High Risk for Infection related to increased susceptibility secondary to compromised immune system

High Risk for Altered Oral Mucous Membrane related to compromised immune system

Neoplastic Disorders

CANCER (Initial Diagnosis)

See also specific types.

Nursing Diagnoses

Anxiety related to unfamiliar hospital environment, uncertainty about cancer treatment outcomes, feelings of loss and grief, feelings of helplessness and/or hopelessness, and fear of death

Grieving of family members/significant others related to changes in life-style or role relationship and fear that patient will die

Powerlessness related to perceived loss or control secondary to uncertainty about prognosis and outcome of cancer treatment

High Risk for Altered Family Process related to (examples) recent cancer diagnosis, treatment plan creating significant changes in life-style, role, or relationships, little experience with losses, nonsupportive family, high anxiety among family members and patient (immmediate

family includes children and adolescents), and financ̲
problems

Decisional Conflict related to choices of treatment modality

High Risk for Self-Concept Disturbance related to changes
in life-style, role responsibilities, and appearance

High Risk for Social Isolation related to fear of rejection or
actual rejection secondary to fear

High Risk for Spiritual Distress related to conflicts centering
around the meaning of life, cancer, spiritual beliefs, and
death

High Risk for Altered Health Maintenance related to
insufficient knowledge of cancer, cancer treatment
options, diagnostic tests, effects of treatment, treatment
plan, and support services

CANCER (General; Applies to Malignancies in Varied Sites and Stages)

Nursing Diagnoses

Altered Oral Mucous Membranes related to (examples)
disease process, therapy, radiation, chemotherapy,
inadequate oral hygiene, and altered nutritional/hydration
status

High Risk for Altered Sexuality Patterns related to
(examples) fear, grieving, changes in body image,
anatomical changes, pain, fatigue (treatments, disease),
or change in role responsibilities

Altered Comfort related to disease process and treatments

Diarrhea related to (examples) disease process,
chemotherapy, radiation, and medications

Colonic Constipation related to (examples) disease
process, chemotherapy, radiation therapy, immobility,
dietary intake, and medications

Self-Concept Disturbance related to (examples) anatomical
changes, role disturbances, uncertain future, disruption of
life-style

(Specify) Self-Care Deficits related to fatigue, pain, or
depression

High Risk for Infection related to altered immune system

Altered Nutrition: Less Than Body Requirements related to
anorexia, fatigue, nausea, and vomiting secondary to
disease process and treatments

High Risk for Injury related to disorientation, weakness,

sensory-perceptual deterioration, and/or skeletal/muscle deterioration

High Risk for Disuse Syndrome related to effects of immobility, altered nutrition status, and altered circulation

High Risk for Fluid Volume Deficit related to (examples) altered ability/desire to obtain fluids, weakness, vomiting, diarrhea, depression, and fatigue

High Risk for Impaired Home Maintenance Management related to (examples) lack of knowledge, lack of resources, (support system, equipment, finances), motor deficits, sensory deficits, cognitive deficits, and emotional deficits

High Risk for Impaired Social Interactions related to fear of rejection or actual rejection of others after diagnosis

Powerlessness related to inability to control situation

Altered Family Process related to (examples) stress of diagnosis/treatments, role disturbances, and uncertain future

Grieving (Family, Individual) related to actual, perceived, or anticipated losses associated with diagnosis

High Risk for Altered Health Maintenance related to insufficient knowledge of disease, misconceptions, treatments, home care, and support agencies

CANCER (End-stage)

See also specific types.

Collaborative Problems

PC: Hypercalcemia
PC: Intracerebral metastasis
PC: Malignant effusions
PC: Narcotic toxicity
PC: Pathological fractures
PC: Spinal cord compression
PC: Superior vena cava syndrome
PC: Negative nitrogen imbalance
PC: Myelosuppression

Nursing Diagnoses

Altered Nutrition: Less Than Body Requirements related to decreased oral intake and increased metabolic rate

Colonic Constipation related to decreased dietary fiber

intake, decreased intestinal mobility secondary to
    narcotic medication, and inactivity
Pain related to inadequate relief from measures
Altered Comfort related to pruritus secondary to dry skin
    and biliary obstruction
Ineffective Airway Clearance related to inability to cough up
    secretions secondary to weakness, increased viscosity,
    and pain
Impaired Physical Mobility related to pain, sedation,
    weakness, fatigue, and edema
High Risk for Injury related to weakness, fatigue, and/or
    confusion
(Specify) Self-Care Deficit related to fatigue, weakness,
    sedation, pain, and/or decreased sensory–perceptual
    capacity
Activity Intolerance related to hypoxia, fatigue, malnutrition,
    and decreased mobility
Grieving related to terminal illness and impending death,
    functional losses, changes in self-concept, and
    withdrawal of others
Hopelessness related to functional losses and/or impending
    death
Self-Concept Disturbance related to dependence on others
    to meet basic needs and decrease in functional ability
Powerlessness related to change from curative status to
    palliative status
Altered Family Processes related to change of member to a
    terminal status and concern over ability to manage home
    care
Spiritual Distress related to fear of death, overwhelming
    grief, belief system conflicts, and unresolved relationship
    conflicts
High Risk for Altered Health Maintenance related to
    insufficient knowledge of pain management and home
    care

COLORECTAL CANCER
(Additional Nursing Diagnoses)

See also *Cancer (General)*.

High Risk for Altered Sexuality Patterns (Male) related to
    inability to have or sustain an erection secondary to
    surgical procedure on perineal structures

High Risk for Altered Health Maintenance related to
insufficient knowledge of ostomy care, supplies, dietary
management, signs and symptoms of complications, and
community services

Surgical Procedures

GENERAL SURGERY
Preoperative Period

Nursing Diagnoses

Fear related to surgical experience, loss of control, and the
unpredictable outcome

Anxiety related to preoperative procedures (surgical permit,
diagnostic studies, Foley catheter, diet and fluid
restrictions, medications, skin preparation, waiting area
for family) and postoperative procedure (disposition
[recovery room, intensive care unit], medications for pain,
coughing–turning–leg exercises, tubes/drain placement,
NPO/diet restrictions, bed rest)

Postoperative Period
Collaborative Problems

PC: Urinary retention
PC: Hemorrhage
PC: Hypovolemia/shock
PC: Renal failure
PC: Pneumonia (stasis)
PC: Peritonitis
PC: Thrombophlebitis
PC: Paralytic ileus
PC: Evisceration
PC: Dehiscence

Nursing Diagnoses

High Risk for Infection related to destruction of first line of
defense against bacterial invasion

High Risk for Altered Respiratory Function related to
postanesthesia state, postoperative immobility, and pain

Impaired Physical Mobility related to pain and weakness
secondary to anesthesia, tissue hypoxia, and insufficient
fluids/nutrients

(Specify) Self-Care Deficits related to limited mobility and
pain

High Risk for Colonic Constipation related to decreased
peristalsis secondary to the effects of anesthesia,
immobility, and pain medication

High Risk for Altered Nutrition: Less Than Body
Requirements related to increased protein/vitamin
requirements for wound healing and decreased intake
secondary to pain, nausea, vomiting, and diet restrictions

High Risk for Altered Health Maintenance related to
insufficient knowledge of home care, incisional care,
signs and symptoms of complications, activity restriction,
and follow-up care

AMPUTATION (Lower Extremity)

Preoperative Period

See *Surgery (General).*

Nursing Diagnoses

Anxiety related to insufficient knowledge of postoperative
routines, postoperative sensations, and crutch-walking

Postoperative Period

Collaborative Problems

PC: Edema of stump
PC: Hemorrhage
PC: Hematoma site

Nursing Diagnoses

High Risk for Disuse Syndrome related to impaired
movement secondary to pain

Grieving related to loss of limb and its effects on life-style

Altered Comfort related to phantom sensations secondary
to nerve stimulation secondary to amputation

High Risk for Injury related to altered gait and hazards of
  assistive devices
High Risk for Impaired Home Maintenance Management
  related to architectural barriers
High Risk for Altered Health Maintenance related to
  insufficient knowledge of adaptions in activities of daily
  living, stump care, prosthesis care, and gait training
High Risk for Body Image Disturbance related to perceived
  negative effects of amputation

ANEURYSM RESECTION (Abdominal Aortic)

See *Surgery (General).*

Preoperative Period
Collaborative Problems

PC: Rupture of aneurysm

Postoperative Period
Collaborative Problems

PC: Distal vessel thrombosis or emboli
PC: Renal failure
PC: Mesenteric ischemia/thrombosis
PC: Spinal cord ischemia

Nursing Diagnoses

High Risk for Infection related to location of surgical incision
High Risk for Altered Sexuality Patterns (Male) related to
  possible loss of ejaculate and erections secondary to
  surgery and/or atherosclerosis
High Risk for Altered Health Maintenance related to
  insufficient knowledge of home care, activity restrictions,
  signs and symptoms of complications, and follow-up
  care

ANORECTAL SURGERY

See also *Surgery (General).*

Preoperative Period (see *Hemorrhoids*
or *Anal Fissure*)

Postoperative Period

Collaborative Problems

PC: Hemorrhage
PC: Urinary retention

Nursing Diagnoses

High Risk for Constipation related to failure to respond to cues for defecation for fear of pain

High Risk for Infection related to surgical incision and fecal contamination

High Risk for Altered Health Maintenance related to insufficient knowledge of wound care, prevention of recurrence, nutritional requirements (diet, fluid), exercise program, and signs and symptoms of complications

ARTERIAL BYPASS GRAFT OF LOWER EXTREMITY

(Aortic, Iliac, Femoral, Popliteal)

See also *Surgery (General)*.
See also *Anticoagulant Therapy*.

Postoperative Period

Collaborative Problems

PC: Thrombosis of graft
PC: Compartmental syndrome
PC: Lymphocele
PC: Disruption of anastomosis

Nursing Diagnoses

High Risk for Infection related to location of surgical incision

Pain related to increased tissue perfusion to previously ischemic tissue

High Risk for Impaired Tissue Integrity related to immobility and vulnerability of heels

High Risk for Altered Health Maintenance related to insufficient knowledge of wound care, signs and symptoms of complications, activity restrictions, and follow-up care

ARTHROPLASTY (Total Hip, Knee, or Ankle Replacement)

Preoperative Period

See also *Surgery (General)*.

Nursing Diagnosis

Anxiety related to lack of knowledge of use of trapeze

Postoperative Period

Collaborative Problems

PC: Fat emboli
PC: Hematoma formation
PC: Infection
PC: Dislocation of joint
PC: Stress fractures
PC: Neurovascular alterations
PC: Synovial herniation
PC: Thromboemboli formation

Nursing Diagnoses

High Risk for Impaired Skin Integrity related to immobility and incision

Activity Intolerance related to fatigue, pain, and impaired gait

Impaired Home Maintenance Management related to postoperative flexion restrictions

High Risk for Colonic Constipation related to activity restriction

High Risk for Injury related to altered gait and assistive devices

High Risk for Altered Health Maintenance related to insufficient knowledge of activity restrictions, use of supportive devices, rehabilitative program, follow-up care, apparel restrictions, signs of complications, supportive services, and prevention of infection

ARTHROSCOPY, ARTHROTOMY, MENISCECTOMY, BUNIONECTOMY

See also *Surgery (General)*.

Preoperative Period

Nursing Diagnoses

Anxiety related to lack of knowledge of crutch-walking and leg exercises

Postoperative Period

Collaborative Problems

PC: Hematoma formation
PC: Neurovascular impairments
PC: Hemorrhage
PC: Effusion

Nursing Diagnoses

High Risk for Altered Health Maintenance related to insufficient knowledge of home care, incision care, activity restrictions, signs of complications, and follow-up care

CAROTID ENDARTERECTOMY

See also *Surgery (General)*.

Postoperative Period

Collaborative Problems

PC: Circulatory
   Thrombosis
   Hypotension
   Hypertension
   Hemorrhage
   Cerebral infarction
PC: Neurological
   Cerebral infarction
   Cranial nerve impairment
      Facial
      Hypoglossal
      Glossopharyngeal
      Vagus
   Local nerve impairment (peri-incisional numbness of skin)
PC: Respiratory obstruction

Nursing Diagnoses

High Risk for Injury related to syncope secondary to
vascular insufficiency

High Risk for Altered Health Maintenance related to
insufficient knowledge of risk factors (smoking, diet,
obesity), activity restrictions, surgical site care, signs of
complications, and follow-up care

CATARACT EXTRACTION

Preoperative Period

Nursing Diagnoses

Fear related to upcoming surgery and potential failure to
regain vision

High Risk for Altered Health Maintenance related to
insufficient knowledge of preoperative routine,
intraoperative experience, and postoperative activities

Postoperative Period

Collaborative Problem

PC: Hemorrhage

Nursing Diagnoses

High Risk for Infection related to increased susceptibility
secondary to surgical interruption of body surface

High Risk for Injury related to visual limitations, unfamiliar
environment, limited mobility, and postoperative eye
patch

High Risk for Social Isolation related to altered visual acuity
and fear of falling

High Risk for Impaired Home Maintenance Management
related to inability to perform activities of daily living
secondary to activity restrictions and visual limitations

High Risk for Altered Health Maintenance related to
insufficient knowledge of activities permitted and
restricted, medications, complications (potential), and
follow-up care

CESAREAN SECTION

See *Surgery (General)*.
See *Postpartum Period*.

CESIUM IMPLANT
Preoperative Period

Nursing Diagnoses

Anxiety related to lack of knowledge of internal radiation, effects of internal radiation, precautions regarding caregivers/visitors, and activity restrictions

Postoperative Period
Collaborative Problems

PC: *Bleeding*
PC: *Infection*
PC: *Pulmonary complications*
PC: *Vaginal stenosis*
PC: *Radiation cystitis*
PC: *Displacement of radioactive source*
PC: *Thrombophlebitis*
PC: *Bowel dysfunction*

Nursing Diagnoses

Anxiety related to fear of radiation and its effects, uncertainty of outcome, feelings of isolation, and pain/or discomfort
Bathing, Toileting Self-Care Deficit related to activity restrictions and isolation
High Risk for Impaired Skin Integrity related to immobility secondary to prescribed activity restrictions
Social Isolation related to precautions necessitated by cesium implant safety precautions
High Risk for Altered Health Maintenance related to insufficient knowledge of home care, reportable signs and symptoms, and activity restrictions

CHOLECYSTECTOMY

See also *Surgery (General)*.

Preoperative Period

Collaborative Problem

PC: Peritonitis

Nursing Diagnoses

High Risk for Altered Respiratory Function related to high abdominal incision and splinting secondary to pain
High Risk for Altered Oral Mucous Membrane related to NPO state and mouth breathing secondary to nasogastric intubation

COLOSTOMY

See also *Surgery (General)*.

Preoperative Period

Nursing Diagnosis

Anxiety related to lack of knowledge of colostomy care and perceived negative effects on life-style

Postoperative Period

Collaborative Problems

PC: Peristomal ulceration/herniation
PC: Stomal necrosis, retraction, prolapse, stenosis, obstruction

Nursing Diagnoses

Grieving related to implications of cancer diagnosis
High Risk for Self-Concept Disturbance related to effects of ostomy on body image
High Risk for Altered Sexuality Patterns related to perceived negative impact of ostomy on sexual functioning and attractiveness
High Risk for Altered Sexuality Patterns related to physiological impotence secondary to damaged sympathetic nerves (male) or inadequate vaginal lubrication
High Risk for Social Isolation related to anxiety over possible odor and leakage from appliance

High Risk for Altered Health Maintenance related to insufficient knowledge of stoma pouching procedure, colostomy irrigation, peristomal skin care, perineal wound care, and incorporation of ostomy care into activities of daily living

CORNEAL TRANSPLANT (Penetrating Keratoplasty)

See also *Surgery (General)*.

Preoperative Period

Nursing Diagnoses

Fear related to surgical experience, loss of control, and unpredictable outcome

Anxiety related to lack of knowledge of preoperative routines, postoperative routines/activities, and postoperative sensations

Postoperative Period

Collaborative Problems

PC: Endophthalmitis
PC: Increased intraocular pressure
PC: Epithelial defects
PC: Graft failure

Nursing Diagnoses

High Risk for Infection related to nonintact ocular defense mechanisms secondary to surgery or previous eye disorder

High Risk for Altered Health Maintenance related to insufficient knowledge of eye care, resumption of activities, medications/medication administration, signs and symptoms of graft rejections, glaucoma, infection, and long-term follow-up care

CORONARY ARTERY BYPASS GRAFT (CABG)

See also *Surgery (General)*.

Preprocedure Period

Nursing Diagnoses

Anxiety related to insufficient knowledge of Pre-CABG routines/care, and post-CABG routine/care

Fear (Individual/Family) related to the client's health status, the need for CABG surgery, and the unpredictable outcome

Postprocedure Period

Collaborative Problems

PC: Cardiovascular insufficiency
PC: Respiratory insufficiency
PC: Renal insufficiency

Nursing Diagnoses

Impaired Physical Mobility related to surgical incisions, chest tubes, and fatigue

Fear related to intensive environment of the critical care unit and potential for complications

Impaired Verbal Communication related to endotracheal tube (temporary)

Altered Family Process related to disruption of family life, fear of outcome (death, disability), and stressful environment (intensive care unit)

High Risk for Self-Concept Disturbance related to the symbolic meaning of the heart and changes in life-style

High Risk for Altered Health Maintenance related to insufficient knowledge of incisional care, pain management (angina, incisions), signs and symptoms of complications, condition, pharmacological care, risk factors, restrictions, stress management techniques, and follow-up care

CRANIAL SURGERY

See also *Surgery (General)*.
See also *Brain Tumor* for preoperative/postoperative care.

Preoperative Period

Nursing Diagnosis

Anxiety related to impending surgery and perceived negative effects on life-style

Postoperative Period

Collaborative Problems

PC: Increased intracranial pressure
PC: Cerebral edema
PC: Hypoxemia
PC: Seizures
PC: Brain hemorrhage, hematomas
PC: Cranial nerve dysfunctions
PC: Cardiac dysrhythmias
PC: Fluid/electrolyte imbalances
PC: Meningitis/encephalitis
PC: Sensory–motor losses
PC: Hypothermia/hyperthermia
PC: Antidiuretic hormone secretion disorders
PC: Cerebrospinal fluid leaks
PC: Hygromas
PC: Brain shifts/herniations
PC: Hydrocephalus
PC: Gastrointestinal bleeding

Nursing Diagnoses

High Risk for Impaired Tissue Integrity: Corneal related to
   inadequate lubrication secondary to tissue edema
High Risk for Altered Health Maintenance related to
   insufficient knowledge of wound care, signs and
   symptoms of complications, restrictions, and follow-up
   care

DILATATION AND CURETTAGE (D&C)

See also *Surgery (General; Preoperative and Postoperative).*

Postoperative Period

Collaborative Problem

PC: Hemorrhage

Nursing Diagnoses

High Risk for Altered Health Maintenance related to
   insufficient knowledge of condition, home care, signs and
   symptoms of complications, and activity restrictions

ENUCLEATION

Preoperative Period

Nursing Diagnoses

Fear related to upcoming surgery, uncertain outcome of surgery, and other factors expressed by individual

Anxiety related to lack of knowledge of preoperative routine, intraoperative activities, and postoperative self-care activities

Postoperative Period

Collaborative Problems

PC: Hemorrhage
PC: Abscess

Nursing Diagnoses

High Risk for Infection related to increased susceptibility secondary to surgical interruption of body surface and use of prosthesis (ocular)

High Risk for Injury related to visual limitations and presence in unfamiliar environment

Grieving related to loss of eye and its effects on life-style

High Risk for Self-Concept Disturbance related to effects of change in appearance on life-style

High Risk for Social Isolation related to changes in body image and altered vision

High Risk for Impaired Home Maintenance Management related to inability to perform activities of daily living secondary to change in visual abilities

High Risk for Altered Health Maintenance related to insufficient knowledge of activities permitted, self-care activities, medications, complications, and plans for follow-up care

FRACTURED HIP

See also *Surgery (General)*.

Preoperative Period

Nursing Diagnoses

Pain related to trauma and muscle spasms
Anxiety related to lack of knowledge of use
   of trapeze

Postoperative Period

Collaborative Problems

PC: Hemorrhage/shock
PC: Pulmonary embolism
PC: Sepsis
PC: Fat emboli
PC: Compartmental syndrome
PC: Peroneal nerve palsy
PC: Displacement of hip joint
PC: Venous stasis/thrombosis
PC: Avascular necrosis of femoral head

Nursing Diagnoses

(Specify) Self-Care Deficit related to prescribed activity
   restriction
High Risk for Colonic Constipation related to immobility
Fear related to anticipated postoperative dependence
High Risk for Impaired Skin Integrity related to immobility
   and urinary incontinence secondary to inability to reach
   toilet quickly enough between urge to void and need to
   void
High Risk for Sensory–Perceptual Alteration related to
   increased age, pain, and immobility
High Risk for Altered Health Maintenance related to
   insufficient knowledge of activity restrictions, assistive
   devices, home care, follow-up care, and supportive
   services

HYSTERECTOMY (Vaginal, Abdominal)

See also *Surgery (General).*

Postoperative Period

Collaborative Problems

PC: Vaginal bleeding (postpacking removal)
PC: Urinary retention (postcatheter removal)
PC: Fistula formation
PC: Deep vein thrombosis
PC: Trauma (ureter, bladder, rectum)

Nursing Diagnoses

High Risk for Infection related to surgical intervention and presence of urinary catheter

High Risk for Self-Concept Disturbance related to implications of loss of body part

High Risk for Altered Sexuality Patterns related to personal significance of loss of body part and implications of loss on life-style

Grieving related to loss of body part and childbearing ability

High Risk for Altered Health Maintenance related to insufficient knowledge of perineal/incisional care, signs of complications, activity restrictions (sexual, activities of daily living, occupational), loss of menses, and follow-up care (routine gynecological examinations)

ILEOSTOMY

Preoperative Period

Nursing Diagnoses

Anxiety related to lack of knowledge of ileostomy care and perceived negative effects on life-style

Postoperative Period

Collaborative Problems

PC: Peristomal Ulceration/Herniation
PC: Stomal Necrosis, Retraction Prolapse, Stenosis, Obstruction
PC: Fluid and Electrolyte Imbalances
PC: Ileal Reservoir Pouchitis
PC: Failed Nipple Valve
PC: Ileonal Pouchitis

Nursing Diagnoses

High Risk for Self-Concept Disturbance related to effects of ostomy on body image

High Risk for Altered Sexuality Patterns related to perceived negative impact of ostomy on sexual functioning and attractiveness, physiological impotence secondary to damaged sympathetic nerves (male) or inadequate vaginal lubrication (female)

High Risk for Social Isolation related to anxiety over possible odor and leakage from appliance

High Risk for Altered Health Maintenance related to insufficient knowledge of stoma pouching procedure, peristomal skin care, perineal wound care, and incorporation of ostomy care into activities of daily living

High Risk for Altered Health Maintenance related to insufficient knowledge of care of ileonal reservoir

High Risk for Altered Health Maintenance related to insufficient knowledge of intermittent intubation of Kock continent ileostomy

LAMINECTOMY

See also *Surgery (General)*.

Preoperative Period

Nursing Diagnoses

Anxiety/Fear related to possibility of postoperative paralysis
Anxiety related to lack of knowledge of postoperative care, positioning, monitoring, and logrolling

Postoperative Period

Collaborative Problems

PC: Neurosensory impairments
PC: Bowel/bladder dysfunction
PC: Paralytic ileus
PC: Cord edema
PC: Skeletal misalignment
PC: Cerebrospinal fluid leakage
PC: Hematoma

ɡh Risk for Injury related to vertigo secondary to postural
    hypotension

Anxiety related to Acute Pain secondary to muscle spasms
    (back, thigh) secondary to irritation of nerves during
    surgery

Impaired Physical Mobility related to treatment restrictions

High Risk for Diversional Activity Deficit related to monotony
    of immobility

(Specify) Self-Care Deficit related to activity restrictions

High Risk for Altered Health Maintenance related to
    insufficient knowledge of activity restrictions,
    immobilization devices, and exercises

MASTECTOMY

See also *Cancer (General)*.
See also *Surgery (General)*.

Preoperative Period

Nursing Diagnoses

Fear related to perceived effects of mastectomy (immediate
    [pain, edema], post-discharge [relationships, work]), and
    prognosis

Postoperative Period

Collaborative Problem

PC: Neurovascular compromises

Nursing Diagnoses

High Risk for Impaired Physical Mobility (shoulder, arm)
    related to lymphedema, nerve/muscle damage, and pain

High Risk for Injury (affected arm) related to compromised
    lymph, motor, and sensory function

High Risk for Self-Concept Disturbance related to perceived
    negative effects of loss of functioning

Grieving related to loss of breast and change in
    appearance

High Risk for Altered Health Maintenance related to
    insufficient knowledge of wound care, exercises, breast

prosthesis, signs and symptoms of complications, hand/arm precautions, community resources, and follow-up care

OPHTHALMIC SURGERY

See also *Surgery (General)*.

Preoperative Period

Nursing Diagnoses

Anxiety related to lack of knowledge of postoperative positioning, postoperative eye care/bandaging, and postoperative activity restrictions

Fear/Anxiety related to having surgery with a local anesthetic, possible loss of vision, and fear of pain during procedure

High Risk for Injury related to impaired vision and unfamiliar environment

Postoperative Period

Collaborative Problems

PC: Wound dehiscence/evisceration
PC: Increased intraocular pressure
PC: Retinal detachment
PC: Dislocation of lens implant
PC: Choroidal hemorrhage
PC: Endophthalmitis
PC: Hyphema
PC: Hypopyon
PC: Blindness

Nursing Diagnoses

High Risk for Infection related to increased susceptibility secondary to interruption of body surfaces

High Risk for Injury related to visual limitations, presence in unfamiliar environment, and presence of eye patches postoperative

High Risk for Feeding, Hygiene Self-Care Deficit related to activity restrictions, visual impairment, or presence of eye patch(es).

Risk for Sensory–Perceptual Alteration related to
insufficient input secondary to impaired vision and/or
presence of unilateral/bilateral eye patches
High Risk for Altered Health Maintenance related to
insufficient knowledge of activities permitted and
restricted, medications, complications (potential), and
plans for follow-up care

OTIC SURGERY (Stapedectomy, Tympanoplasty, Myringotomy, Tympanic Mastoidectomy)

See also *Surgery (General)*.

Preoperative Period

Nursing Diagnoses

Anxiety/Fear related to possibility of greater loss of hearing
after surgery

Postoperative Period

Collaborative Problems

PC: Hemorrhage
PC: Facial paralysis
PC: Infection
PC: Impaired hearing/deafness

Nursing Diagnoses

Impaired Communication related to decreased hearing
High Risk for Social Isolation related to embarrassment of
not being able to hear in a social setting
High Risk for Injury related to vertigo
High Risk for Altered Health Maintenance related to
insufficient knowledge of signs and symptoms of
complications (facial nerve injury, vertigo, tinnitus, gait
disturbances, and ear discharge), ear care,
contraindications, and follow-up care

RADICAL NECK DISSECTION (Laryngectomy)
Preoperative Period

See also *Surgery (General)*.

See also *Cancer (General)*.
See also *Tracheostomy*.

Nursing Diagnoses

Anxiety related to lack of knowledge of: postoperative disposition (intensive care unit), method to communicate, and tracheostomy

Postoperative Period

Collaborative Problems

PC: *Hypoxemia*
PC: *Flap rejection*
PC: *Hemorrhage*
PC: *Carotid artery rupture*
PC: *Cranial nerve injury*
PC: *Infection*

Nursing Diagnoses

High Risk for Impaired Physical Mobility: Shoulder, Head related to removal of muscles, nerves, flap graft reconstruction, trauma secondary to surgery
High Risk for Self-Concept Disturbance related to change in appearance
High Risk for Altered Health Maintenance related to insufficient knowledge of condition, home care, contraindications (lifting), signs and symptoms of complications (swelling, pain, difficulty swallowing, purulent sputum), follow-up care, identification card/medallion, esophageal breathing, and community services (American Cancer Society)

RADICAL VULVECTOMY

See also *Surgery (General)*.
See also *Anticoagulant Therapy*.

Preoperative Period

Nursing Diagnoses

Anxiety related to lack of knowledge of preoperative/postoperative routines and perceived negative effects on life-style

Postoperative Period

Collaborative Problems

PC: Hemorrhage/shock
PC: Urinary retention
PC: Sepsis
PC: Pulmonary embolism
PC: Thrombophlebitis

Nursing Diagnoses

Grieving related to loss of body function and its effects on life-style

High Risk for Altered Sexuality Patterns related to perceived negative impact of surgery on sexual functioning and attractiveness

High Risk for Altered Health Maintenance related to insufficient knowledge of home care, wound care, self-catheterization, and community services

RENAL SURGERY (General, Percutaneous Nephrostomy/Extracorporeal Renal Surgery, Nephrectomy)

See also *Surgery (General)*.

Collaborative Problems

PC: Hemorrhage
PC: Shock
PC: Paralytic ileus
PC: Pneumothorax
PC: Fistulae
PC: Renal insufficiency
PC: Pyelonephritis
PC: Ureteral stent dislodgement
PC: Pneumothorax secondary to thoracic approach

Nursing Diagnoses

High Risk for Altered Respiratory Function related to pain on breathing and coughing secondary to location of incision

High Risk for Altered Health Maintenance related to insufficient knowledge of nephrostomy care and signs and symptoms of complications

o

RENAL TRANSPLANT

See also *Corticosteroid Therapy*.
See also *Surgery (General)*.

Collaborative Problems

PC: *Hemodynamic instability*
PC: *Hypervolemia/hypovolemia*
PC: *Hypertension/hypotension*
PC: *Renal failure (donor kidney)*
    Examples:
      Ischemic damage prior to implantation
      Hematoma
      Rupture of anastomosis
      Bleeding at anastomosis
      Renal vein thrombosis
      Renal artery stenosis
      Blockage of ureter (kinks, clots)
      Kinking of ureter, renal artery
PC: *Rejection of donor tissue*
PC: *Excessive immunosuppression*
PC: *Electrolyte imbalances (potassium, phosphate)*
PC: *Deep vein thrombosis*
PC: *Sepsis*

Nursing Diagnoses

High Risk for Infection related to altered immune system secondary to medications

High Risk for Altered Oral Mucous Membrane related to increased susceptibility to infection secondary to immunosuppression

High Risk for Self-Concept Disturbance related to transplant experience and potential for rejection

Fear related to possibility of rejection and dying

High Risk for Noncompliance related to complexity of treatment regimen (diet, medications, record-keeping, weight, blood pressure, urine testing) and euphoria (post-transplant)

High Risk for Altered Health Maintenance related to insufficient knowledge of prevention of infection, activity progression, dietary management, daily recording (intake, output, weights, urine testing, blood pressure, temperature), pharmacological therapy, daily urine testing

(protein), signs and symptoms of rejection/infection,
avoidance of pregnancy, follow-up care, and community
resources

THORACIC SURGERY

See also *Surgery (General)*.
See also *Mechanical Ventilation*.

Preoperative Period

Nursing Diagnoses

Anxiety/Fear related to possible respiratory difficulty after
surgery
Anxiety related to lack of knowledge of drainage devices
and mechanical ventilation

Postoperative Period

Collaborative Problems

PC: *Atelectasis*
PC: *Pneumonia*
PC: *Respiratory insufficiency*
PC: *Pneumothorax*
PC: *Hemorrhage*
PC: *Pulmonary embolus*
PC: *Subcutaneous emphysema*
PC: *Mediastinal shift*
PC: *Acute pulmonary edema*
PC: *Thrombophlebitis*

Nursing Diagnoses

Ineffective Airway Clearance related to difficulty in coughing
secondary to pain
Activity Intolerance related to reduction in exercise capacity
secondary to loss of alveolar ventilation
Impaired Physical Mobility related to arm/shoulder muscle
trauma secondary to surgery, position restrictions, and
drainage tubes
Grieving related to loss of body part and its perceived effects
on life-style
    h Risk for Altered Health Maintenance related to insufficient
     owledge of condition, pain management, shoulder/arm

exercises, incisional care, breathing exercises, splinting, prevention of infection, nutritional needs, rest versus activity, respiratory toilet, and follow-up care

TONSILLECTOMY

See also *Surgery (General)*.

Collaborative Problems

PC: Airway obstruction
PC: Aspiration
PC: Bleeding

Nursing Diagnoses

High Risk for Fluid Volume Deficit related to decreased fluid intake secondary to pain on swallowing

High Risk for Altered Nutrition: Less Than Body Requirements related to decreased intake secondary to pain on swallowing

High Risk for Altered Health Maintenance related to insufficient knowledge of rest requirements, nutritional needs, signs and symptoms of complications, pain management, positioning, and activity restrictions

TRANSURETHRAL RESECTION

(Prostate [Benign Hypertrophy or Cancer], Bladder Tumor)

See also *Surgery (General)*.

Preoperative Period

Nursing Diagnoses

Anxiety related to lack of knowledge of postoperative procedures (Foley catheter, genitourinary irrigation, nephrostomy/pyelostomy tubes), activity restrictions, and oral fluid requirements

Postoperative Period
Collaborative Problems

PC: Oliguria/anuria

PC: Hemorrhage
PC: Perforated bladder (intraoperative)
PC: Hyponatremia
PC: Sepsis
PC: Occlusion of drainage devices
PC: Prostatectomy

Nursing Diagnoses

Altered Comfort related to back/leg pains secondary to bladder spasms or clot retention

High Risk for Altered Sexuality Patterns related to fear of impotence resulting from surgical intervention

High Risk for Altered Health Maintenance related to insufficient knowledge of fluid requirements, activity restrictions, catheter care, urinary control, and follow-up care

UROSTOMY

See also *Surgery (General)*.

Preoperative Period

Nursing Diagnosis

Anxiety related to lack of knowledge of urostomy care and perceived negative effects on life-style

Postoperative Period
Collaborative Problems

PC: Internal urine leakage
PC: Urinary tract infection
PC: Peristomal ulceration/herniation
PC: Stomal necrosis, retraction, prolapse, stenosis, obstruction

Nursing Diagnoses

High Risk for Self-Concept Disturbance related to effects of ostomy on body image

High Risk for Altered Sexuality Patterns related to perceived negative impact of ostomy on sexual functioning and attractiveness

High Risk for Altered Sexuality Patterns related to erectile
dysfunction (male) or inadequate vaginal lubrication
(female)

High Risk for Social Isolation related to anxiety over possible
odor and leakage from appliance

High Risk for Altered Health Maintenance related to
insufficient knowledge of stoma pouching procedure,
colostomy irrigation, peristomal skin care, perineal wound
care, incorporation of ostomy care into activities of daily
living, and intermittent self-catheterization of Kock
continent urostomy

Obstetrical/ Gynecological Conditions

Obstetrical Conditions

PRENATAL PERIOD (General)

Nursing Diagnoses

Altered Comfort related to nausea/vomiting secondary to
elevated estrogen levels, decreased blood sugar, or
decreased gastric motility

Altered Comfort related to pressure on cardiac sphincter
from enlarged uterus

Colonic Constipation related to decreased gastric motility
and pressure of uterus on lower colon

Activity Intolerance related to fatigue and dyspnea
secondary to pressure of enlarging uterus on diaphragm
and increased blood volume

High Risk for Altered Oral Mucous Membranes related to
hyperemic gums secondary to estrogen and
progesterone levels

Fear related to the possibility of having an imperfect baby

High Risk for Infection related to increased vaginal
secretions secondary to hormonal changes

High Risk for Injury related to syncope/hypotension secondary to peripheral venous pooling

Altered Comfort related to constipation and increased pressure of enlarging uterus

High Risk for Self-Concept Disturbance related to effects of pregnancy on biopsychosocial patterns

High Risk for Altered Parenting (mother, father) related to (examples) knowledge deficit, unwanted pregnancy, powerlessness, or feelings of incompetence

High Risk for Altered Health Maintenance related to insufficient knowledge of (examples) effects of pregnancy on body systems (cardiovascular, integumentary, gastrointestinal, urinary, pulmonary, musculoskeletal), psychosocial domain, sexuality/sexual function, family unit (spouse, children), fetal growth and development, nutritional requirements, hazards of smoking, excessive alcohol intake, drug abuse, excessive caffeine intake, and excessive weight gain, signs and symptoms of complications (vaginal bleeding, cramping, gestational diabetes, excessive edema, preeclampsia), preparation for childbirth (classes, printed references)

ABORTION, INDUCED

Preprocedure Period

Nursing Diagnoses

Anxiety related to lack of knowledge of (specify) options available, procedure, postprocedure care, normalcy of emotions

Postprocedure Period

Collaborative Problems

PC: Hemorrhage
PC: Infection

Nursing Diagnoses

High Risk for Ineffective Individual Coping related to unresolved emotional responses (guilt) to societal, moral, religious, and familial opposition

High Risk for Altered Family Processes related to effects of procedure on relationships (disagreement regarding decisions, previous conflicts [personal, marital], or adolescent identity problems)

High Risk for Altered Health Maintenance related to insufficient knowledge of self-care (hygiene, breast care), nutritional needs, expected bleeding, cramping, signs and symptoms of complications, resumption of sexual activity, contraception, sex education as indicated, comfort measures, expected emotional responses, follow-up appointment, and community resources

ABORTION, SPONTANEOUS

Nursing Diagnoses

Fear related to possibility of subsequent abortions
Grieving related to loss of pregnancy

EXTRAUTERINE PREGNANCY

(Ectopic Pregnancy)

Collaborative Problems

PC: Hemorrhage
PC: Shock
PC: Sepsis
PC: Acute pain

Nursing Diagnoses

Grieving related to loss of fetus
Fear related to possibility of not being able to carry subsequent pregnancies

HYPEREMESIS GRAVIDARUM

Collaborative Problems

PC: Dehydration
PC: Negative nitrogen balance

Nursing Diagnoses

High Risk for Altered Nutrition: Less Than Body Requirements related to loss of nutrients and fluid secondary to vomiting

Anxiety related to possible ambivalent feeling toward pregnancy and parenthood

PREGNANCY-INDUCED HYPERTENSION

See also *Prenatal Period.*
See also *Postpartum Period.*

Collaborative Problems

PC: Hypertension
PC: Seizures
PC: Proteinuria
PC: Visual disturbances
PC: Coma
PC: Renal failure
PC: Cerebral edema
PC: Fetal compromise

Nursing Diagnoses

Activity Intolerance related to compromised oxygen supply
Fear related to the effects of condition on self, pregnancy, and infant
High Risk for Impaired Skin Integrity related to generalized edema secondary to impaired renal function
High Risk for Injury related to vertigo, visual disturbances, or seizures
High Risk for Altered Health Maintenance related to insufficient knowledge of dietary restrictions, signs and symptoms of complications, conservation of energy, pharmacological therapy, and comfort measures for headaches and backaches

UTERINE BLEEDING DURING PREGNANCY
(Placenta Previa, Abruptio Placentae, Uterine Rupture, Nonmalignant Lesions, Hydatidiform Mole)

See also *Postpartum Period.*

Collaborative Problems

PC: Hemorrhage
PC: Shock
PC: Disseminated intravascular coagulation

PC: *Renal failure*
PC: *Fetal death*
PC: *Anemia*
PC: *Sepsis*

Nursing Diagnoses

Fear related to effects of bleeding on pregnancy and infant
Impaired Physical Mobility related to increased bleeding in
    response to activity
Grieving related to anticipated loss of pregnancy and loss
    of expected child
Fear related to possibility of subsequent future
    complications of pregnancy

INTRAPARTUM PERIOD (General)

Collaborative Problems

PC: *Hemorrhage (placenta previa, abruptio placentae)*
PC: *Fetal distress*
PC: *Hypertension*
PC: *Uterine rupture*

Nursing Diagnoses

Altered Comfort related to uterine contractions during labor
Fear related to unpredictability of uterine contractions and
    possibility of having an impaired baby
High Risk for Altered Health Maintenance related to
    insufficient knowledge of relaxation/breathing exercises,
    positioning and procedures (preparations [bowel, skin],
    frequent assessments, anesthesia [regional, inhalation])

POSTPARTUM PERIOD (General, Mastitis [Lactational], Fetal/Newborn Death)

General Postpartum Period

Collaborative Problems

PC: *Hemorrhage*
PC: *Uterine atony*
PC: *Retained placental fragments*
PC: *Lacerations*
PC: *Hematomas*
PC: *Urinary retention*

Nursing Diagnoses

High Risk for Infection related to bacterial invasion secondary to trauma during labor, delivery, and episiotomy

High Risk for Ineffective Breastfeeding related to inexperience and/or engorged breasts

Altered Comfort related to trauma to perineum during labor and delivery, hemorrhoids, engorged breasts, and involution of uterus

High Risk for Colonic Constipation related to decreased intestinal peristalsis (postdelivery) and decreased activity

High Risk for Altered Parenting related to (examples) inexperience, feelings of incompetence, powerlessness, unwanted child, disappointment with child, or lack of role models

Stress Incontinence related to tissue trauma during delivery

High Risk for Sleep Pattern Disturbance related to maternity department's routines and demands of newborn

High Risk for Situational Low Self-Esteem related to changes that persist after delivery (skin, weight, and life-style)

High Risk for Altered Health Maintenance related to insufficient knowledge of postpartum routines, hygiene (breast, perineum), exercises, sexual counseling (contraception), nutritional requirements (infant, maternal), infant care, stresses of parenthood, adaptation of fathers, sibling relationships, parent/infant bonding, postpartum emotional responses, sleep/rest requirements, household management, community resources, management of discomforts (breast, perineum), and signs and symptoms of complications

Mastitis (Lactational)

Collaborative Problem

PC: Abscess

Nursing Diagnoses

Altered Comfort related to inflammation of breast tissue

High Risk for Ineffective Breastfeeding related to interruption secondary to inflammation

High Risk for Altered Health Maintenance related to insufficient knowledge of need for breast support, breast hygiene, breastfeeding restrictions, and signs and symptoms of abscess formation

Fetal/Newborn Death

Nursing Diagnoses

Altered Family Processes related to emotional trauma of loss on each family member

Grieving related to loss of child

Fear related to the possibility of future fetal deaths

CONCOMITANT MEDICAL CONDITIONS (Cardiac Disease [Prenatal, Postpartum], Diabetes [Prenatal, Postpartum])

Cardiac Disease

See also *Cardiac Disorders.*
See also *Prenatal Period.*
See also *Postpartum Period.*

Collaborative Problems

PC: Congestive heart failure
PC: Pregnancy-associated hypertension
PC: Eclampsia
PC: Valvular damage

Nursing Diagnoses

Fear related to effects of condition on self, pregnancy, and infant

Activity Intolerance related to increased metabolic requirements (pregnancy) in presence of compromised cardiac function

Impaired Home Maintenance Management related to impaired ability to perform role responsibilities during and after pregnancy

High Risk for Altered Family Processes related to disruption of activity restrictions and fears of effects on life-style

High Risk for Altered Health Maintenance related to insufficient knowledge of dietary requirements, prevention of infection, conservation of energy, signs and symptoms of complications, and community resources

Diabetes (Prenatal)

See also *Prenatal Period*.
See also *Diabetes Mellitus*.
See also *Postpartum Period*.

Collaborative Problems

PC: Hypoglycemia/hyperglycemia
PC: Hydramnios
PC: Acidosis
PC: Pregnancy-associated hypertension

Nursing Diagnoses

High Risk for Impaired Skin Integrity related to excessive
 skin stretching secondary to hydramnios
High Risk for Infection: Vaginal related to susceptibility to
 monilial infection
Altered Comfort: Headaches related to cerebral edema or
 hyperirritability
High Risk for Altered Health Maintenance related to
 insufficient knowledge of effects of pregnancy on
 diabetes, effects of diabetes on pregnancy, nutritional
 requirements, insulin requirements, signs and symptoms
 of complications, and need for frequent blood/urine
 samples

Diabetes (Postpartum)

See also Postpartum Period (General).

Collaborative Problems

PC: Hypoglycemia
PC: Hyperglycemia
PC: Eclampsia
*PC: Hemorrhage (secondary to uterine atony from
 excessive amniotic fluid)*
PC: Hypertension

Nursing Diagnoses

Anxiety related to separation from infant secondary to the
 need for special care needs of infant
High Risk for Infection: Perineal area related to depleted

host defenses and depressed leukocytic phagocytosis
secondary to hyperglycemia

High Risk for Altered Health Maintenance related to
insufficient knowledge of risks of future pregnancies, birth
control methods, types contraindicated, and special care
requirements for infant

Gynecological Conditions

ENDOMETRIOSIS

Collaborative Problems

PC: Hypermenorrhea
PC: Polymenorrhea

Nursing Diagnoses

Chronic Pain related to response of displaced endometrial
tissue (abdominal, peritoneal) to cyclic ovarian hormonal
stimulation

Altered Sexuality Patterns related to painful intercourse or
infertility

Anxiety related to unpredictable nature of disease

High Risk for Altered Health Maintenance related to
insufficient knowledge of condition, myths,
pharmacological therapy, and potential for pregnancy

REPRODUCTIVE TRACT INFECTIONS (Vaginitis,
Endometritis, Pelvic Cellulitis, Peritonitis)

Collaborative Problems

PC: Septicemia
PC: Abscess formation
PC: Pneumonia
PC: Pulmonary embolism

Nursing Diagnoses

Altered Comfort related to malaise, increased temperature
secondary to infectious process

High Risk for Fluid Volume Deficit related to inadequate
intake, fatigue, pain, and fluid losses secondary to
elevated temperature

393

High Risk for Ineffective Individual Coping: Depression
related to chronicity of condition and lack of definitive
diagnosis/treatment

Altered Comfort related to malaise, fever secondary to
infectious process

High Risk for Altered Health Maintenance related to
insufficient knowledge of condition, nutritional
requirements, signs and symptoms of recurrence/
complications, and sleep/rest requirements

Neonatal Conditions

NEONATE, NORMAL

Collaborative Problems

PC: Hypothermia
PC: Hypoglycemia
PC: Hyperbilirubinemia
PC: Bradycardia

Nursing Diagnoses

High Risk for Infection related to vulnerability of infant, lack
of normal flora, environmental hazards, and open wound
(umbilical cord, circumcision)

High Risk for Ineffective Airway Clearance related to
oropharynx secretions

High Risk for Impaired Skin Integrity related to susceptibility
to nosocomial infection and lack of normal skin flora

Ineffective Thermoregulation related to newborn extrauterine
transition

High Risk for Altered Health Maintenance related to
insufficient knowledge of (specify) (see Postpartum
Period)

NEONATE, PREMATURE

See also *Family of High-Risk Neonate.*

Collaborative Problems

PC: *Cold stress*
PC: *Apnea*
PC: *Bradycardia*
PC: *Hypoglycemia*
PC: *Acidosis*
PC: *Hypocalcemia*
PC: *Sepsis*
PC: *Seizures*
PC: *Pneumonia*
PC: *Hyperbilirubinemia*

Nursing Diagnoses

High Risk for Altered Nutrition: Less Than Body
Requirements related to diminished sucking

High Risk for Colonic Constipation related to decreased
intestinal motility and immobility

High Risk for Aspiration related to immobility and increased
secretions

High Risk for Infection related to vulnerability of infant, lack
of normal flora, environmental hazards, and open wounds
(umbilical cord, circumcision)

High Risk for Impaired Skin Integrity related to susceptibility
to nosocomial infection (lack of normal skin flora)

Ineffective Thermoregulation related to newborn transition to
extrauterine environment

NEONATE, POSTMATURE

(Small for Gestational Age [SGA],
Large for Gestational Age [LGA])

Collaborative Problems

PC: *Asphyxia at birth*
PC: *Meconium aspiration*
PC: *Hypoglycemia*
PC: *Polycythemia (SGA)*
PC: *Edema (generalized, cerebral)*
PC: *Central nervous system depression*
PC: *Renal tubular necrosis*
PC: *Impaired intestinal absorption*
PC: *Birth injuries (LGA)*

Nursing Diagnoses

High Risk for Impaired Skin Integrity related to absence of
protective vernix and prolonged exposure to amniotic
fluid (LGA)

High Risk for Altered Nutrition: Less Than Body
Requirements related to swallowing and sucking
difficulties

NEONATE WITH SPECIAL PROBLEM (Congenital
Infections—Cytomegalovirus [CMV], Rubella,
Toxoplasmosis, Syphilis, Herpes)

See also *High-Risk Neonate.*
See also *Family of High-Risk Neonate.*
See also *Developmental Problems/Needs* under
Pediatric Disorders.

Collaborative Problems

PC: *Hyperbilirubinemia*
PC: *Hepatosplenomegaly*
PC: *Anemia*
PC: *Hydrocephalus*
PC: *Microcephaly*
PC: *Mental retardation*
PC: *Congenital heart disease (rubella)*
PC: *Cataracts (rubella)*
PC: *Retinitis*
PC: *Thrombocytopenic purpura (rubella)*
PC: *Sensory-motor deafness (CMV)*
PC: *Periostitis (syphilis)*
PC: *Seizures*

Nursing Diagnoses

High Risk for Infection Transmission related to contagious
nature of organism

High Risk for Injury related to uncontrolled tonic/clonic
movements

High Risk for Altered Nutrition: Less Than Body Requirements
related to poor sucking reflex

NEONATE OF A DIABETIC MOTHER

See also *Neonate, Normal.*
See also *Family of High-Risk Neonate.*

Collaborative Problems

PC: *Hypoglycemia*
PC: *Hypocalcemia*
PC: *Polycythemia*
PC: *Hyperbilirubinemia*
PC: *Sepsis*
PC: *Acidosis*
PC: *Birth injury (macrosomia)*
PC: *Hyaline membrane disease*
PC: *Respiratory distress syndrome*
PC: *Venous thrombosis*

Nursing Diagnoses

High Risk for Fluid Volume Deficit related to increased
urinary excretion and osmotic diuresis

HIGH-RISK NEONATE

See also *Family of High-Risk Neonate.*

Collaborative Problems

PC: *Hypoxemia*
PC: *Shock*
PC: *Respiratory distress*
PC: *Seizures*
PC: *Hypotension*
PC: *Septicemia*

Nursing Diagnoses

High Risk for Altered Nutrition: Less Than Body
Requirements related to poor sucking reflex secondary to
(specify)
High Risk for Injury related to uncontrolled tonic/clonic
movements or hyperirritability
High Risk for Infection related to vulnerability of infant, lack
of normal flora, environmental hazards, open wounds
(umbilical cord, circumcision), and invasive lines

High Risk for Altered Respiratory Function related to
oropharyngeal secretions

High Risk for Impaired Skin Integrity related to susceptibility
to nosocomial infection secondary to lack of normal skin
flora

Ineffective Thermoregulation related to newborn transition to
extrauterine environment

FAMILY OF HIGH-RISK NEONATE

Nursing Diagnoses

Grieving related to realization of present or future loss for
family and/or child

Altered Family Processes related to effect of extended
hospitalization on family (role responsibilities, finances)

Anxiety related to unpredictable prognosis

High Risk for Altered Parenting related to inadequate
bonding secondary to parent–child separation or failure
to accept impaired child

HYPERBILIRUBINEMIA (Rh Incompatibility,
ABO Incompatibility)

See also *Family of High-risk Neonate.*
See also *Neonate, Normal.*

Collaborative Problems

PC: *Anemia*
PC: *Jaundice*
PC: *Kernicterus*
PC: *Hepatosplenomegaly*
PC: *Hydrops fetalis (cardiac failure, hypoxia, anasarca,
and pericardial, pleural, and peritoneal effusions)*
PC: *Renal failure (phototherapy complications,
hyperthermia/hypothermia, dehydration,
priapism, "bronze baby" syndrome)*

Nursing Diagnoses

High Risk for Impaired Tissue Integrity: Corneal
related to exposure to phototherapy light and continuous
wearing of eye pads

High Risk for Impaired Skin Integrity related to diarrhea, urinary excretions of bilirubin, and exposure to phototherapy light

NEONATE OF NARCOTIC-ADDICTED MOTHER

See also *Family of High-Risk Neonate.*
See also *Neonate, Normal.*
See also *Substance Abuse for Mother.*

Collaborative Problems

PC: Hyperirritability/seizures
PC: Withdrawal
PC: Hypocalcemia
PC: Hypoglycemia
PC: Sepsis
PC: Dehydration
PC: Electrolyte imbalances

Nursing Diagnoses

High Risk for Altered Nutrition: Less Than Body Requirements related to uncoordinated and ineffective sucking and swallowing reflexes
High Risk for Impaired Skin Integrity related to generalized diaphoresis and marked rigidity
Diarrhea related to increased peristalsis secondary to hyperirritability
Sleep Pattern Disturbance related to hyperirritability
High Risk for Injury related to frantic sucking of fists
High Risk for Injury related to uncontrolled tremors or tonic/clonic movements
Sensory–Perceptual Alterations related to hypersensitivity to environmental stimuli

RESPIRATORY DISTRESS SYNDROME

See also *High-risk Neonate.*
See also *Mechanical Ventilation.*

Collaborative Problems

PC: Hypoxemia

399

PC: *Atelectasis*
PC: *Acidosis*
PC: *Sepsis*
PC: *Hyperthermia*

Nursing Diagnoses

Activity Intolerance related to insufficient oxygenation of tissues secondary to impaired respirations

High Risk for Infection related to vulnerability of infant, lack of normal flora, environmental hazards (personnel, other newborns, parents), and open wounds (umbilical cord, circumcision)

High Risk for Impaired Skin Integrity related to susceptibility to nosocomial infection and lack of normal skin flora

SEPSIS (Septicemia)

See also *Newborn*.
See also *Family of High-Risk Neonate*.

Collaborative Problems

PC: *Anemia*
PC: *Respiratory distress*
PC: *Hypothermia/hyperthermia*
PC: *Hypotension*
PC: *Edema*
PC: *Seizures*
PC: *Hepatosplenomegaly*
PC: *Hemorrhage*
PC: *Jaundice*
PC: *Meningitis*
PC: *Pyarthrosis*

Nursing Diagnoses

High Risk for Impaired Skin Integrity related to edema and immobility

Altered Nutrition: Less Than Body Requirements related to poor sucking reflex

Diarrhea related to intestinal irritation secondary to infecting organism

High Risk for Injury related to uncontrolled tonic/clonic movements and hematopoietic insufficiency

Pediatric/Adolescent Disorders*

DEVELOPMENTAL PROBLEMS/NEEDS RELATED TO CHRONIC ILLNESS

(*e.g.,* Permanent Disability, Multiple Handicaps, Developmental Disability [Mental/Physical], Life-Threatening Illness)

Nursing Diagnoses

Grieving (Parental) related to anticipated losses secondary to condition

Altered Family Processes related to adjustment requirements for situation; (examples) time, energy (emotional, physical), financial, and physical care

High Risk for Impaired Home Maintenance Management related to inadequate resources, housing, or impaired caregiver(s)

High Risk for Parental Role Conflict related to separations secondary to frequent hospitalizations

High Risk for Social Isolation (Child/Family) related to the disability and the requirements of the caregiver(s)

High Risk for Altered Parenting related to abuse, rejection, overprotection secondary to inadequate resources or coping mechanisms

Decisional Conflict related to illness, health-care interventions, and parent–child separation

(Specify) Self-Care Deficit related to illness limitations or hospitalization

High Risk for Altered Growth and Development related to impaired ability to achieve developmental tasks

* For additional pediatric medical diagnoses, see the adult diagnoses and also Developmental Problems/Needs; for example:

Diabetes mellitus	Neoplastic disorders
Anorexia nervosa (psychiatric disorders)	Fractures
	Congestive heart failure
Spinal cord injury	Pneumonia
Head trauma	

secondary to restrictions imposed by disease, disability, or treatments

ACQUIRED IMMUNODEFICIENCY SYNDROME (Child)

See also *Acquired Immunodeficiency Syndrome (Adult).*
See also *Developmental Problems/Needs Related to Chronic Illness*

Nursing Diagnoses

High Risk for Infection transmission related to exposure to stool and other secretions during diaper changes or failure of child to follow handwashing procedure after toileting

Altered Nutrition: Less Than Body Requirements related to lactose intolerance, need for double the usual recommended daily allowance, anorexia secondary to oral lesions, and malaise

Altered Growth and Development related to decreased muscle tone secondary to encephalopathy

Impaired Physical Mobility related to hypotonia or hypertonia secondary to cortical atrophy

Altered Family Processes related to the impact of the child's condition on role responsibilities, siblings, finances, and negative responses of relatives, friends, and community

High Risk for Altered Health Maintenance related to insufficient knowledge of modes of transmission, risks of live virus vaccines, avoidance of infections, school attendance, and community resources

ASTHMA

See also *Developmental Problems/Needs.*

Collaborative Problems

PC: Hypoxemia
PC: Corticosteroid therapy
PC: Respiratory acidosis

Nursing Diagnoses

Ineffective Airway Clearance related to bronchospasm and increased pulmonary secretions

Fear related to breathlessness and recurrences

High Risk for Altered Health Maintenance related to insufficient knowledge of condition, environmental hazards (smoking, allergens, weather), prevention of infection, breathing/relaxation exercises, signs and symptoms of complications, pharmacological therapy, fluid requirements, behavioral modification, and daily diary recording

CELIAC DISEASE

See also *Developmental Problems/Needs.*

Collaborative Problems

PC: Severe malnutrition/dehydration
PC: Anemia
PC: Altered blood coagulation
PC: Osteoporosis
PC: Electrolyte imbalances
PC: Metabolic acidosis
PC: Shock
PC: Delayed growth

Nursing Diagnoses

High Risk for Altered Nutrition: Less Than Body Requirements related to malabsorption, dietary restrictions, and anorexia

Diarrhea related to decreased absorption in small intestines secondary to damaged villi resulting from toxins from undigested gliadin

High Risk for Fluid Volume Deficit related to fluid loss in diarrhea

High Risk for Altered Health Maintenance related to insufficient knowledge of dietary management, restrictions, and requirements

CEREBRAL PALSY*

See also *Developmental Problems/Needs.*

Collaborative Problems

PC: Contractures
PC: Seizures
PC: Respiratory infections

Nursing Diagnoses

High Risk for Injury related to inability to control movements
High Risk for Potential Altered Nutrition: Less Than Body
  Requirements related to sucking difficulties (infant) and
  dysphagia
(Specify) Self-Care Deficit related to sensory-motor
  impairments
Impaired Verbal Communication related to impaired ability
  to speak words related to facial muscle involvement
High Risk for Fluid Volume Deficit related to difficulty
  obtaining or swallowing liquids
High Risk for Diversional Activity Deficit related to effects of
  limitations on ability to participate in recreational activities
High Risk for Altered Health Maintenance related to
  insufficient knowledge of disease, pharmacological
  regimen, activity program, education, community
  services, and orthopedic appliances

CHILD ABUSE (Battered Child Syndrome, Child Neglect)

See also *Fractures, Burns.*
See also *Failure to Thrive.*

Collaborative Problems

PC: Failure to thrive
PC: Malnutrition

---

* Because disabilities associated with cerebral palsy can be varied (hemiparesis, quadriparesis, diplegia, monoplegia, triplegia, paraplegia), the nurse will have to specify the child's limitations clearly in the diagnostic statements.

PC: *Drug or alcohol addiction (older child)*
PC: *Venereal disease*

Nursing Diagnoses

Ineffective Family Coping: Disabling related to presence of factors that contribute to child abuse: (examples) lack of or unavailability of extended family, economic conditions (inflation, unemployment); lack of role model as a child, high-risk children (unwanted, of undesired gender or appearance, physically or mentally handicapped, hyperactive, terminally ill), and high-risk parents (single, adolescent, emotionally disturbed, alcoholic, drug-addicted, or physically ill)

Ineffective Individual Coping (Child Abuser) related to (examples) history of abuse by own parents and lack of warmth and affection from them, social isolation (few friends or outlets for tensions), marked lack of self-esteem, with low tolerance for criticism, emotional immaturity and dependency, distrust of others, inability to admit need for help, high expectations for/of child (perceiving child as a source of emotional gratification), and unrealistic desire for child to give pleasure

Ineffective Individual Coping (nonabusing parent) related to passive and compliant response to abuse

Fear related to possibility of placement in a shelter or foster home

Fear (parental) related to responses of others, possible loss of child, and criminal prosecution

High Risk for Altered Nutrition: Less Than Body Requirements related to inadequate intake secondary to lack of knowledge or neglect

High Risk for Altered Health Maintenance related to insufficient knowledge of parenting skills (discipline, expectations), constructive stress management, signs and symptoms of abuse, high-risk groups, child protection laws, and community services

CLEFT LIP AND PALATE

See also *Developmental Problems/Needs*.
See also *Surgery (General)*.

Preoperative Period

Nursing Diagnosis

High Risk for Altered Nutrition: Less Than Body
Requirements related to inability to suck secondary to
cleft lip

Postoperative Period

Collaborative Problems

PC: Respiratory distress
PC: Failure to thrive (organic)

Nursing Diagnoses

Impaired Physical Mobility related to restricted activity
secondary to use of restraints
High Risk for Impaired Verbal Communication related to
impaired muscle development, insufficient palate
function, faulty dentition, or hearing loss
High Risk for Aspiration related to impaired sucking
High Risk for Altered Health Maintenance related to
insufficient knowledge of condition, feeding and
suctioning techniques, surgical site care, risks for otitis
media (dental/oral problems), and referral to speech
therapist

COMMUNICABLE DISEASES

See also *Developmental Problems/Needs.*

Nursing Diagnoses

Altered Comfort related to pruritus, fatigue, malaise, sore
throat, elevated temperature
High Risk for Infection Transmission related to contagious
agents
High Risk for Fluid Volume Deficit related to increased fluid
loss secondary to elevated temperature or insufficient oral
intake secondary to malaise
High Risk for Altered Nutrition: Less Than Body
Requirements related to anorexia and sore throat or pain
on chewing (mumps)

Altered Comfort: Photophobia related to disorder
High Risk for Ineffective Airway Clearance related to
increased mucus production (whooping cough)
High Risk for Altered Health Maintenance related to
insufficient knowledge of condition, transmission,
prevention, immunizations, and skin care

CONGENITAL HEART DISEASE

See also *Developmental Problems/Needs Related to
Chronic Illness.*

Collaborative Problems

PC: *Congestive heart failure*
PC: *Pneumonia*
PC: *Hypoxemia*
PC: *Cerebral thrombosis*
PC: *Digoxin toxicity*

Nursing Diagnoses

Activity Intolerance related to insufficient oxygenation
secondary to heart defects
High Risk for Altered Nutrition: Less Than Body
Requirements related to inadequate sucking, fatigue, and
dyspnea
High Risk for Altered Health Maintenance related to
insufficient knowledge of condition, prevention of
infection, signs and symptoms of complications, digoxin
therapy, nutrition requirements, and community services

CONVULSIVE DISORDERS

See also *Developmental Problems/Needs.*
See also *Mental Disabilities, if indicated.*

Collaborative Problem

PC: *Respiratory arrest*

Nursing Diagnoses

High Risk for Injury related to uncontrolled movements of
seizure activity

Anxiety related to embarrassment and fear of seizure episodes

High Risk for Ineffective Individual Coping: Aggression related to restrictions, parental overprotection, parental indulgence

High Risk for Altered Health Maintenance related to insufficient knowledge of condition/cause, pharmacological therapy, treatment during seizures, and environmental hazards (water, driving, heights)

CRANIOCEREBRAL TRAUMA

Collaborative Problems

PC: Increased intracranial pressure
PC: Hemorrhage
PC: Tentorial herniation
PC: Cranial nerve dysfunction

Nursing Diagnoses

Altered Comfort related to compression/displacement of cerebral tissue

High Risk for Injury related to uncontrolled tonic/clonic movements during seizure episode and/or somnolence

High Risk for Altered Health Maintenance related to insufficient knowledge of condition, signs and symptoms of complications, post-traumatic syndrome, activity restrictions, and follow-up care

CYSTIC FIBROSIS

See also *Developmental Problems/Needs.*

Collaborative Problems

PC: Bronchopneumonia, atelectasis
PC: Paralytic ileus

Nursing Diagnoses

Ineffective Airway Clearance related to mucopurulent secretions

High Risk for Altered Nutrition: Less Than Body Requirements related to need for increased calories and

protein secondary to impaired intestinal absorption, loss
of fat, and fat-soluble vitamins in stools

Constipation/Diarrhea related to excessive or insufficient
pancreatic enzyme replacement

Activity Intolerance related to dyspnea secondary to
mucopurulent secretions

High Risk for Altered Health Maintenance related to
insufficient knowledge of condition (genetic transmission),
risk of infection, pharmacological therapy (side effects,
ototoxicity, renal toxicity), equipment, nutritional therapy,
salt replacement requirements, breathing exercises,
postural drainage, exercise program, and community
resources (Cystic Fibrosis Foundation)

DOWN SYNDROME

See also *Developmental Problems/Needs.*
See also *Mental Disabilities, if indicated.*

Nursing Diagnoses

High Risk for Altered Respiratory Function related to
decreased respiratory expansion secondary to
decreased muscle tone, inadequate mucus drainage,
and mouth-breathing

High Risk for Impaired Skin Integrity related to rough, dry
skin surface and flaccid extremities

High Risk for Colonic Constipation related to decreased
gastric motility

Altered Nutrition: Less Than Body Requirements (infant)
related to sucking difficulties secondary to large,
protruding tongue

High Risk for Altered Nutrition: Greater Than Body
Requirements related to increased caloric consumption
secondary to boredom in the presence of limited physical
activity

(Specify) Self-Care Deficits related to physical limitations

High Risk for Altered Health Maintenance related to
insufficient knowledge of condition, home care,
education, and community services

FAILURE TO THRIVE (Nonorganic)

See also *Developmental Problems/Needs.*

Collaborative Problems

PC: Metabolic dysfunction
PC: Dehydration

Nursing Diagnoses

Ineffective Individual Coping (caregiver) related to failure to respond to child's needs (emotional/physical) secondary to caregiver's emotional problems

Altered Nutrition: Less Than Body Requirements related to inadequate intake secondary to the lack of emotional and sensory stimulation or lack of knowledge of caregiver

Sensory–Perceptual Alterations related to history of insufficient sensory input from primary caregiver

Sleep Pattern Disturbance related to anxiety and apprehension secondary to parental deprivation

Altered Parenting related to (examples) lack of knowledge of parenting skills, impaired caregiver, impaired child, lack of support system, lack of role model, relationship problems, unrealistic expectations for child, unmet psychological needs

Impaired Home Maintenance Management related to difficulty of caregiver with maintaining a safe home environment

High Risk for Altered Health Maintenance related to insufficient knowledge of growth and development requirements, feeding guidelines, risk for child abuse, parenting skills, and community agencies

GLOMERULAR DISORDERS (Glomerulonephritis: Acute, Chronic; Nephrotic Syndrome: Congenital, Secondary, Idiopathic)

See also *Developmental Problems/Needs.*
See also *Corticosteroid Therapy.*

Collaborative Problems

PC: Anasarca (generalized edema)
PC: Hypertension
PC: Azotemia
PC: Septicemia
PC: Malnutrition
PC: Ascites

PC: Pleural effusion
PC: Hypoalbuminemia

Nursing Diagnoses

High Risk for Infection related to increased susceptibility during edematous phase and lowered resistance secondary to corticosteroid therapy

High Risk for Impaired Skin Integrity related to (examples) immobility, lowered resistance, edema, or frequent application of collection bags

Altered Nutrition: Less Than Body Requirements related to dietary restrictions, anorexia secondary to fatigue, malaise, and pressure on abdominal structures (edema)

Fatigue related to circulatory toxins, fluid and electrolytic imbalance

Diversional Activity Deficit related to hospitalization and impaired ability to perform usual activities

High Risk for Altered Health Maintenance related to insufficient knowledge of condition, etiology, course, treatments, signs and symptoms of complications, pharmacological therapy, nutritional/fluid requirements, prevention of infection, home care, follow-up care, and community services

HEMOPHILIA

See also *Developmental Problems/Needs.*

Collaborative Problem

PC: Hemorrhage

Nursing Diagnoses

Pain related to joint swelling and limitations secondary to hemarthrosis

High Risk for Impaired Physical Mobility related to joint swelling and limitations secondary to hemarthrosis

High Risk for Altered Oral Mucous Membranes related to trauma from coarse food and insufficient dental hygiene

High Risk for Altered Health Maintenance related to insufficient knowledge of condition, contraindications (*e.g.,* aspirin), genetic transmission, environmental hazards, and emergency treatment to control bleeding

HYDROCEPHALUS

See also *Developmental Problems/Needs Related to Chronic Illness.*

Collaborative Problems

PC: Increased intracranial pressure
PC: Sepsis (postshunt procedure)

Nursing Diagnoses

High Risk for Impaired Skin Integrity related to impaired ability to move head secondary to size

High Risk for Injury related to inability to support large head and strain on neck

High Risk for Altered Nutrition: Less Than Body Requirements related to vomiting secondary to cerebral compression and irritability

High Risk for Altered Health Maintenance related to insufficient knowledge of condition, home care, signs and symptoms of infection, increased intracranial pressure, and emergency treatment of shunt

INFECTIOUS MONONUCLEOSIS (Adolescent)

Collaborative Problems

PC: Enlarged spleen
PC: Hepatic dysfunction

Nursing Diagnoses

Activity Intolerance related to fatigue secondary to infectious process

Altered Comfort related to throat, malaise, and headaches

High Risk for Altered Nutrition: Less Than Body Requirements related to sore throat and malaise

Grieving related to restrictions of disease and treatments on life-style

High Risk for Infection Transmission related to contagious condition

High Risk for Altered Health Maintenance related to insufficient knowledge of condition, communicable nature, diet therapy, risks of alcohol ingestion (with

hepatic dysfunction), signs and symptoms of
complications (hepatic, splenic, neurological,
hematological), and activity restrictions

LEGG–CALVÉ–PERTHES DISEASE

See also *Developmental Problems/Needs.*

Collaborative Problem

PC: *Permanent deformed femoral head*

Nursing Diagnoses

Pain related to joint dysfunction
High Risk for Impaired Skin Integrity related to
  immobilization devices (casts, braces)
(Specify) Self-Care Deficits related to pain and
  immobilization devices
High Risk for Altered Health Maintenance related to
  insufficient knowledge of disease, weight-bearing
  restrictions, application/maintenance of devices, and pain
  management at home

LEUKEMIA

See also *Chemotherapy.*
See also *Radiation Therapy.*
See also *Cancer (General).*
See also *Developmental Problems/Needs.*

Collaborative Problems

PC: *Hepatosplenomegaly*
PC: *Increased intracranial edema*
PC: *Metastasis (brain, lungs, kidneys, gastrointestinal
      tract, spleen, liver)*
PC: *Hypermetabolism*
PC: *Hemorrhage*
PC: *Dehydration*
PC: *Myelosuppression*
PC: *Lymphadenopathy*
PC: *Central nervous system involvement*
PC: *Electrolyte imbalance*

Nursing Diagnoses

High Risk for Infection related to altered immune system secondary to leukemic process and side effects of chemotherapeutic agents

High Risk for Social Isolation related to effects of disease and treatments on appearance and fear of embarrassment

High Risk for Injury related to bleeding tendencies secondary to leukemic process and side effects of chemotherapy

Powerlessness related to inability to control situation

High Risk for Altered Sexual Patterns related to fear secondary to potential for infection and injury

High Risk for Altered Growth and Development related to impaired ability to achieve developmental tasks secondary to limitations of disease and treatments

MENINGITIS (Bacterial)

See also *Developmental Problems/Needs*.

Collaborative Problems

PC: Peripheral circulatory collapse
PC: Disseminated intravascular coagulation
PC: Increased intracranial pressure/hydrocephalus
PC: Visual/auditory nerve palsies
PC: Paresis (hemi-, quadri-)
PC: Subdural effusions
PC: Respiratory distress
PC: Seizures
PC: Fluid/electrolyte imbalances

Nursing Diagnoses

High Risk for Injury related to seizure activity secondary to infectious process

Altered Comfort related to nuchal rigidity, muscle aches, and immobility

Sensory–Perceptual Alteration: Visual, Auditory related to increased sensitivity to external stimuli secondary to infectious process

Impaired Physical Mobility related to intravenous infusion, nuchal rigidity, and restraining devices

High Risk for Impaired Skin Integrity related to immobility
High Risk for Altered Comfort related to effects of infectious
  processes
High Risk for Altered Health Maintenance related to
  insufficient knowledge of condition, antibiotic therapy,
  and diagnostic procedures

MENINGOMYELOCELE

See also *Developmental Problems/Needs.*

Collaborative Problems

PC: Hydrocephalus/shunt infections
PC: Increased intracranial pressure
PC: Urinary tract infections

Nursing Diagnoses

Reflex Incontinence related to sensory-motor dysfunction
High Risk for Infection related to vulnerability of
  meningomyelocele sac
High Risk for Impaired Skin Integrity related to sensory-
  motor impairments and orthopedic appliances
(Specify) Self-Care Deficit related to sensory-motor
  impairments
High Risk for Injury: Fractures, Membrane Tears, related to
  pathological condition
Impaired Physical Mobility related to lower limb impairments
Grieving (parental) related to birth of infant with defects
High Risk for Altered Health Maintenance related to
  insufficient knowledge of condition, home care,
  orthopedic appliances, self-catheterization, activity
  program, and community services

MENTAL DISABILITIES

See *Developmental Problems/Needs.*

Nursing Diagnoses

(Specify) Self-Care Deficit related to sensory–motor deficits
Impaired Communication related to impaired receptive skills
  or impaired expressive skills
High Risk for Social Isolation (family, child) related to fear
  and embarrassment of child's behavior/appearance

415

High Risk for Altered Health Maintenance related to insufficient knowledge of condition, child's potential, home care, community services, and education

MUSCULAR DYSTROPHY (Duchenne)

See also *Developmental Problems/Needs.*

Collaborative Problems

PC: Seizures
PC: Respiratory infections
PC: Metabolic failure

Nursing Diagnoses

High Risk for Injury related to inability to control movements

High Risk for Altered Nutrition: Less Than Body Requirements related to sucking difficulties (infant) and dysphagia

(Specify) Self-Care Deficits related to sensory-motor impairments

Impaired Verbal Communication related to impaired ability to speak words secondary to facial muscle involvement

High Risk for Impaired Physical Mobility related to muscle weakness

High Risk for Altered Nutrition: More Than Body Requirements related to increased caloric consumption secondary to boredom in presence of decreased metabolic needs secondary to limited physical activity

Grieving (parental) related to progressive, terminal nature of disease

Impaired Swallowing related to sensory-motor deficits

High Risk for Hopelessness related to progressive nature of disease

High Risk for Diversional Activity Deficit related to effects of limitations on ability to participate in recreational activities

High Risk for Altered Health Maintenance related to insufficient knowledge of disease, pharmacological regimen, activity program, education, and community services

OBESITY

See also *Developmental Problems/Needs.*

Nursing Diagnoses

Ineffective Individual Coping related to increased food consumption in response to stressors

Altered Health Maintenance related to the need for exercise program, nutrition counseling, and behavioral modification

Self-Concept Disturbance related to feelings of self-degradation and response of others (peers, family, others) to obesity

Altered Family Processes related to responses to and effects of weight loss therapy on parent/child relationship

High Risk for Impaired Social Interaction related to inability to initiate and maintain relationships secondary to feelings of embarrassment and negative responses of others

High Risk for Altered Health Maintenance related to insufficient knowledge of condition, etiology, course, risks, therapies available, destructive versus constructive eating patterns, and self-help groups

OSTEOMYELITIS

See also *Developmental Problems/Needs.*

Collaborative Problems

PC: Infective emboli
PC: Side effects of antibiotic therapy (hematological, renal, hepatic)

Nursing Diagnoses

Altered Comfort related to swelling, hyperthermia, and infectious process of bone

Diversional Activity Deficit related to impaired mobility and long-term hospitalization

High Risk for Altered Nutrition: Less Than Body Requirements related to anorexia secondary to infectious process

High Risk for Colonic Constipation related to immobility

High Risk for Impaired Skin Integrity related to mechanical irritation of cast/splint

High Risk for Injury: Pathological Fractures related to disease process

High Risk for Altered Health Maintenance related to insufficient knowledge of condition, wound care, activity restrictions, signs and symptoms of complications, pharmacological therapy, and follow-up care

PARASITIC DISORDERS

See also *Developmental Problems/Needs.*

Nursing Diagnoses

High Risk for Altered Nutrition: Less Than Body Requirements related to anorexia, nausea, vomiting, and deprivation of host nutrients by parasites

Impaired Skin Integrity related to pruritus secondary to emergence of parasites (pinworms) onto perianal skin, lytic necrosis, and tissue digestion

Diarrhea related to parasitic irritation to intestinal mucosa

Altered Comfort: Abdominal Pain related to parasitic invasion of small intestines

High Risk for Infection Transmission related to contagious nature of parasites

High Risk for Altered Health Maintenance related to insufficient knowledge of condition, mode of transmission, and prevention of reinfection

POISONING

See also *Dialysis,* if indicated.
See also *Unconscious Individual.*

Collaborative Problems

PC: Respiratory alkalosis
PC: Metabolic acidosis
PC: Hemorrhage
PC: Fluid/electrolyte imbalance
PC: Burns (acid/alkaline)
PC: Aspiration
PC: Blindness

Nursing Diagnoses

Altered Comfort related to heat production secondary to poisoning (*e.g.,* salicylate)

High Risk for Injury related to (examples) tonic/clonic movement, bleeding tendencies

Fear related to invasive nature of treatments (gastric lavage, dialysis)

Anxiety (parental) related to uncertainty of situation and feelings of guilt

Potential for Injury related to lack of awareness of environmental hazards

High Risk for Altered Health Maintenance related to insufficient knowledge of condition, treatments, home treatment of accidental poisoning, and poison prevention (storage, teaching, poisonous plants, locks)

RESPIRATORY TRACT INFECTION (Lower)

See also *Developmental Problems/Needs.*
See also *Adult Pneumonia.*

Collaborative Problems

PC: Hyperthermia
PC: Respiratory insufficiency
PC: Septic shock
PC: Paralytic ileus

Nursing Diagnoses

Altered Comfort related to hyperthermia, malaise, and respiratory distress

High Risk for Altered Nutrition: Less Than Body Requirements related to anorexia secondary to dyspnea and malaise

Anxiety related to breathlessness and apprehension

High Risk for Fluid Volume Deficit related to insufficient intake secondary to dyspnea and malaise

Altered Comfort related to malaise and fever secondary to infectious process

High Risk for Altered Health Maintenance related to insufficient knowledge of condition, prevention of recurrence, and treatment

RHEUMATIC FEVER

See also *Developmental Problems/Needs.*

Collaborative Problem

PC: Endocarditis

Nursing Diagnoses

Diversional Activity Deficit related to prescribed bed rest

Altered Nutrition: Less Than Body Requirements related to anorexia

Altered Comfort related to arthralgia

High Risk for Injury related to choreic movements

High Risk for Noncompliance related to difficulty of maintaining preventive drug therapy when illness is resolved

High Risk for Altered Health Maintenance related to insufficient knowledge of condition, signs and symptoms of complications, long-term antibiotic therapy, prevention of recurrence, and risk factors (surgery, *e.g.,* dental)

RHEUMATOID ARTHRITIS (Juvenile)

See also *Developmental Problems/Needs.*
See also *Corticosteroid Therapy.*

Collaborative Problems

PC: *Pericarditis*
PC: *Iridocyclitis*

Nursing Diagnoses

Impaired Physical Mobility related to pain and restricted joint movement

Pain related to swollen, inflamed joints and restricted movement

Fatigue related to chronic inflammatory process

High Risk for Altered Health Maintenance related to insufficient knowledge of condition, pharmacological therapy, exercise program, rest versus activity, myths, and community resources

REYE'S SYNDROME

See also *Unconscious Individual,* if indicated.

Collaborative Problems

PC: *Renal failure*
PC: *Increased intracranial pressure*
PC: *Fluid/electrolyte imbalance*

PC: *Hepatic failure*
PC: *Shock*
PC: *Seizures*
PC: *Coma*
PC: *Respiratory distress*
PC: *Diabetes insipidus*

Nursing Diagnoses

Anxiety (parental) related to diagnosis and uncertain prognosis

High Risk for Injury related to uncontrolled tonic/clonic movements

High Risk for Infection related to invasive monitoring procedures

Altered Comfort related to hyperpyrexia and malaise secondary to disease process

Fear related to separation from family, sensory bombardment (intensive care, treatments), and unfamiliar experiences

Altered Family Process related to critical nature of syndrome, hospitalization of child, and separation of family members

Grieving related to actual, anticipated, or possible death of child

High Risk for Impaired Skin Integrity related to immobility

High Risk for Altered Health Maintenance related to insufficient knowledge of condition, treatment, and complications

SCOLIOSIS

See also *Developmental Problems/Needs*.

Nursing Diagnoses

Impaired Physical Mobility related to restricted movement secondary to braces

High Risk for Impaired Skin Integrity related to mechanical irritation of brace

High Risk for Noncompliance related to chronicity and complexity of treatment regimen

High Risk for Injury: Falls related to restricted range of motion

High Risk for Altered Health Maintenance related to insufficient knowledge of condition, treatment, exercises, environmental hazards, care of appliances, follow-up care, and community services

SICKLE CELL ANEMIA

See also *Developmental Problems/Needs* if the individual is a child.

Collaborative Problems

PC: Sickling crisis
PC: of Transfusion therapy
PC: Thrombosis and infarction
PC: Cholelithiasis

Nursing Diagnoses

Altered Peripheral Tissue Perfusion related to viscous blood and occlusion of microcirculation
Pain related to viscous blood and tissue hypoxia
(Specify) Self-Care Deficit related to pain and immobility of exacerbations
High Risk for Altered Health Maintenance related to insufficient knowledge of hazards, signs and symptoms of complications, fluid requirements, and hereditary factors

TONSILLITIS

See also *Tonsillectomy,* if indicated.

Collaborative Problems

PC: Otitis media
PC: Rheumatic fever (β-hemolytic streptococci)

Nursing Diagnoses

High Risk for Fluid Volume Deficit related to inadequate fluid intake secondary to pain
High Risk for Altered Health Maintenance related to insufficient knowledge of condition, treatments, nutritional/fluid requirements, and signs and symptoms of complications

WILMS' TUMOR

See also *Developmental Problems/Needs.*
See also *Nephrectomy.*
See also *Cancer (General).*

Collaborative Problems

PC: Metastases to liver, lung, bone, brain
PC: Sepsis
PC: Tumor rupture

Nursing Diagnoses

Anxiety (child) related to (examples) age-related concerns
(separation, strangers, pain), response of others to visible
signs (alopecia), and uncertain future

Anxiety (parental) related to (examples) unknown
prognosis, painful procedures, treatments
(chemotherapy), and feelings of inadequacy

Grieving related to actual, anticipated, or possible death of
child

Spiritual Distress related to nature of disease and its
possible disturbances on belief systems

High Risk for Altered Health Maintenance related to
insufficient knowledge of condition, prognosis, treatments
(side effects), home care, nutritional requirements, follow-
up care, and community services

Psychiatric Disorders

AFFECTIVE DISORDERS (Depression)

Nursing Diagnoses

Grooming Self-Care Deficit related to decreased interest in
body, inability to make decisions, and feelings of
worthlessness

Ineffective Individual Coping related to internal conflicts
(guilt, low self-esteem) or feelings of rejection

Impaired Social Interactions related to alienation from others by constant complaining, rumination, or loss of pleasure from relationships

Ineffective Individual Coping: Excessive Physical Complaints (without organic etiology) related to inability to express emotional needs directly

Social Isolation related to inability to initiate activities to reduce isolation secondary to low energy levels

Dysfunctional Grieving related to unresolved grief, prolonged denial, and repression

Chronic Low Self-Esteem related to feelings of worthlessness and failure

Ineffective Family Coping related to marital discord and role conflicts secondary to effects of chronic depression

Powerlessness related to unrealistic negative beliefs about self-worth or abilities

Altered Thought Processes related to negative cognitive set (overgeneralizing, polarized thinking, selected abstraction, arbitrary inference)

Altered Sexuality Patterns related to decreased sex drive, loss of interest and pleasure

Diversional Activity Deficit related to a loss of interest or pleasure in usual activities and low energy levels

Impaired Home Maintenance Management related to inability to make decisions or concentrate

Potential for Self-Harm related to feelings of hopelessness and loneliness

Sleep Pattern Disturbance related to difficulty in falling asleep or early morning awakening secondary to emotional stress

Colonic Constipation related to sedentary life-style, insufficient exercise, or inadequate diet

High Risk for Altered Nutrition: More Than Body Requirements related to increased intake versus decreased activity expenditures secondary to boredom and frustrations

High Risk for Altered Nutrition: Less Than Body Requirements related to anorexia secondary to emotional stress

High Risk for Altered Health Maintenance related to insufficient knowledge of condition, behavior modification, therapy options (pharmacological, electroshock), and community resources

ANOREXIA NERVOSA

Collaborative Problems

PC: Anemia
PC: Hypotension
PC: Dysrhythmias

Nursing Diagnoses

Altered Nutrition: Less Than Body Requirements related to anorexia and self-induced vomiting following eating and laxative abuse

Self-Concept Disturbance related to inaccurate perception of self as obese

High Risk for Fluid Volume Deficit related to vomiting and excessive weight loss

Sleep Pattern Disturbance related to fears and anxiety concerning weight status

Activity Intolerance related to fatigue secondary to malnutrition

Ineffective Individual Coping related to self-induced vomiting, denial of hunger, and insufficient food intake secondary to feelings of loss of control and inaccurate perceptions of body states

Ineffective Family Coping related to marital discord and its effect on family members

High Risk for Impaired Skin Integrity related to dry skin secondary to malnourished state

Colonic Constipation related to insufficient food and fluid intake

Impaired Social Interactions related to inability to form relationships with others or fear of trusting relationships with others

Fear related to implications of a maturing body and dissatisfaction with relationships with others

ANXIETY AND ADJUSTMENT DISORDERS

(Phobias, Anxiety States, Traumatic Stress Disorders, Adjustment Reactions)

See also *Substance Abuse Disorders,* if indicated.

Nursing Diagnoses

Ineffective Individual Coping related to irrational avoidance of objects or situations

Impaired Social Interactions related to effects of behavior and actions on forming and maintaining relationships

Ineffective Individual Coping related to dependence on drugs

Anxiety related to irrational thoughts or guilt

Social Isolation related to irrational fear of social situations

Ineffective Individual Coping related to avoidance of objects or situations secondary to a numbing of responsiveness following a traumatic event

Sleep Pattern Disturbance related to recurrent nightmares

Self-Concept Disturbance related to feelings of guilt

Ineffective Individual Coping related to altered ability to constructively manage stressors secondary to (examples) physical illness, marital discord, business crisis, natural disasters, or developmental crisis

High Risk for Altered Health Maintenance related to insufficient knowledge of condition, pharmacological therapy, and legal system regarding violence

BIPOLAR DISORDER (Mania)

Nursing Diagnoses

Defensive Coping related to exaggerated sense of self-importance and abilities secondary to feelings of inadequacy and inferiority

Impaired Social Interaction related to overt hostility, overconfidence, or manipulation of others

High Risk for Violence to Others related to impaired reality testing, impaired judgment, or inability to control behavior

Sleep Pattern Disturbance related to hyperactivity

Altered Thought Processes related to flight of ideas, delusions, or hallucinations

Impaired Verbal Communication related to pressured speech

High Risk for Fluid Volume Deficit related to altered sodium excretion secondary to lithium therapy

Noncompliance related to feelings of no longer requiring medication

High Risk for Altered Health Maintenance related to
insufficient knowledge of condition, pharmacological
therapy, and follow-up care

CHILDHOOD BEHAVIORAL DISORDERS
(Attention Deficit Disorders, Learning Disabilities)

Nursing Diagnoses

Impaired Social Interactions related to inattention,
impulsivity, or hyperactivity

Grieving (parental) related to anticipated losses secondary
to condition

Altered Family Process related to adjustment requirements
for situation: (examples) time, energy, money, physical
care, and prognosis

High Risk for Violence related to impaired ability to control
aggression

High Risk for Impaired Home Maintenance Management
related to inadequate resources, inadequate housing, or
impaired caregivers

High Risk for Social Isolation (child, family) related to
disability and requirements for caregivers

High Risk for Altered Parenting: Abuse, Rejection, or
Overprotection related to inadequate resources or
inadequate coping mechanisms

Self-Concept Disturbance related to effects of limitations on
achievement of developmental tasks

OBSESSIVE–COMPULSIVE DISORDER

Nursing Diagnoses

(Specify) Self-Care Deficit related to ritualistic obsessions
interfering with performance of activities of daily living

Noncompliance related to poor concentration and poor
impulse control secondary to obsessive thought patterns

Social Isolation related to fear of vulnerability associated
with need for closeness and embarrassment over
ritualistic behavior

Anxiety related to the perceived threat of actual or
anticipated events

PARANOID DISORDERS

Nursing Diagnoses

Impaired Social Interactions related to feelings of mistrust and suspicions of others

Ineffective Denial related to inability to accept own feelings and responsibility for actions secondary to low self-esteem

High Risk for Altered Nutrition: Less Than Body Requirements related to reluctance to eat secondary to fear of poisoning

Altered Thought Processes related to inability to evaluate reality secondary to feelings of mistrust

Social Isolation related to fear and mistrust of situations and others

PERSONALITY DISORDERS

Examples:

Schizoid	Histrionic
Antisocial	Passive–aggressive
Borderline	Paranoid
Narcissistic	Schizotypal
Avoidant	Dependent
Compulsive	

Nursing Diagnoses

Ineffective Individual Coping: Passive Dependence related to subordinating one's needs to decisions of others

Ineffective Individual Coping:

Inappropriate intense anger

Poor impulse control

Marked mood shifts

Habitual disregard for social norms related to altered ability to meet responsibilities (role, social)

Impaired Social Interaction related to inability to maintain enduring attachments secondary to negative responses

Ineffective Individual Coping related to resistance (procrastination, stubbornness, intentional inefficiency) in responses to responsibilities (role, social)

SCHIZOPHRENIC DISORDERS

Nursing Diagnoses

High Risk for Violence to Others or Self-Harm related to responding to delusional thoughts or hallucinations

Impaired Verbal Communication related to incoherent/ illogical speech pattern, poverty of content of speech, and side-effects of medications

Impaired Social Interactions related to preoccupation with egocentric and illogical ideas and extreme suspiciousness

Impaired Home Maintenance Management related to impaired judgment, inability to self-initiate activity, and loss of skills over long course of illness

SOMATOFORM DISORDERS (Somatization, Hypochondriasis, Conversion Reactions)

See also *Affective Disorders,* if indicated.

Nursing Diagnoses

Impaired Social Interactions related to effects of multiple somatic complaints on relationships

Ineffective Individual Coping related to unrealistic fear of having a disease despite reassurance to contrary

Ineffective Individual Coping: Depression related to belief of not getting proper care or sufficient response from others for complaints

Ineffective Family Coping related to chronicity of illness

Noncompliance related to impaired judgments and thought disturbances

Dressing/Grooming Self-Care Deficit related to loss of skills and lack of interest in body and appearance

Diversional Activity Deficit related to apathy, inability to initiate goal-directed activities, and loss of skills

Self-Concept Disturbance related to feelings of worthlessness and lack of ego boundaries

High Risk for Altered Health Maintenance related to insufficient knowledge of condition, pharmacological therapy, tardive dyskinesia, occupational skills, and follow-up care

SUBSTANCE ABUSE DISORDERS

Collaborative Problems

PC: Delirium tremens
PC: Autonomic hyperactivity
PC: Seizures
PC: Alcohol hallucinosis
PC: Hypertension (alcohol, opiates, heroin)
PC: Sepsis (IV drug use)

Nursing Diagnoses

Altered Nutrition: Less Than Body Requirements related to anorexia

High Risk for Fluid Volume Deficit related to abnormal fluid loss secondary to vomiting and diarrhea

High Risk for Injury related to disorientation, tremors, or impaired judgment

High Risk for Self-harm related to disorientation, tremors, or impaired judgment

High Risk for Violence related to (examples) impulsive behavior, disorientation, tremors, or impaired judgment

Sleep Pattern Disturbances related to irritability, tremors, and nightmares

Anxiety related to loss of control, memory losses, and fear of withdrawal

Ineffective Individual Coping: Anger, Dependence, or Denial related to inability to constructively manage stressors without drugs/alcohol

Self-Concept Disturbance related to guilt, mistrust, or ambivalence

Impaired Social Interactions related to (examples) emotional immaturity, irritability, high anxiety, impulsive behavior, or aggressive responses

Social Isolation related to loss of work or withdrawal from others

Altered Sexuality Patterns related to impotence/loss of libido secondary to altered self-concept and substance abuse

Ineffective Family Coping related to disruption in marital dyad and inconsistent limit setting

High Risk for Altered Health Maintenance related to insufficient knowledge of condition, treatments available, high-risk situations, and community resources

Diagnostic and Therapeutic Procedures

ANGIOPLASTY (Percutaneous, Transluminal, Coronary, Peripheral)

Preprocedure Period
Nursing Diagnoses

Anxiety related to insufficient knowledge of procedure (equipment, sensations), preparation, and postprocedure care

Fear related to procedure, outcome, and possible need for cardiac surgery

Postprocedure Period
Collaborative Problems

PC: Dysrhythmias (coronary)
PC: Acute coronary occlusion (clot, spasm, collapse)
PC: Myocardial infarction (coronary)
PC: Arterial dissection or rupture
PC: Hemorrhage/hematoma (site)
PC: Paresthesia distal to site
PC: Arterial thrombosis
PC: Embolization (peripheral)

Nursing Diagnoses

Impaired Physical Mobility related to prescribed immobility and restricted movement of involved extremity

High Risk for Altered Health Maintenance related to insufficient knowledge of condition, home activities, site care, medications, and signs and symptoms of complications

ANTICOAGULANT THERAPY
Collaborative Problem

PC: Hemorrhage

Nursing Diagnoses

High Risk for Altered Health Maintenance related to insufficient knowledge of administration schedule, identification medallion/card, contraindications (food, medications), signs and symptoms of bleeding, and potential hazards (surgery, pregnancy, dental extraction, shaving)

ARTERIOGRAM

Preprocedure Period

Nursing Diagnoses

Anxiety related to lack of knowledge of procedure (equipment, possible sensations), preparation, and postcare

Postprocedure Period

Collaborative Problems

PC: Hematoma formation
PC: Hemorrhage
PC: Stroke
PC: Thrombosis (arterial site)
PC: Urinary retention
PC: Renal failure
PC: Paresthesia
PC: Embolism
PC: Allergic reaction

Nursing Diagnoses

High Risk for Altered Health Maintenance related to insufficient knowledge of activity restrictions and signs and symptoms of complications

CARDIAC CATHETERIZATION

Preprocedure Period

Nursing Diagnoses

Anxiety related to lack of knowledge of procedure (purpose, appearance of laboratory, positioning, equipment, length, possible sensations), preparation (NPO, premedication), and postprocedure care (frequent versus activity restriction)

Postprocedure Period

Collaborative Problems

PC: *Systemic (hypovolemia/hypervolemia, allergic reaction)*
PC: *Cardiac (dysrhythmias, myocardial infarction, perforation)*
PC: *Cerebrovascular accident (CVA)*
PC: *Neurovascular (hematoma formation [site], hemorrhage [site], paresis, or paresthesia)*

Nursing Diagnoses

Altered Comfort related to tissue trauma and prescribed postprocedure immobilization
High Risk for Altered Health Maintenance related to insufficient knowledge of site care, signs and symptoms of complications, and follow-up care

CASTS

Collaborative Problems

PC: *Pressure (edema, mechanical)*
PC: *Compartmental syndrome*
PC: *Ulcer formation*
PC: *Infection*

Nursing Diagnoses

High Risk for Injury related to hazards of crutch-walking and impaired mobility secondary to cast
High Risk for Impaired Skin Integrity related to pressure of cast on skin surface
High Risk for Impaired Home Maintenance Management related to the restrictions imposed by cast on performing activities of daily living and role responsibilities
(Specify) Self-Care Deficits related to limitation of movement secondary to cast
High Risk for Altered Respiratory Function related to imposed immobility or restricted respiratory movement secondary to cast (body)

Diversional Activity Deficit related to boredom and inability to perform usual recreational activities

High Risk for Altered Health Maintenance related to insufficient knowledge of crutch-walking, cast care, exercise program, and signs and symptoms of complications

CESIUM IMPLANT

Preprocedure Period

Nursing Diagnoses

Anxiety related to scheduled internal radiation insertion and the effects of internal radiation and insufficient knowledge of postprocedure restrictions

Postprocedure Period

Collaborative Problems

PC: Bleeding
PC: Infection
PC: Pulmonary Complications
PC: Vaginal Stenosis
PC: Radiation Cystitis
PC: Displacement of Radioactive Source
PC: Thrombophlebitis
PC: Bowel Dysfunction

Nursing Diagnoses

Anxiety related to fear of radiation and its effects, uncertainty of outcome, feelings of isolation, and pain or discomfort

Self-Care Deficit: bathing, toileting related to activity restrictions and isolation

High Risk for Impaired Skin Integrity related to immobility secondary to prescribed activity restrictions

Social Isolation related to precautions necessitated by cesium implant safety precautions

High Risk for Altered Health Maintenance related to insufficient knowledge of home care, reportable signs and symptoms, activity restrictions, and follow-up care

CHEMOTHERAPY

See also *Cancer (General)*.

Collaborative Problems

PC: Necrosis/phlebitis at intravenous site
PC: Thrombocytopenia
PC: Anemia
PC: Leukopenia
PC: Peripheral nerve toxicosis
PC: Anaphylaxis
PC: Pulmonary fibrosis
PC: Central nervous system toxicity
PC: Congestive heart failure
PC: Electrolyte imbalance
PC: Extravasation of vesicant drugs
PC: Hemorrhagic cystitis
PC: Myelosuppression
PC: Renal insufficiency
PC: Renal calculi

Nursing Diagnoses

High Risk for Fluid Volume Deficit related to gastrointestinal fluid losses secondary to vomiting

High Risk for Infection related to altered immune system secondary to effects of cytotoxic agents or disease process

High Risk for Altered Family Processes related to interruptions imposed by treatment and schedule on patterns of living

High Risk for Altered Sexuality Patterns related to amenorrhea and sterility (temporary/permanent) secondary to effects of chemotherapy on testes/ovaries

High Risk for Injury related to bleeding tendencies

Anxiety related to prescribed chemotherapy, insufficient knowledge of chemotherapy, and self-care measures

Fatigue related to effects of anemia, malnutrition, persistent vomiting, and sleep pattern disturbance

High Risk for Colonic Constipation related to autonomic nerve dysfunction secondary to Vinca alkaloid administration and inactivity

Diarrhea related to intestinal cell damage, inflammation, and increased intestinal mobility

Altered Comfort: Nausea/Vomiting related to gastrointestinal cell damage, stimulation of vomiting center, fear, and anxiety

High Risk for Impaired Skin Integrity related to persistent diarrhea, malnutrition, prolonged sedation, and fatigue

Altered Nutrition: Less Than Body Requirements related to anorexia, taste changes, persistent nausea/vomiting, and increased metabolic rate

Altered Oral Mucous Membrane related to dryness and epithelial cell damage secondary to chemotherapy

Self-Concept Disturbance related to change in life-style, role, alopecia, and weight loss of gain

CORTICOSTEROID THERAPY

Collaborative Problems

PC: Peptic ulcer
PC: Avascular necrosis
PC: Diabetes mellitus
PC: Osteoporosis
PC: Hypertension
PC: Thromboembolism
PC: Hypokalemia

Nursing Diagnoses

High Risk for Fluid Volume Excess: Edema related to sodium and water retention

High Risk for Infection related to immunosuppression secondary to excessive adrenocortical hormones

High Risk for Altered Nutrition: More Than Body Requirements related to increased appetite

Situational Low Self-Esteem related to appearance changes (*e.g.,* abnormal fat distribution, increased production of androgens)

High Risk for Altered Health Maintenance related to insufficient knowledge of administration schedule, indications for therapy, side effects, signs and symptoms of complications, hazards of adrenal insufficiency, potential causes of adrenal insufficiency (injuries, surgery, vomiting, abrupt cessation of therapy), emergency kit, dietary requirements, and prevention of infection

ELECTROCONVULSIVE THERAPY (ECT)

Preprocedure Period

Nursing Diagnoses

High Risk for Noncompliance related to preprocedure food/
fluid restrictions secondary to memory deficits and
confusion

Anxiety related to anticipated treatment and unknown
prognosis

Anxiety related to lack of knowledge of preprocedure/
postprocedure, sensations expected, and food, fluid
restrictions

Postprocedure Period

Collaborative Problems

PC: Hypertension
PC: Dysrhythmias

Nursing Diagnoses

High Risk for Injury related to uncontrolled tonic/clonic
movements and disorientation, confusion post-treatment

Altered Comfort: Headaches, Muscle Aches, Nausea
related to seizure activity and tissue trauma secondary to
electrical current

High Risk for Aspiration related to post-ECT somnolence

Anxiety related to memory losses and disorientation
secondary to effects of ECT on cerebral function

ELECTRONIC FETAL MONITORING
(Internal)

See also *Intrapartum Period (General)*.

Preinsertion

Nursing Diagnoses

Anxiety related to need for internal electronic fetal
monitoring and lack of information

Postinsertion

Collaborative Problems

PC: Fetal scalp laceration
PC: Perforated uterus

Nursing Diagnosis

Impaired Physical Mobility related to restrictions secondary to monitor cords

ENTERAL NUTRITION

Collaborative Problems

PC: Hypoglycemia/hyperglycemia
PC: Hypervolemia
PC: Hypertonic dehydration
PC: Electrolyte and trace mineral imbalances
PC: Mucosal erosion

Nursing Diagnoses

High Risk for Infection related to gastrostomy incision and enzymatic action of gastric juices on skin

Altered Comfort: Cramping, Distention, Nausea, Vomiting related to type of formula, rate, or temperature

Diarrhea related to adverse response to formula, rate, or temperature

High Risk for Aspiration related to position of tube and of individual

Altered Comfort related to incision and tension on gastrostomy tube

High Risk for Self-Concept Disturbance related to inability to taste or swallow food/fluids

High Risk for Altered Health Maintenance related to insufficient knowledge of nutritional indications/requirements, home care, and signs and symptoms of complications (infections, diarrhea, mechanical problems)

EXTERNAL ARTERIOVENOUS SHUNTING

Collaborative Problems

PC: Thrombosis
PC: Bleeding

Nursing Diagnoses

High Risk for Altered Health Maintenance related to insufficient knowledge of catheter care, precautions, emergency measures, prevention of infection, and activity limitations

Anxiety related to upcoming shunt insertion

HEMODIALYSIS

See also *Chronic Renal Failure*.

Collaborative Problems

PC: *Fluid imbalances (disequilibrium syndrome)*
PC: *Electrolyte imbalance (potassium, sodium)*
PC: *Nausea/vomiting*
PC: *Transfusion reaction*
PC: *Aneurysm*
PC: *Hemorrhage*
PC: *Vascular access (fistulas, graft, shunts, venous catheters)*
PC: *Bleeding*
PC: *Dialysate leakage*
PC: *Clots*
PC: *Infection*
PC: *Hepatitis B*
PC: *Fever/chills*
PC: *Hemolysis*
PC: *Seizures*
PC: *Hyper-/hypotension*
PC: *Dialysis disequilibrium syndrome*
PC: *Air embolism*
PC: *Sepsis*
PC: *Hyperthermia*

Nursing Diagnoses

High Risk for Injury to (Vascular) Access Site related to vulnerability

High Risk for Infection related to direct access to bloodstream secondary to vascular access

Powerlessness related to need for treatments to live despite effects on life-style

Altered Family Processes related to the interruptions of treatment schedule on role responsibilities

High Risk for Altered Health Maintenance related to insufficient knowledge of rationale of treatment, care of site, precautions, emergency treatments (disconnected, bleeding, clotting), pretreatment instructions, and daily assessments (bruit, blood pressure, weights)

High Risk for Infection Transmission related to frequent contacts with blood and high risk for hepatitis B

HEMODYNAMIC MONITORING

See also Medical Conditions for the specific medical diagnosis.

Collaborative Problems

PC: Sepsis
PC: Hemorrhage (site)
PC: Bleeding back
PC: Vasospasm
PC: Tissue ischemia/hypoxia
PC: System interference
PC: Thrombosis/thrombophlebitis
PC: Pulmonary embolism, air embolism
PC: Arterial spasm

Nursing Diagnoses

High Risk for Infection related to direct access to bloodstream

Impaired Physical Mobility related to position restrictions during monitoring

High Risk for Altered Health Maintenance related to insufficient knowledge of purpose, procedure and associated care

Anxiety related to impending procedure, loss of control, and unpredictable outcome

HICKMAN CATHETER

Collaborative Problems

PC: Air embolism
PC: Nonpatent catheter

Nursing Diagnoses

High Risk for Infection related to direct access to bloodstream

High Risk for Impaired Home Maintenance Management related to lack of knowledge of catheter management

LONG-TERM VENOUS CATHETER

Collaborative Problems

PC: Pneumothorax
PC: Hemorrhage
PC: Embolism/Thrombosis
PC: Sepsis
PC: Catheter Malfunction

Nursing Diagnoses

Anxiety related to upcoming insertion of catheter and insufficient knowledge of procedure

High Risk for Altered Health Maintenance related to insufficient knowledge of home care, signs and symptoms of complications, and community resources

High Risk for Infection related to catheter's direct access to bloodstream

INTRA-AORTIC BALLOON PUMPING

Preprocedure Period

Nursing Diagnoses

Anxiety related to lack of knowledge of procedure (preparations) and nursing care

Intraprocedure/Postprocedure Period

Collaborative Problems

PC: Arterial insufficiency/thrombosis
PC: Sepsis/infection
PC: Peripheral neuropathy/claudication
PC: Thrombocytopenia
PC: Bleeding
PC: Emboli

PC: Gastrointestinal bleeding
PC: Disseminated intravascular coagulation
PC: Dysrhythmias

Nursing Diagnoses

Impaired Physical Mobility related to prescribed immobility
and restricted movement of involved extremity
High Risk for Infection related to direct access to
bloodstream
High Risk for Colonic Constipation related to immobility and
restricted movement of involved limb
Fear related to treatments, environment, and risk of death
Altered Family Processes related to the critical nature of
situation and uncertain prognosis

MECHANICAL VENTILATION

See also *Tracheostomy.*

Collaborative Problems

PC: Acidosis/alkalosis
PC: Airway obstruction/atelectasis
PC: Tracheal necrosis
PC: Infection
PC: Gastrointestinal bleeding
PC: Tension pneumothorax
PC: Oxygen toxicity
PC: Respiratory insufficiency
PC: Atelectasis
PC: Decreased cardiac output

Nursing Diagnoses

Impaired Verbal Communication related to inability to speak
secondary to intubation
High Risk for Disuse Syndrome related to imposed
immobility
High Risk for Infection related to disruption of skin layer
secondary to tracheostomy
Altered Family Processes related to critical nature of
situation and uncertain prognosis
Anxiety/Fear related to condition, treatments, environment,
and risk of death

High Risk for Sensory–Perceptual Alterations related to
   excessive environmental stimuli and decreased input of
   meaningful stimuli secondary to treatment and critical
   care unit

High Risk for Ineffective Airway Clearance related to
   increased secretions secondary to tracheostomy,
   obstruction of inner cannula, or displacement of
   tracheostomy tube

Powerlessness related to dependency on respirator, inability
   to talk, and loss of mobility

High Risk for Ineffective Breathing Patterns related to
   weaning attempts, respiratory muscle fatigue secondary
   to mechanical ventilation, increased work of breathing,
   supine position, protein–calorie malnutrition, inactivity,
   and fatigue

High Risk for Self-Concept Disturbance related to
   mechanical ventilation, dependence on achieving
   developmental tasks, and life-style

PACEMAKER INSERTION

Preprocedure Period

Nursing Diagnoses

Fear related to impending pacemaker insertion and
   prognosis

Postprocedure Period

Collaborative Problems

PC: Cardiac (perforation, dysrhythmias)
PC: Pacemaker malfunction
PC: Rejection of unit
PC: Pressure necrosis of skin over unit
PC: Site (hemorrhage)

Nursing Diagnoses

Altered Comfort related to pain at insertion site and
   prescribed postprocedure immobilization

Self-Concept Disturbance related to perceived loss of
   health and dependence on pacemaker

Impaired Physical Mobility related to incisional site pain,
   activity restrictions, and fear of lead displacements

443

High Risk for Infection related to operative site

High Risk for Altered Health Maintenance related to insufficient knowledge of site care, signs and symptoms of skin complications, electromagnetic interference (microwave ovens, arc welding equipment, gasoline engines, electric motors, antitheft devices, power transmitters), pacemaker function (daily pulse taking, signs of impending battery failure), activity restrictions, and follow-up care

PERITONEAL DIALYSIS

Collaborative Problems

PC: Fluid imbalances
PC: Electrolyte imbalances
PC: Hemorrhage
PC: Negative nitrogen balance
PC: Bowel/bladder perforation
PC: Hyperglycemia
PC: Peritonitis
PC: Hypo-/hypervolemia
PC: Uremia
PC: Inflow/outflow problems

Nursing Diagnoses

High Risk for Infection related to direct access to peritoneal cavity, need to disconnect catheter for treatment, and growth medium potential of the dialysate (high glucose concentration)

High Risk for Injury to catheter site related to vulnerability

High Risk for Impaired Breathing Patterns related to immobility and pressure on diaphragm during dwell time

Altered Comfort related to rapid instillation, pressure from fluid, excessive suction during outflow, and/or extreme temperature of solution (hot or cold)

High Risk for Altered Nutrition: Less Than Body Requirements related to anorexia secondary to abdominal distention during dialysis, protein loss in dialysate, or vomiting

High Risk for Fluid Volume Excess related to fluid retention secondary to catheter problems (kinks, blockages) and/or position

Altered Family Processes related to interruptions of treatment schedule on role responsibilities

Powerlessness related to need for treatment to live despite effects on life-style

Impaired Home Maintenance Management related to lack of knowledge of treatment procedure

High Risk for Altered Health Maintenance related to insufficient knowledge of home care, self-care activities, protection of catheter, activity needs, prescribed diet, control of fluid intake/output, medication regimen, signs and symptoms of complications, follow-up visits, and daily recording (intake, output, blood pressure, weights)

RADIATION THERAPY (External)

Preprocedure Period

Nursing Diagnoses

Anxiety related to lack of knowledge of procedure and site-related, local/systemic effects of therapy (skin, gastrointestinal, neurological, oral membranes)

Postprocedure Period

Collaborative Problems

PC: Increased intracranial pressure
PC: Myelosuppression
PC: Malabsorption
PC: Pleural effusion
PC: Fluid/electrolyte imbalances
PC: Cerebral edema
PC: Inflammation
PC: Renal calculi

Nursing Diagnoses

Anxiety related to prescribed radiation therapy and insufficient knowledge of treatments and self-care measures

Altered Comfort related to stimulation of the vomiting center and damage to the gastrointestinal mucosa cells secondary to radiation

Fatigue related to systemic effects of radiation therapy

Altered Comfort related to damage to sebaceous and sweat glands secondary to radiation

High Risk for Altered Oral Mucous Membrane related to dry mouth and/or inadequate oral hygiene

Impaired Skin Integrity related to effects of radiation on epithelial and basal cells and effects of diarrhea on perineal area

Altered Nutrition: Less Than Body Requirements related to decreased oral intake, reduced salivation, mouth discomfort, dysphasia, nausea/vomiting, and increased metabolic rate

Self-Concept Disturbance related to alopecia, skin changes, weight loss, sterility, and changes in role, relationships, and life-styles

Grieving related to changes in life-style, role, finances, functional capacity, body image, and health losses

High Risk for Altered Sexuality Patterns related to fatigue, weakness, pain, self-concept changes, grief, impotence, and dyspareunia

Altered Family Processes related to imposed changes in family roles, relationships, and responsibilities

Diarrhea related to increased peristalsis secondary to irradiation of abdomen/lower back

High Risk for Infection related to moist skin reaction

Activity Intolerance related to fatigue secondary to treatments or transportation

High Risk for Altered Health Maintenance related to insufficient knowledge of skin care and signs of complications

TRACHEOSTOMY

Preoperative Period

Nursing Diagnoses

Anxiety related to lack of knowledge of impending surgery and implications of condition on life-style (chronic)

Postoperative Period

Collaborative Problems

PC: Hypoxemia
PC: Hemorrhage
PC: Tracheal edema

Nursing Diagnoses

High Risk for Ineffective Airway Clearance related to increased secretions secondary to tracheostomy, obstruction of inner cannula, or displacement of tracheostomy tube

High Risk for Infection related to excessive pooling of secretions and bypassing of upper respiratory defenses

Impaired Verbal Communications related to inability to produce speech secondary to tracheostomy

High Risk for Altered Sexuality Patterns related to change in appearance, fear of rejection

High Risk for Altered Health Maintenance related to insufficient knowledge of tracheostomy care, hazards, and signs and symptoms of complications

TRACTION

See also *Fractures.*

Collaborative Problems

PC: Thrombophlebitis
PC: Renal calculi
PC: Urinary tract infection
PC: Neurovascular compromise

Nursing Diagnoses

High Risk for Impaired Skin Integrity related to imposed immobility

High Risk for Infection related to susceptibility to microorganism secondary to skeletal traction pins

High Risk for Colonic Constipation related to decreased peristalsis secondary to immobility and analgesics

High Risk for Altered Respiratory Function related to imposed immobility and pooling of respiratory secretions

TOTAL PARENTERAL NUTRITION
(Hyperalimentation Therapy)

Collaborative Problems

PC: Sepsis
PC: Hypoglycemia/hyperglycemia

PC: *Air embolism*
PC: *Osmotic diuresis*
PC: *Perforation*
PC: *Pneumothorax, hydrothorax, hemothorax*

Nursing Diagnoses

High Risk for Infection related to catheter's direct access to bloodstream

High Risk for Impaired Skin Integrity related to continuous skin surface irritation secondary to catheter and adhesive

High Risk for Self-Concept Disturbance related to inability to ingest food

High Risk for Altered Oral Mucous Membrane related to inability to ingest food/fluid

High Risk for Altered Health Maintenance related to insufficient knowledge of home care, signs and symptoms of complications, catheter care, and follow-up care (laboratory studies)

High Risk for Activity Intolerance related to deconditioning secondary to immobility

Appendix

Adult Screening Admission Assessment Guide

The screening admission assessment form directs the nurse to collect data to assess functional health patterns* of the individual and to screen for the presence of actual, potential, or possible nursing diagnoses. When the person has a medical problem, the nurse will also have to assess for data in order to collaborate with the physician in monitoring the problem.

As with any printed assessment tool, the nurse must determine whether to collect or defer collecting certain data.

The admission interview form can be structured to allow for deferring the collection of data. The following codes illustrate the defer options:

1 = N/A, not applicable: applies to sections that are not suitable

2 = Unable to acquire: applies to items or sections that need to be assessed but cannot be addressed at this time. For example, a confused patient may be unable to provide the needed information

3 = Not a priority: applies to items or sections that are not appropriate at this time

4 = Other: applies to items or sections that are not assessed for reasons other than 2 or 3. For example, the admission interview may be discontinued in order to transport the patient for emergency surgery. This option requires an explanatory note in the chart.

If desired, the admission assessment form can be marked to indicate selected items that must always be assessed unless, of

---

* The functional health patterns have been adapted from Gordon M: Nursing Diagnosis: Application and Process. New York, McGraw-Hill, 1982.

course, the situation is an Option 2—unable to acquire. An example of an admission assessment form appears on the following pages. The form contains several characteristics that facilitate its use for the defer options and has a format that allows for checking options rather than writing them. Some data collection is not facilitated by checking choices, such as support system, emotional status, sexual concerns, etc.

As the nurse interviews the person, significant data may surface. The nurse should then ask other questions (focus assessment) to determine the presence of a pattern. For further information, the reader is referred to Section II of *Nursing Diagnosis: Application to Clinical Practice,* 4th ed., by Lynda Juall Carpenito (Philadelphia, JB Lippincott, 1991).

For example, the client reports during the initial interview that she has a problem with incontinence. The nurse should then ask specific questions utilizing the focus assessment for Altered Patterns of Urinary Elimination to determine which diagnosis of incontinence is present. After the nurse has identified the related factors, the plan of care can be initiated.

NURSING ADMISSION
SCREENING ASSESSMENT

Date _____ Arrival Time _____ Contact Person _____ Phone _____

ADMITTED FROM: ____ Home alone   ____ Home with relative   ____ Long-term care
             ____ Homeless   ____ Home with _____   ____ facility
             ____ ER   ____ (Specify)   ____ Other _____

MODE OF ARRIVAL: ____ Wheelchair   ____ Ambulance   ____ Stretcher

REASON FOR HOSPITALIZATION: _____
_____

LAST HOSPITAL ADMISSION: Date _____ Reason _____
_____

PAST MEDICAL HISTORY: _____
_____

MEDICATION (Prescription/Over-the-Counter)	DOSAGE	LAST DOSE	FREQUENCY

HEALTH MAINTENANCE–PRESCRIPTION PATTERN

USE OF:

Tobacco: ____ None   ____ Quit (date)   ____ Pipe   ____ Cigar   ____ <1 pk/day
                ____ 1–2 pks/day   ____ >2 pks/day   Pks/year history _____

Alcohol: ____ None   ____ Type/amount   ____ /day   ____ /wk   ____ /month

Other Drugs: ____ No   ____ Yes   Type _____   Use _____

Allergies (drugs, food, tape, dyes): _____   Reaction _____

ACTIVITY/EXERCISE PATTERN

SELF-CARE ABILITY:

0 = Independent   1 = Assistive device   2 = Assistance from others
3 = Assistance from person and equipment   4 = Dependent/Unable

	0	1	2	3	4
Eating/Drinking					
Bathing					
Dressing/Grooming					
Toileting					
Bed Mobility					
Transferring					
Ambulating					
Stair Climbing					
Shopping					
Cooking					
Home Maintenance					

ASSISTIVE DEVICES: ____ None ____ Crutches ____ Bedside commode ____ Walker
                      ____ Cane ____ Splint/Brace ____ Wheelchair ____ Other ____

CODE: (1) Non-applicable   (2) Unable to acquire
        (3) Not a priority at this time   (4) Other (specify in notes)

Side One

451

NUTRITION/METABOLIC PATTERN

Special Diet/Supplements _____

Previous Dietary Instruction: ____ Yes ____ No

Appetite: ____ Normal ____ Increased ____ Decreased ____ Decreased taste sensation
____ Nausea ____ Vomiting ____ Stomatitis

Weight Fluctuations Last 6 Months: ____ None _____ lbs. Gained/Lost

Swallowing Difficulty (Dysphagia): ____ None ____ Solids ____ Liquids

Dentures: ____ Upper (_ Partial _ Full) ____ Lower (_ Partial _ Full)
With Patient ____ Yes ____ No

History of Skin/Healing Problems: ____ None ____ Abnormal Healing ____ Rash
____ Dryness ____ Excess Perspiration

ELIMINATION PATTERN

Bowel Habits: ____ # BMs/day ____ Date of last BM ____ Within normal limits
____ Constipation ____ Diarrhea ____ Incontinence
____ Ostomy: Type ____ Appliance ____ Self-care ____ Yes ____ No

Bladder Habits: ____ WNL ____ Frequency ____ Dysuria ____ Nocturia ____ Urgency
____ Hematuria ____ Retention

Incontinency: ____ No ____ Yes ____ Total ____ Daytime ____ Nighttime
____ Occasional ____ Difficulty delaying voiding
____ Difficulty reaching toilet

Assistive Devices: ____ Intermittent catheterization
____ Indwelling catheter ____ External catheter
____ Incontinent briefs ____ Penile implant type _____

SLEEP/REST PATTERN

Habits: ____ hrs/night ____ AM nap ____ PM nap
Feel rested after sleep ____ Yes ____ No

Problems: ____ None ____ Early waking ____ Insomnia ____ Nightmares

COGNITIVE–CONCEPTUAL PATTERN

Hearing: ____ WNL ____ Impaired (_ Right _ Left) ____ Deaf (_ Right _ Left)
____ Hearing Aid ____ Tinnitus

Vision: ____ WNL ____ Eyeglasses ____ Contact lens
____ Impaired ____ Right ____ Left
____ Blind ____ Right ____ Left
____ Cataract ____ Right ____ Left
____ Glaucoma
____ Prosthetis ____ Right ____ Left

Vertigo: ____ Yes ____ No

Discomfort/Pain: ____ None ____ Acute ____ Chronic ____ Description _____

Pain Management: _____

COPING STRESS TOLERANCE/SELF-PERCEPTION/SELF-CONCEPT PATTERN

Major concerns regarding hospitalization or illness (financial, self-care): _____

Major loss/change in past year: ____ No ____ Yes _____

Emotional State: Pleasant ____ Calm ____ Anxious ____ Present Mood: Calm ____

Other _____

CODE: (1) Non-applicable (2) Unable to acquire
(3) Not a priority at this time (4) Other (specify in notes)

Side Two

SEXUALITY/REPRODUCTIVE PATTERN
LMP: _____
Menstrual Problems: ____ Yes ____ No _____
Last Pap Smear: _____
Monthly Self-Breast/Testicular Exam: ____ Yes ____ No
Sexual Concerns R/T Illness: _____
_____

ROLE-RELATIONSHIP PATTERN
Occupation: _____
Employment Status: ____ Employed ____ Short-term disability
                 ____ Long-term disability ____ Unemployed
Support System: ____ Spouse ____ Neighbors/Friends ____ None
             ____ Family in same residence ____ Family in separate residence
             ____ Other _____
Family concerns regarding hospitalization: _____
_____

VALUE-BELIEF PATTERN
Religion: ____ Roman Catholic ____ Protestant ____ Jewish ____ Other
Religious Restrictions: ____ No ____ Yes (Specify) _____
Request Chaplain Visitation at This Time: ____ Yes ____ No

PHYSICAL ASSESSMENT (Objective)

1. CLINICAL DATA
Age _____ Height _____ Weight _____ (Actual/Approximate)
Temperature _____
Pulse: ____ Strong ____ Weak ____ Regular ____ Irregular
Blood Pressure: Right Arm ____ Left Arm ____ Sitting ____ Lying ____
General Appearance: Groomed ____ Unkempt ____ Thin ____ Well-nourished ____

            Obese ____

2. RESPIRATORY/CIRCULATORY
Rate _____
Quality: ____ WNL ____ Shallow ____ Rapid ____ Labored ____ Other _____
Cough: ____ No ____ Yes/Describe _____
Auscultation:
  Upper rt lobes ____ WNL ____ Decreased ____ Absent ____ Abnormal sounds ____
  Upper lt lobes ____ WNL ____ Decreased ____ Absent ____ Abnormal sounds ____
  Lower rt lobes ____ WNL ____ Decreased ____ Absent ____ Abnormal sounds ____
  Lower lt lobes ____ WNL ____ Decreased ____ Absent ____ Abnormal sounds ____
Right Pedal Pulse: ____ Strong ____ Weak ____ Absent
Left Pedal Pulse: ____ Strong ____ Weak ____ Absent

3. METABOLIC-INTEGUMENTARY
SKIN:
  Color: ____ WNL ____ Pale ____ Cyanotic ____ Ashen ____ Jaundice ____ Other ____
  Temperature: ____ WNL ____ Warm ____ Cool
  Turgor: ____ WNL ____ Poor
  Edema: ____ No ____ Yes/Description/location _____
  Lesions: ____ None ____ Yes/Description/location _____
  Bruises: ____ None ____ Yes/Description/location _____
  Reddened: ____ No ____ Yes/Description/location _____
  Pruritus: ____ No ____ Yes/Description/location _____
  Tubes: Specify _____
MOUTH:
  Gums: ____ WNL ____ White plaque ____ Lesions ____ Other _____
  Teeth: ____ WNL ____ Other _____
ABDOMEN:
  Bowel Sounds: ____ Present ____ Absent

Side Three

4. NEURO/SENSORY

Mental Status: ____ Alert ____ Receptive aphasia ____ Poor historian
____ Oriented ____ Confused ____ Combative ____ Unresponsive
Speech: ____ Normal ____ Slurred ____ Garbled ____ Expressive aphasia
Spoken language_____ Interpreter _____
Pupils: ____ Equal ____ Unequal

Left: • • • • • • ● ●

Right: • • • • • • ● ●

Reactive to light:
Left: ____ Yes ____ No/Specify _____
Right: ____ Yes ____ No/Specify _____

Eyes: ____ Clear ____ Draining ____ Reddened ____ Other _____

5. MUSCULAR–SKELETAL

Range of Motion: ____ Full ____ Other _____
Balance and Gait: ____ Steady ____ Unsteady
Hand Grasps: ____ Equal ____ Strong ____ Weakness/Paralysis (__ Right __ Left)
Leg Muscles: ____ Equal ____ Strong ____ Weakness/Paralysis (__ Right __ Left)

DISCHARGE PLANNING

Lives: Alone ____ With _____ No known residence _____
Intended Destination Post Discharge: ____ Home ____ Undetermined ____ Other _____
Previous Utilization of Community Resources:
____ Home care/Hospice ____ Adult day care ____ Church groups ____ Other _____
____ Meals on Wheels ____ Homemaker/Home health aide ____ Community support group
Post-discharge Transportation:
____ Car ____ Ambulance ____ Bus/Taxi
____ Unable to determine at this time
Anticipated Financial Assistance Post-discharge?: ____ No ____ Yes _____
Anticipated Problems with Self-care Post-discharge?: ____ No ____ Yes _____
Assistive Devices Needed Post-discharge?: ____ No ____ Yes _____
Referrals: (record date)
Discharge Coordinator _____ Home Health _____
Social Service _____ V.N.A. _____
Other Comments: _____-
_____

SIGNATURE/TITLE _____ DATE _____

Side Four

Index

Nursing diagnoses appear in **boldface.**